A Cure for the Crisis
IRISH HEALTHCARE IN CONTEXT

Dr Bill Tormey

BLACKWATER PRESS

Editor
Antoinette Walker

Design & Layout
Melanie Gradtke

Cover Design
Melanie Gradtke

ISBN
1-84131-629-6

© Dr Bill Tormey, 2003

Produced in Ireland by Blackwater Press, c/o Folens Publishers, Hibernian Industrial Estate, Greenhills Road, Tallaght, Dublin 24.

All rights reserved. No part of this publication may be reproduced or transmitted in any form or by any means electronic, mechanical, photocopying, recording, or otherwise without prior written permission from the Publisher.

The book is sold subject to the conditions that it shall not, by way of trade or otherwise, be lent, re-sold, hired out or otherwise circulated without the Publisher's prior consent in any form or cover other than that in which it is published and without similar conditions including this condition being imposed on the subsequent purchaser.

To all the people who have come to see me for medical care over nearly three decades, and the people who have inspired me in medicine; these include successive editors of the New England Journal of Medicine, *Prof F Muldowney, the late Dr PJ Blaney, Prof Austin Darragh, the late Prof Brian Morgan, Dr WG Davis, Dr Harry Counihan, Profs Mick Farrell, Shane O'Neill and Gerry McElvaney, and my medical colleagues in Dublin, whom I do not wish to embarrass by naming.*

Acknowledgements

I am indebted to Prof Shane O'Neill for reviewing relevant parts of the manuscript and to Dr Rory O'Donnell for reviewing the first draft. My thanks goes to Antoinette Walker for her logical reshaping of the text and for her subsequent diligence in editing my mistakes. To John O'Connor of Blackwater Press, who, like myself, can claim to be ex-Marian College, I say thanks.

Contents

Acknowledgements v

Part 1 ⁓ Introduction

1. Marks for overall impression 1
2. National Health Strategy 7
3. Are there no improvements in the health service despite the huge investment? 18

Part 2 ⁓ The Cast

4. Health service employment............................ 20
5. The Health Boards................................... 27
6. The General Medical Services (GMS) 35
7. Nursing... 43
8. Self-preservation for administrators 55

Part 3 ⁓ At Crisis Point

9. Waiting lists and treatment plans..................... 63
10. Pay and expenditure vs cutbacks..................... 69
11. Private health insurance 73
12. Medical indemnity.................................. 78
13. Prescription medicines 87
14. Impact of advances in technology 96

Part 4 ⁓ The Global Picture

15. Life expectancy in Europe and beyond............... 100
16. National Health Service (NHS) 106
17. Best healthcare system: France 118
18. Healthcare systems of selected countries 121
19. Ireland: medical incomes and party policies.......... 126

Part 5 ⁓ Health and the Nation

20. Health inequalities................................. 134
21. Immigrants and the Irish 138

22. Disturbed children 145
23. People with disabilities. 147
24. Depression and suicide 150
25. Drugs of abuse and recreational drug use. 153
26. Alcohol and tobacco 161
27. Mental Health Act Ireland 171
28. Exercise and obesity 175
29. Cardiovascular Strategy: Building Healthier Hearts. 179
30. Screening for disease 193

Part 6 ⌇ Professional Issues

31. Irish medical morale and job satisfaction. 206
32. Consultants: gongs and chairs 208
33. Scientists in medicine. 211
34. Continuing medical education/continuing
    professional development. 213
35. Salaries and economic incentives 219
36. Medical errors 225
37. Organ retention inquiry 232
38. Aberrant clinical behaviour. 238
39. Whistle blowing in the Irish health service 247

Part 7 ⌇ The Future

40. Change: liberalisation of the medical system. 256
41. Competition in the medical market. 259
42. Healthcare rationing. 266
43. Could healthcare collapse?. 270
44. Action plan for Ireland. 273

Glossary 301
References. 305
Selected bibliography 321
Index 324

1

Marks for overall impression

The most overwhelming feature of medicine in the 21st century is the phenomenal pace of change. The investigations and therapeutics of 10 years ago have now been supplanted to an enormous extent. Often therapies that one would think are intuitively crazy have turned out to be spot on; for example, the use of betablockers, ACE inhibitors, angiotensin receptor blockers and spironolactone in heart failure. Other therapies such as albumin infusions in intensive care have been refuted. Statins, SSRIs in psychiatry, antibodies such as abciximab and sirolimus with stents, etanercept and infliximab in Crohn's disease and rheumatoid arthritis, new cancer chemotherapy, virtual colonoscopy, spiral CT, MRI scanners, PET scanners and other physical methods have had a huge impact.

So much so that the patent lobbies have been making a huge fortune. Look no further than to the stock performances of pharmaceutical companies for proof. This industry is essentially driven by a massive research effort in the United States (US). The US government fulfilled a five-year commitment to double the budget of the National Institutes of Health (NIH). The 2002 annual spend is now $28 billion which exceeds the biomedical research spending of all other governments combined. Thirty-one per cent is spent on clinical research, whereby currently the NIH partly or wholly supports more than 5,000 clinical trials. This effectively fast tracks a huge volume of research from the laboratory into clinical practice. It benefits patients but also quickly escalates costs. Not surprisingly, there is a constant struggle to keep up and ensure that world-class healthcare is, in fact, first class. Thus, medical inflation easily outpaces the consumer price index. In Ireland we are only too well aware of this consequence. Needless to say, if the Irish people refuse to pay the resultant cost, then they cannot expect a truly world-class service. Ultimately, we get what we vote for.

A Cure for the Crisis

My impression and prejudice is that medicine as a profession is in crisis. Nonetheless, the standard of technical medical care is continuously improving and treatment outcomes for major diseases are demonstrably better. The obvious excellence of many of my colleagues sometimes leaves me in awe. Those that I deal with personally in Beaumont Hospital, James Connolly Memorial Hospital, Blanchardstown, the Mater Hospital, The Children's Hospital, Temple Street and Our Lady's Hospital for Sick Children, Crumlin are excellent. This was not always my view but fortunately time passes as do retirement dates. However, I have no wish to embarrass those who should have real gongs by naming them.

Certainly, the calibre of the medical profession today prompts many questions, exposing the good and the bad. Have I major respect for my colleagues' abilities? Yes. Are their "arrogant, boring, pretentious prats" in hospital medicine? Yes, there are. Are there far fewer entertaining characters than in the recently retired cohort? Yes, medicine and medics seem blander and more unidimensional, like all other professions. Are consultants motivated by money? Medics are no different to other professionals. However, I couldn't imagine someone 20 years ago in a kind of clipped squeal uttering the sentiment "I love my job so much I'd work for nothing", while sitting in the consultant's common room. Personally, I love medicine but will only work for nothing for people on low or no incomes and for friends where I consider doing anything for them to be an honour and a privilege. Is the profession male dominated? Thankfully, medicine is being changed by the number of women at consultant level. They are different and often have different priorities, especially having to be more family-orientated. Are public relations ventures a good thing? The propensity for consultants to get involved in public relations campaigns for themselves is indeed noticeable. This is both good and bad because often there is much closed-door cynicism among other consultants at what Mary/Joe Bloggs is now at. In many cases it is not mere professional jealousy. Has the status of consultants in hospitals been eroded? Yes, the status has slowly but obviously diminished over the past 25 years while the hospital administrator has flourished. Do consultants experience some appalling nonsense from administrators? Yes, they do.

In every hospital the successful interaction between administration, medical, nursing and paramedical staff is crucial to improve patient care and outcomes. However, in the current climate this can be far from the case with roles constantly shifting and evolving.

Marks for overall impression

Administrators

When the Northern Area Health Board (NAHB) took over James Connolly Memorial Hospital, Blanchardstown from the unlamented Eastern Health Board (EHB), my first experience of the new administration was not a "Hello, I/we would like to meet you" but a letter telling us that a "Management Consultancy" would inspect us. I vaguely remember sending off a fairly terse reply. Dealing with laboratory issues with EHB officials in Blanchardstown, one was left in no doubt that THE MAN had come to decide what would or would not happen there. The situation was particularly acute as James Connelly Memorial is greatly disadvantaged by not having its own board and is not as autonomous as it should be, unlike Beaumont, St James's or Tallaght hospitals.

Over the years the actions of administrators have exasperated and frustrated consultants' exercise of their duties and responsibilities. So inexcusably bad is the *modus operandi* of some administrators that they should answer to an Oireachtas Committee for their policies and actions. Administrators often play Mickey Mouse power games, frustrate doctors and try to turn them into middle-grade civil servants. When some consultants are given administrative power, rather than being agents for progress, they turn native instead. Certainly they can easily influence the administrative executive to give those they may dislike, or consider a nuisance, a "hard time".

Undoubtedly, the growth in the numbers of administrative staff in Irish hospitals is startling. There are posts to watch posts, to manage other line managers, with many on job sharing. If a brush were run through a whole load of them, I don't believe the hospital's core service would be affected in any way. There is an amusing pretend policy called "consultants in management". Indeed, the whole objective of much of administration is to keep consultants away from management as much as possible.

General nursing staff

The next army in hospitals is the general nursing staff. Time was when the ward sister was all-powerful in her (as it nearly always was) bailiwick. She organised admissions, co-ordinated social workers getting patients home or placed, spoke to relatives and made sure that the appropriate doctor did the same, attended ward rounds and took part in the scheduling of investigations and treatments, got outlying patients of

A Cure for the Crisis

"her team" moved into the ward as soon as a bed became available, made sure that the staff nurses and students kept proper reports and notes and reported to the consultant if she was unhappy about the junior doctors. In simple terms – a formidable person! These people were not all nuns but many were and they did a fantastic job.

The situation has changed somewhat over time. Now, patients in some specialties are all over the hospital. Many consultants have difficulty getting senior nurses to attend ward rounds. The role of student nurses has changed where they are now academic to a degree. While no one would deny further education for nurses, is this development wise or necessary? Where there used to be a matron and a deputy to do rounds of the whole hospital every day, now following the Commission on Nursing Report the nomenclature has changed. There is a director of nursing (formerly, the matron), a deputy director of nursing (deputy matron), divisional nurse managers (assistant matrons), clinical nurse managers with three grades (ward sisters). Grade I used to be the junior ward sisters. In Beaumont Hospital, there are 900 nursing posts with a total of over 1,000 nurses because of job sharing and, despite the employment of 150 overseas nurses, there are still 50 vacant posts.

There is one person for the top two nursing posts and seven divisional nurse managers. These senior nurses manage about 170 nurses each. This protects the director of nursing from having to spend all day every day touring the whole hospital, which she tells me would be impossible. One of these divisional nurse managers supervises medicine, another surgery, and the others neurosciences, Accident & Emergency (A&E) and Outpatients, Radiology, Theatre and the CSSD (Central Sterile Supply Department). Clinical nurse specialists are separate again. Some have interesting titles; for example, tissue viability nurse, motor neuron disease nurse, infectious diseases nurse. I have come across asthma nurses, epilepsy nurses and the now common triage liaison nurse in A&E.

In an institution the size of Beaumont Hospital, it is necessary to have a chain of management but whether the ward sister could be made more autonomous and the hospital operate with less divisional managerial nurses is debatable. Listening to the Irish Nurses Organisation (INO), one gets the impression that they see themselves as running the hospitals. During an industrial dispute, they took it upon themselves to decide who they would allow be admitted to hospitals. This presumption was instantly rejected by the doctors.

4

Marks for overall impression

NCHDs

The non-consultant hospital doctors (NCHDs) or junior doctors are in training posts in the teaching hospitals. In Beaumont, there are 246 NCHDs. Until recently, NCHDs were poorly paid. Now the income figures per year for those at Beaumont are in the following ranges – interns who are pre-full registration €50,000–€55,000; €70,000 for senior house officers; €80,000 for middle grade registrars; and €120,000–€130,000 for specialist registrars. These figures are the total for salaries, on-call overtime payments and a training allowance. Even with this, it is often difficult to get junior doctors to cover others on-call when a crisis arises.

NCHDs will have less direct patient exposure than their predecessors. This will encourage superspecialisation and further increase costs. The measurable effects of learning curves must be factored into quantifiable clinically acceptable outcomes, otherwise there would be no training and services would collapse.

Human resources

Personnel, now known as Human Resources (HR), is another area that has seen a profusion of staff. Aside from the cost implication of employing them, what role do they actually play? Where does the role of Human Resources staff interact with the managerial role of supervisory nurses? Are all these Human Resources people necessary? There were only about five in Beaumont Hospital when Jervis Street and the Richmond Hospitals amalgamated in 1987. Over a decade later there are excessive layers of checks and balances with people "marking" others and often being very slow to make a decision. New layers of managers have been placed as a buffer between the CEO and consultants running departments or staff providing direct patient services. This convolutes decision making and retards the speed of change. These people are well meaning but would a commercial enterprise be run in such a manner? I think not. Administration sclerosis is becoming endemic.

Another feature is the proliferation of clerical staff supervisors. Secretaries in clinical departments and in pathology departments should be answerable to the consultant staff and the senior medical laboratory scientist rather than clerical staff supervisors. Recruitment panels should be organised by Human Resources for interviews. I believe that there are layers of redundant supervisory staff. A good department secretary, properly motivated and working as a valued part of the department team, does not need extraneous pseudosupervision. Needless to say, this arrangement would save money.

Irish healthcare in context

This book attempts to place in a world context a coherent set of proposals for the Irish health services. The Prospectus, Brennan and Hanly Reports and Maev-Ann Wren's *Unhealthy State – Anatomy of a Sick Society* can be read in concert and as a contrast. Controversy and contradictions in some of the major disease burdens are discussed in an explanatory manner without trying to be comprehensive. Clearly, every country has a different healthcare system. No rich country's health service is free of controversy, financially secure and organisationally robust. We must therefore openly and honestly address rationing and discuss and resolve what should be a minimum standard of health provision for everyone. Openness, accountability, fairness and realism must be the founding principles. Empty political points scoring serves no one's long-term interest. Untimately, there is no correct template that could be imported to resolve our issues.

2

National Health Strategy

The Irish Government's blueprint for building a world-class health service is encapsulated in its National Health Strategy launched in 2001 at a cost of IR£10 billion (€12.7 billion). With costs escalating year on year, the Minister for Health and Children, Mr Micheál Martin TD, was (and is) committed to spending another €1.1 billion to implement the first phase of the Strategy. However, Budget 2003 provided for only an additional €2.8 million, so the Strategy was effectively binned. Mark Hennessy writing in *The Irish Times* reported that the Government's much-touted Health Strategy scheduled to cost €10 billion over 10 years had effectively been put to one side for several years. What is clear is that neither the Minister nor the public are happy to say the least. This is shameful because the Strategy is largely coherent and offers much across the board, despite being flawed in certain areas, as will be made clear. That improved healthcare is a number one priority among Irish people is evident from the level of debate witnessed in the media in the aftermath of Budget 2003, which is worth recounting here. The picture that emerges is of a government whose commitment to the health services is severely lacking, characterised by faulty accounting and internal divisions between the Department of Finance and Department of Health.

Headlines and analysis

"Screwed by liars" was the banner headline that screamed from the front page of the *The Irish Star* newspaper after the Minister for Finance, Mr Charlie McCreevy TD revealed the Budget Estimates for 2003. This occurred in spite of his pledge endlessly replayed on TV that "no cutbacks whatsoever" were planned in May before the 2002 General Election.

In their agreed programme for government in June 2002, the Fianna Fáil/Progressive Democrat (PD) Government promised to implement their National Health Strategy, which included the creation of 3,000 new hospital beds and the allocation of 200,000 extra medical cards to those on low incomes. What their Estimates reveal is a 6 per cent increase of €587 million which allows for an additional 709 beds over the winter period and no increase in medical card numbers. According to Minister McCreevy, the Exchequer was spending €9 billion on health, which was above the EU average. The cost of the General Medical Services (GMS) has nearly doubled over the last two years and would cost €1.4 billion in 2003.

The Irish Star editorial under the headline "God help Ireland" castigated the Government's postion in no uncertain terms:

> **This is a government of liars and cheats.** They frittered away our money, conned us before the May election and now they're adding insult to injury by screwing us big time.... **This is a Government without soul.** [their emphasis]

Health spending will rise by 6 per cent. The 200,000 medical cards for the lowest income group will not be delivered, despite being promised in the National Health Strategy and in the programme for government:

> Is it any wonder that people are turning away in disgust from politics?.... This latest assault by the Government upon the people of Ireland is despicable. The damage must be undone. ... God help Ireland.

On the same page, a banner headline with "Loser McCreevy, you are the enemy of the people" in a piece by Terry McGeehan was equally scathing in its criticism.

The response of *The Irish Times* was more sanguine: "McCreevy gets tough before budget" and "Increases in indirect taxes to follow cutbacks in spending". The list of provisions and cutbacks were as follows:

- Private beds in public hospitals to cost 10 per cent more and generate €15 million.
- Possible means testing for Drug Refund Scheme to be introduced.
- 31 per cent increase in General Medical Service scheme budget.
- The total budget will be €8.9 billion.
- 70 per cent of health budget is spent on pay.
- An additional 109 hospital beds and the cost of the additional 600 extra provided in 2002 to be covered.
- Heart–lung transplants to start in the Mater Hospital.
- Budget of €31 million for the Treatment Purchase Fund to take 7,000 people off hospital waiting lists.

National Health Strategy

- €60 million compensation for HIV and hepatitis C patients.
- €10 million for general practitioner (GP) co-ops across the country.
- €29 million extra for cancer services, which would not allow radio-therapy in Waterford but would allow the development of centres of excellence to treat breast cancer.
- BreastCheck would be extended over a two-year period.
- €514 million for hospital building projects, including many which are in progress.
- €26 million extra for acute hospitals with the appointment of additional cardiologists.
- €15 million extra for services to the elderly.
- €2.7 million for adult homelessness.
- €1.5 million for youth homelessness.
- €7.5 million for childcare services.
- €7 million extra for the Cardiovascular Strategy.
- Services for developments for the mentally handicapped cut by €24.5 million.

Numbers incorrect

Figures cited by Minister Martin came under close scrutiny and were found to be inaccurate. He claimed that the cost of providing services to private patients in public hospitals is far greater than the charges levied on the health insurance companies. "In the interests of equity, it is government policy to gradually eliminate the subsidy [to health insurance companies]," he said. In response, Fine Gael's spokesperson on Health, Olivia Mitchell TD, claimed that an extra €380 million was needed to maintain current levels of hospital activity and not the €26 million budgeted.

Similarly, Dr Muiris Houston writing in *The Irish Times* noted that health inflation was running at 10 per cent but that the increase offered was 6 per cent, i.e. in real terms there would be cuts. The Estimates allow for a 31 per cent increase in the cost of the General Medical Services (GMS) scheme. However, Dr Houston pointed out that the extension of medical cards to the over-70s calculated to add 30,000 medical cards to the list was, in fact, a major underestimate. Dr Houston's lack of cynicism was evidenced by his final paragraph which read "but for those of us expecting to see early evidence of reduced inequality and improved access to the public health system, yesterday's figures are the equivalent of a scalpel driven through the heart of *Quality and Fairness – a Health System for You.*"

Ongoing strife between the Departments of Finance and Health has led to confusion over figures quoted. Leinster House sources suggested that McCreevy's thinly veiled attack on Martin may be the result of Fianna Fáil internal politics, or a way of deflecting criticism of the public spending cuts away from himself and the Taoiseach. Obviously, some propagandist whispering against the Minister for Health by the Department of Finance occurred when *The Sunday Times* (17 November 2002) reported that Martin's Department had produced three separate and contradictory lists of capital development projects. A recent check revealed that there were an extra 3,759 new workers in the health services over the number sanctioned. In addition, Minister Martin reportedly claimed that the introduction of new and expensive cancer drugs had accounted for the sharp rise in the GMS bill! To squander even more of the taxpayer's money, an audit of 50 different health agencies was being undertaken by Prospectus Consultants while another audit of medical manpower by Hanly was commissioned.

Blame game

Distributing blame for the escalating problems in the Irish healthcare system has exercised the minds of experts. UCD economist Moore McDowell wrote an interesting article in the *Irish Independent* (19 November 2003) in which he held Micheál Martin responsible for an explosion in spending during his time in health and education.

> If anyone is to blame for an explosion in spending that has succeeded in increasing employment and incomes in the public sector with little or no improvement in services, it is Mr Martin. He failed to hold the line with teachers...which gave us benchmarking. Over the last couple of years he has increased health spending by 50 per cent with no tangible results. And he couldn't even count the number of people in the country over 70 years of age before handing out more medical cards!

Central to the crisis in Irish healthcare is the question of restructuring the health boards. McDowell then points out that nine years earlier in 1994 the Department of Health concluded that the country did not need more than three health boards and could get by with two. However, since

National Health Strategy

then we have gone from eight to eleven. On the same night, Micheál Martin, appearing on RTÉ television, said that the Department was doing a review audit and suggested that the number of health boards would be culled. He also noted that reform in health organisation was needed because there were about 50 agencies at present providing services covered in his brief. In fact, there has been a 43 per cent increase in the number of administrators in the past decade. Moore McDowell opined that it was little wonder that an extra 35,000 people were employed in the health area and invited McCreevy to insist that Martin reduce the number of health boards by half in 2003 and have a maximum of four by the end of 2004. It should be possible to get rid of about half of the administrative staff in the process. McDowell also suggested that McCreevy should insist that Minister Martin pay for private operations on public patients, if and only when all the public surgical beds provided are being used for surgical purposes.

The logic of Moore McDowell's argument is compelling but factually incorrect when he trots out the mantra that the large public investment has not improved the health service. Of course it has, but the effects *should* have been more visible. This raises the question of where exactly has all the money gone? The Minister on RTÉ's *Morning Ireland* accounted for it with 70 per cent of the budget going on pay, but he was "not so sure a large saving will be made by reducing health boards".

Issues such as who will oversee hospitals, medical manpower, waiting lists/hospital beds, and medical card eligibility continue to dog the Department. In terms of the former, the Minister is in favour of a National Hospitals Authority to govern the running of hospitals as specified in the Health Strategy, following a report by Deloitte & Touche. Second, the Medical Manpower National Task Force is charged with trying to negotiate a consultant-provided rather than a consultant-led strategy, which would guarantee a higher standard of medical care than currently exists.

In terms of waiting lists, the Minister also promised that the extra 450 beds for 2002 in the Health Strategy would be exceeded and the total extra beds that year would be 709. When challenged on the plight of a family on €229 per week with children who do not have a medical card, he admitted that the resources were elsewhere but asserted that there was an extra €230 million spent on the GMS in the previous year. However, credit must go to Mr Martin for fighting off a Department of Finance proposal of 20 September 2002 to charge GMS patients a €1 fee-per-item on prescriptions to generate €24 million in revenue. That would have meant the abandonment of free drugs for the lowest income group. That wheeze, which would have been political suicide, was revealed in the *Sunday Tribune* in January 2003.[1]

Hospital budget problems reverberate nationwide

Building a world-class health service as envisaged in the National Health Strategy is doomed because hospitals are constrained by unrealistic budgets. Dublin hospitals were looking at a €100 million deficit even before they faced into 2003. To maintain services, the hospitals budgets would need to increase by €380 million, whereas the actual increase planned was €26 million. Even with increased charges on VHI/BUPA of €15 million, the income shortfall to hospitals will be a staggering €339 million. However, figures released in November 2002 as part of the Health Strategy Review showed just 272 extra beds were in place with the health boards guaranteeing the remainder early in the 2003. Who do you believe? It's easy to be abusive but these wildly inconsistent claims by the public health apparatus suggest that communication is poor and no one knows exactly what is happening. That said, I do not believe Minister Martin is confabulating but the action of his Department in issuing inaccurate information to the public is inexcusable. I see no advantage for the Minister in getting the numbers wrong.[2]

While all hospitals throughout the country are beset with budget problems, I have highlighted the case of four hospitals, which in my opinion, are suffering from chronic underfunding in light of their particular specialities and status.

National Maternity Hospital, Holles Street, Dublin

The annual budget of €40 million is insufficient to treat the increasing number of high-risk pregnancies and premature babies born at the National Maternity Hospital (NMH). A premature baby born at 26–28 weeks gestation may need 10 weeks in a neonatal unit at a cost of €15,000 per week. That totals €150,000. Like Beaumont Hospital, the NMH has to pay other hospitals for services such as the confirmation of haemoglobinopathies, etc. In addition, the NMH gets referrals of complicated cases from all over the country. In 2001, 8,142 babies were born there, while 100 high-risk pregnancies and 37 premature babies were admitted on transfer from other hospitals. They needed an extra €4 mil-

National Health Strategy

lion in 2003 to cover this cost, which usually necessitates single-patient nursing, daily ultrasound and X-rays. Complicated referrals consume about 10 per cent of their budget. Their Caesarean section rate is 14 per cent and there were no maternal deaths in 2001. The changing demographic pattern in Ireland has also added to the financial burden. In 2001, 3,000 refugees gave birth in the three Dublin maternity hospitals.

Funding for sick children at Crumlin

Despite being a public hospital, Our Lady's Hospital for Sick Children, Crumlin is chronically underfunded. It had an allocation of €60 million but spent about €62.9 million in 2002 and carried a deficit of €1.5 million from 2001. Such is the level of State underinvestment that the hospital has had to engage in private fundraising to build new units and renovate existing buildings. Successful Irish people in the construction industry in Britain and the famous footballer Niall Quinn have been major benefactors. Thanks to their efforts, new neurology and gastroenterology building units are due for completion in 2003. The Niall Quinn donation, in particular, will be used to build a new unit for infectious diseases, including HIV. A new play therapy centre was opened in November 2002 again from fundraising efforts. The benefactor was Musgrave SuperValu-Centra, who presented €250,000 each to the hospital and the Irish Cancer Society (i.e. €500,000) towards the joint development of the new facility. The money raised for the two charities came from the Musgrave Triathlon in Cork in September 2002 in which more than 500 people, including that great athlete and ambassador Eamonn Coghlan, took part. According to a report in the *Irish Examiner,* Eamonn emphasised the importance of the play therapy centre: "Play is the only normal element in a very abnormal situation in which these children find themselves."[3] Since time immemorial hospitals have been the beneficiaries of fundraising to support various healthcare initiatives; however, it should not fall to charities to fund major infrastructural projects.

James Connolly Memorial Hospital, Blanchardstown

Strategic long-term investment in James Connolly Memorial Hospital (JCMH) is being overlooked. At present the hospital is being redeveloped from money substantially coming from land sales in the grounds, which I believe to be shortsighted. There are only 189 acute beds at the hospital and this figure is not being increased in the rebuilding programme – an

A Cure for the Crisis

incredible omission. A bed utilisation survey in JCMH in 1999/2000 showed that there is a need for at least 80 additional beds. The chance of building two additional wards of 62 beds is slipping away.

A Comhairle na nOspidéal report recommended the downgrading of the A&E Department with major trauma transferred to the Mater and Beaumont Hospitals instead. The catchment area quoted of 75,000 is less than the population of greater Blanchardstown, which is still growing rapidly. By 2011 the catchment population is likely to be 290,000. This looks like another fine mess from the establishment! There are only 37 consultants at the hospital which, because of part-timers, only works out at 24 wholetime equivalents. Thus for a catchment area population of 260,000 (6.8 per cent of the national population), JCMH has 1.5 per cent of consultant numbers. And the situation is deteriorating as more consultants are appointed elsewhere.

A mere IR£300,000 was set aside for equipment and service developments in 2001 when the figure needed was €2.5 million. The chest pain unit is funded by the Cardiovascular Strategy for staff, but there is a minor capital requirement of €1.5 million. Another €4.5 million needs to be spent on medical manpower, radiology support services to relieve bottlenecks and improve GP services, and new dieticians where the waiting list is six months. Admittedly, there have been dramatic improvements in cardiology and radiology, but there is a need for €70 million to bring the rest of the hospital up to standard.

Part of the problem is that a change to the cumbersome governance structure – with JCMH reporting to the Northern Area Health Board, in turn reporting to the ERHA and then ultimately to the Department of Health – is badly needed. The seriousness of the situation is such that Dr Eamonn Leen, as chairman of the Medical Board, set out a detailed and compelling case for the strategic development of JCMH in a memo to each candidate in the hospital catchment area standing in the General Election to Dáil Éireann in 2002.

The problems are compounded by the presence of so many consultants having their private practice offsite in the Bons Secours Hospital, Glasnevin. This safety valve has, in my view, dampened down clinical revolt at the hospital. Efficiency would be served by the provision of consultants' suites or a clinic on campus. Senior medical staff have a powerful incentive to move to the Mater, St Vincent's or Beaumont when the opportunity arises and many have done so.

Beaumont Hospital and "administrationism"

The budget contraints imposed on Beaumont Hospital have detrimentally impacted on patient services, prompting public advocacy by doctors regarding cutbacks. Such advocacy has in turn incurred the wrath and censure of hospital administration. Certain meetings held in Beaumont Hospital in December 2002 are a case in point. The chief executive officer (CEO) called meetings with consultants to reveal the financial allocation for 2003. The discourse displayed the chasm that exists between "administrationism" and the doctors as service providers. The bottom lines were that in 2001 Beaumont spent €160 million, whereas the budget for that year was €148 million. In 2002, the budget was €170 million and the deficit at year-end was €8 million. For 2003, the projected deficit will be €12 million which cumulates to €20 million. Expenditure will be about €191 million, allowing for 5 per cent inflation in drug costs, which is a gross underestimate.

Inevitably, the hospital's response to such budget deficits is more cutbacks. However, the CEO was informed by the hospital consultants that they would not cut patient services. Dr Liam Grogan and Prof Shane O'Neill said that they would enter the public arena as advocates should patients' welfare be put in jeopardy. Contrary to the perceived view, consultants were demand driven and did not generate bogus extra work. In fact, Dr Grogan deals with 10 per cent of the oncology burden in the country and clearly should have at least one other colleague.

The CEO declared that the outlook was the worst ever. A reminder that we were a hugely rich country and that €20 million was a mere trifle in budget terms was disregarded. I informed him that doctors and administrators can, in the end, be on opposite sides when individual patient care is concerned. Anxious to keep within budget, hospital administrators seem to have scant regard for the professional obligations of medics. The doctor has the ethical duty to look after patients to the highest standards. Indeed, the courts have held doctors responsible even in trying resource circumstances.

A discussion on the number of discharged patients occupying beds in Beaumont followed. The figure cited was 45–50 with another 30 in rehabilitation. With 102 per cent bed occupancy, efficiency in keeping specialty services in core wards was compromised. In some wards, there were patients under five or six consultants' services. This makes the role of the ward sister (unit nurse manager) very difficult. Beaumont has 106

A Cure for the Crisis

private beds with 65 per cent occupancy but many private patients were in public beds. Thus, the hospital was forgoing potential income due to this administrative bed mismatch.

Another case of hospital mismanagement was underutilising bed capacity. In 2002, Beaumont received a financial bonus from the Hospital Inpatient Enquiry (HIPE) data, which is a measure of case complexity. Dr Richard Costello in an audit of the Respiratory Medicine Service concluded that there was 20 per cent underreported activity in Beaumont, i.e. more income had been foregone.

Gross mismanagement also occurred in a public–private partnership venture within the hospital. Details of this deal were unknown to nearly all hospital staff. The hospital suffered a €2 million loss from fines from the car park company over four years because of a penalty clause in the deal which meant that any non-staff cars parked in the grounds attracted a cash penalty paid for by the hospital. According to the Comptroller and Auditor General, Mr John Purcell, the State had lost a potential revenue of between €8.9 million to €13 million. I remain very unimpressed with the management that inflicted that deal on the hospital.

To increase income, the CEO announced that the hospital would charge for other services, such as pathology in the private clinic that heretofore had been regarded as onsite. The introduction of an increased handling charge for the administration of recoverable salaries was also mentioned. This is where the consultants get a research or "soft money" grant to hire staff who then work on their teams in Beaumont to mutual benefit. Next, neurologist Dr Joan Moroney protested at the recent removal of the second MRI (magnetic resonance imaging) scanner from the hospital, which would mean patients occupying a hospital bed while awaiting an MRI scan for up to 15 days. This move is clearly ill advised. The CEO said that there were legal reasons why this happened but did not elaborate. Rheumatologist Dr Paul O'Connell pointed out that new drugs in rheumatology allowed patients to have short-stay and outpatient treatment for conditions where formerly they would have been inpatients for some time. For example, the drug infliximab is infused into people with severe rheumatoid arthritis for one day every two months. Formerly, these patients would have been in hospital for up to two weeks twice yearly for less effective therapy.

The CEO admitted that he was opposed to any public advocacy by doctors regarding cutbacks. It was his objective to achieve as many savings

National Health Strategy

as possible in the hospital; consequently, the hospital would be favourably regarded by the Department of Health. His idea was that the establishment of the new Hospitals Agency would determine the role of Beaumont. However, this is not how excellence in hospitals develops. Such a move would diminish the role of doctors in the treatment of patients and runs counter to their duty of care. Indeed, the Medical Council mandates doctors to be public advocates for their patients.

Prof O'Neill informed the CEO that he had met two Ministers for Health on a formal basis, where the case for capital development at Beaumont had been put. The Ministers seemed sympathetic and signalled agreement, yet nothing happened. In Prof O'Neill's view, being "a good boy" no longer achieved anything for Beaumont Hospital. Methods would have to become more robust. He cited the Mater Hospital's autumn public protests as a successful precedent. Not surprisingly, this irked the CEO who responded by saying that the health authorities were angry at the Mater's protests with the result that no extra money was achieved, having succeeded in alienating the governing decision-makers instead. He contradicted information to the contrary, as reported in the *Irish Medical Times* and quoted by Prof O'Neill.

I believe that Beaumont Hospital should get its house in order by hiring financial people to quantify the cost of each clinical service and the major diseases therein. Then it should campaign for a national system which ensures that the money follows the patient. Then the administration's justifiable complaint that Beaumont subsidises other public health agencies would be answered. At the meeting, there was uniform solidarity amongst the consultants to look for savings where possible, while noting that pay was about 70 per cent of the hospital's expenditure. Possible savings of zero to €2 million were claimed, but these were "pie in the sky" without specifics.

A week later an editorial in *The Irish Times* regarding the Denise Livingstone case in Monaghan General Hospital highlighted the tensions that exist between doctors and health authorites:

> A clear conflict emerges between the local health board and independent medical experts about the treatment of Denise Livingstone, exposing the incompatibility between the administrators of the health system and the medical imperative to put the patient first. This tension rather than the apportionment of blame is the key finding of the reports published by the Minister for Health, Mr Martin.[4]

These words echo the situation in Beaumont Hospital perfectly.

3

Are there no improvements in the health service despite the huge investment?

One would be forgiven for thinking that the quality of healthcare in Ireland is akin to third-world standards judging from its portrayal in the media. The two media sages, Eamon Dunphy and Fintan O'Toole, mutually agreed the obvious truism that the health services were getting worse on *The Last Word* on Today FM in November 2002. A quick glance at the facts would prove otherwise. The State's hospitals treated 870,000 patients in 2000 compared with 960,000 in 2002. There was a 15 per cent increase in the number of prescriptions written over this period. Half the increase of 6 per cent in health spending next year will be spent on drugs with pharmaceutical prices up 15 per cent on average. Our Lady's Hospital for Sick Children, Crumlin admitted 14,719 to the end of September 2002, up 1,349 on 2001. Outpatient attendances were up 2,443 to 47,719 in the same period. Admittedly, the population growth in Ireland has placed an added burden on patient services, where there are undeniably longer queues such as in A&E Departments, etc. and waiting times for elective procedures, such as hip replacements, are lengthened.

In 1996, public health spending was €3.2 billion which had risen to €8.4 billion by 2002, a 162 per cent increase in six years. This is 17.5 per cent per year and is way ahead of inflation. In Britain, health spending is about £68 billion (€107 billion) on the National Health Service (NHS). This averages €1,725 per head of population. The British consider this level inadequate and intend to greatly increase spending in the immediate future. Public sector health spending per head in the Republic averages €2,125 per head. This is 23 per cent ahead of the British at present.

In the *Evening Herald* (21 November 2002), Dan White made a few apposite comments. He described the effects of capacity restraint on services. The Government cannot increase the supply of health services simply by increasing the volume spending. It takes time to plan and build new beds and hospitals. It takes years to increase the supply of doctors, nurses and other health professionals. In contrast, it takes a

Are there no improvements in the health service despite the huge investment?

blink of the eye to increase the number of administrators and health boards. If the Government increases health spending at a greater rate than can be absorbed in capacity increase, then the price will go up, i.e. medical inflation.

The Wanless Report on the NHS calculated that real increases in health spending should be kept at about 7 per cent per year. It is likely that the huge increase in health spending here has lead to inflationary thinking in health services and consequent money wasting. White rightly suggests that competition should be enforced on the health sector to improve value for money.

Not surprisingly, value for money is also occupying the mind of the Minister for Finance. In September 2002, Charlie McCreevy wrote to Micheál Martin expressing his "dismay" and "considerable alarm" at the failure of increased spending to bring about expected improvements in the standard of services for patients. One area that is consuming budgets is drugs bills. The figures for the cost explosion for oncology drugs countrywide are frightening and underline the difficulties of budget control for drugs. See Table 3.1 for the oncology drugs costs in respective health boards. See also Chapter 30 on "screening for disease" for some evidence of outcome improvements.

Table 3.1 Oncology drug costs

Health Board	2000 (€)	2001 (€)	2002 (€)
ERHA	10 million		15 million
North Western	245,889		1,899,000
North Eastern	730,771		1,355,494
Midland		450,000	
Western		271,000*	730,000*
UCHG			2.6 million
Southern	930,000		1.8 million†
Mid Western		1,539,077	1,729,300
South Eastern		936,000	1 million

*Portiuncula Hospital, Ballinasloe only
†The Southern Health Board appointed two new oncologists since 2001
UCHG: University College Hospital Galway

4

Health service employment

Much of the recent investment in the health service has gone towards creating a multi-layered health board bureaucracy. Relatively small hospitals which were once administered by two senior health board personnel now require up to ten times that number of managers in order to function.

Irish Times editorial, 23 December 2002

Administration rules OK

There is no simple answer to the question, "what is the best way to provide social services?" In an age of increasing bureaucratisation, the health service is always likely to soak up large numbers of people because accreditation, management meetings and futile circles of indecision and contradiction can always ensure that everyone is busy providing patient services. Just in case there is any doubt, however, "Patient Services" is a title spread around like confetti to confer pseudovalidity to expressions of group therapy.

The figures cited for those employed in the health service are open to scrutiny. By 2002, there were over 96,000 people working in the public health sector, almost 30,000 more than the 1997 total when Fianna Fáil and the Progressive Democrats (PDs) took office. The budget increased from €3 billion to €8.3 billion over this period. Given that level of investment, the impact on patients should have been much greater and it is obvious that something is wrong. But who really knows how many are employed? Trinity College Dublin (TCD) economist Dr Sean Barrett speaking at a post-Budget 2003 conference said that the Department of Health had stated that there were 90,000 people working in the public health sector, but the Department of Finance had put the figure at 96,000. Clearly, there is neither consensus nor communication between the respective Departments. That said, the Department of Health's recently released Personnel Census for 2002 did adjust the figure to approximately

Health service employment

96,000. Moreover, there are an additional 3,800 unauthorised posts in the health service above the recommended ceiling. There is an intention to cut 1,000 permanent or over 1,200 temporary jobs in health as part of the reduction of 5,000 public sector jobs ordered in the Budget.

Table 4.1 Staff increases (1997–2002)

Year	1997	2001		2002	
	No.	No.	Percentage increase (%)	No.	Percentage increase (%)
Nurses	27,346	31,429	+15	33,395	+6
Medical/Dental	4,976	6,285	+26	6,775	+8
Administrative	8,844	14,714	+66	15,690	+7

Source: Dept of Health & Children Personnel Census, 1997, 2001, 2002

A close look at the staff increases since 1997 beggars belief (see Table 4.1). Does anyone think that employing an extra 4,083 nurses and an extra 1,309 doctors needed an extra 5,870 administrators to keep them at the coalface in 2001. Bearing in mind that 96,000 were employed in total, another 43,572 people are also employed in the health sector. Similarly in 2002, 976 administrators were required for an extra 1,966 nurses and 490 doctors. Quite an army!

Policy chaos

Beyond all doubt there is policy chaos regarding health at the heart of the Fianna Fáil/PD coalition. The front page of *The Sunday Tribune* on 8 December 2002 stated that the Finance Minister had backed down on plans to slash up to 5,000 health service jobs:

> The Department of Finance withdrew [a] statement.... confirming that thousands of unauthorised posts created by health boards without official sanction in the last 18 months be eliminated on top of the government's plans announced in the budget to scale back public sector numbers.... sources close to the health minister insisting .... that the finance plan to slash 5,000 health service posts would not go ahead.

McCreevy was trying to cull 1,200 jobs plus the 3,800 unauthorised jobs in the health service until Martin blocked the move. The Department of Finance has now officially accepted the 3,800 jobs and will cut the 5,000 public sector jobs from across the entire public sector. *The Sunday*

Tribune also noted the *volte-face* of McCreevy's position. "Sources also accepted that the new position was not altogether in line with comments made by the minister [McCreevy] earlier in the week."

Two days later, the *Irish Independent* (12 December) reported that the Department of Health had indicated that there was no basis to believe it was going to be asked to find 1,650 job losses or any other number suggested. Nonetheless, in the same paper on the same page, the Minister admitted that there would be job losses within the healthcare sector, but refused to speculate on reports suggesting the cutbacks could reach 5,000 jobs. If that's not chaos, what is?

Table 4.2 Numbers employed in the Public Health Service (2001–2002)

Public health service	2001 (No.)	2002 (No.)
Management/Administration	14,714	15,690
Medical/Dental	6,285	6,775
Nursing	31,429	33,395
Health and social care professionals	9,228	12,577
General support staff	13,803	13,729
Other patient and client care	17,537	13,513
Total	92,996	95,679

Source: Dept of Health & Children Personnel Census, 2001, 2002

Cheap, easily fired, mainly female home helps, etc. were the losers – so were their clients, while administration still blooms.

Medical manpower

By international standards and in light of EU legislation, medical manpower in Ireland is far from adequate or satisfactory. There were 1,650 consultants in public hospitals in January 2001, which was an increase of 120 in one year. The details are contained in the excellent report of the Forum on Medical Manpower published in January 2001. The Task Force on Medical Staffing will lead to a doubling or trebling of consultants in the next 5 to 10 years. In accordance with the European Working Time Directive, working hours of junior doctors in hospitals will have to be reduced to 58 hours by 2004, 56 hours by 2007 and 48 hours by 2010. To achieve a 48-hour NCHD working week, the Task Force claims that an extra 3,500 consultants will be necessary. The Irish Hospital Consultants' Association (IHCA) in 1999 suggested an increase of 775 posts by 2007, if the Department of Health intended to provide a consultant-delivered service rather

Health service employment

than a consultant-led service as at present. Not surprisingly, the figures are shooting upwards each time a formal group considers the issue.

In terms of general practitioners (GPs), there are about 2,600 in the country at present. However, their job satisfaction levels are far from encouraging. A recent survey of newly qualified GPs shows that 20 per cent have left general practice within five years of qualifying. An Irish Medical Organisation (IMO) survey in 2002 found that nearly one-third of doctors would not enter medicine if they were starting their careers again. Moreover, about 10 per cent of Irish junior doctors leave the profession within six years of graduation. Nonetheless, this is not deterring those entering the profession. The number of Irish junior doctors working in the health service was 1,849 in 2002, which is a record. Essentially, this is an increase from 1,574 in 1984. Overall, the approved complement of junior doctor posts increased from 1,795.5 in 1984 to 3,897.5 in 2002 (+117 per cent). These posts have been filled overwhelmingly by non-national junior doctors whose numbers have increased from 242 in 1984 to 2,088 by 2002. Since 1993, consultant numbers have increased by 390 posts, whereas the number of NCHDs has increased by 900. This has continued the system where there are about two junior doctors to each consultant. In contrast, the UK ratio is about 25 per cent less. The ratio of approved NCHD posts to consultant posts was 1.57:1 in 1984 but is now 2.39:1 in 2002. Clearly, the number of consultant posts needs to be increased, as consultants should do more frontline work. The census figures for junior doctors for 1 October 2002 as published by the Postgraduate Medical and Dental Board are shown in Table 4.3.

Table 4.3 Census figures for NCHDs, 2002

Grade	Approved	Irish		Foreign		Totals		Total
		Male	Female	Male	Female	Male	Female	
Intern	460.00	153.00	173.0	83.0	53.0	236.0	226.0	462.0
H/officer	1,666.75	317.25	405.0	781.0	180.0	1,098.2	583.0	1,683.2
Registrar	1,165.80	1667.10	174.7	744.5	111.5	911.6	286.2	1,193.8
Senior/ SpR registrar	605.00	876.35	220.0	114.0	20.5	353.0	240.5	593.5
Total	3,897.55	876.35	972.7	1,722.5	365.0	2,598.9	1,337.7	3,932.5

Source: Postgraduate Medical and Dental Board, 2002

A Cure for the Crisis

The approved complement means the posts are authorised and funded by the Department of Health. However, the figures do not include the third-year registrar posts in the general practice specialist training schemes. Ireland is also very reliant on foreign medical graduates. Fifty-three per cent of junior doctors in our hospitals are non-nationals, including 72 per cent of all registrars and 23 per cent of all senior registrars/specialist registrars. The percentage of non-nationals in registrar posts varies from a low of 51 per cent in Dublin to 96 per cent in the North West and Midlands. Only in the voluntary hospitals and in Dublin are about half the registrars Irish. In six regions less than 20 per cent of registrars are Irish.

Changing profile

Poor pay, long hours, increased workloads, poor career prospects and stress have all been blamed for the decline in the number of native Irish medical students both male and female. Feminisation is also taking place because girls are outperforming boys in the Leaving Certificate and objective academic merit is ruling medical school intake. Feminisation of general practice in Ireland is well under way. It will have serious consequences for service provision because it is likely to lead to less hours worked per head, assuming that there is no sex difference on patient throughput. My mad generation of early-dying doctors is being replaced by a more sanguine and sensible bunch! Modern doctors want their holidays, time off and uninterrupted by calls, paid study leave and time for sport and recreation.

In 2002, 61 females and 18 males entered the GP training schemes. Eighty-four per cent of Irish College of General Practitioners (ICGP) members under the age of 29 are female and 65 per cent of the 30–34-year age group are female. At present, 65 per cent of all GPs are female. The ICGP has flagged the need for the number of GP training places to rise from the current 79 to 150 in the immediate future to cater for GP retirements over the next decade. The figures in Table 4.4 show the rise of the female workforce in medicine.

Health service employment

Table 4.4 Rise of female workforce in medicine

Workforce	Male (%)	Female (%)
Irish junior doctors, 1984	61	39
Irish junior doctors, 2002	47	53
Medical students	38	62
Consultant surgeons	96	4
A&E	90	10
Gynaecologists	85	15
Radiologists	82	18
Appointed in 1990	75	25
Appointed in 2001	59	41

Source: Postgraduate Medical and Dental Board, 2002

Training in A&E medicine – the "ah sure, it'll do" culture

Daily news features of ever-increasing queues in A&E Departments have highlighted the need for additional consultants in accident and emergency medicine. Nonetheless in 2003, there were 22 smaller hospitals without full-time A&E consultants. Either the public wants properly trained doctors looking after them or they do not. If they do, it costs.

The Royal College of Surgeons in Ireland (RCSI) is the training body that accredits posts and recognises the time spent as suitable for the requirements of professional training programmes. Once the accreditation is not forthcoming, hospitals can no longer employ junior doctors in training posts. The College must ensure that standards are maintained throughout the country with rolling inspections done on facilities available at every department. To keep hospitals at Bantry, Mallow, Ennis, Clonmel, Nenagh, Kilkenny and Dundalk open, it is necessary to hire 50 consultants before mid-2004. Junior doctors in training must have consultant supervision. The bottom line is, how can you train in a profession unless supervised? It certainly does not bode well for the future in providing an equitable health service. However, doctors are no longer prepared to see the unacceptable and less than adequate passed off in silence only to rebound in a new cultural environment a decade down the road.

The unacceptable status of medical manpower was cogently put in an *Irish Examiner* editorial on 7 January 2003:

> The latest controversy underscores the urgency of radically overhauling a health system where bureaucracy is endemic and where management operates in state-of-the-art offices while hospitals and other services are tottering. In recent years three times more administrators were recruited than health professionals.

A Cure for the Crisis

With the college authorities carrying out a rolling inspection of the country's hospitals, foreshadowing the possible withdrawal of junior doctors, they have effectively put the gun to the head of Health Minister Micheál Martin.

Medical schools

At present there are only about 340 medical school places for Irish/EU students. Of this number, only 48 per cent of undergraduates in our five medical schools are nationals. In UCD, there are currently 108 national and 77 non-EU places. This leaves Ireland with an unbridgeable manpower gap unless changes are introduced. The Higher Education Authority (HEA) pays medical schools €7,135 to €9,000 per EU student per year. Non-EU students pay €21,300 per student per year in four of the five medical schools, namely TCD, UCD, UCG and UCC. The fifth, the RCSI, charges €32,000. Non-EU students contribute about €32.4 million to medical schools in the State.

By way of contrast, in Scotland the average grant per student per year is €36,430, while at Queen's University Belfast the capitation is €34,976. However, fees for non-EU students in Belfast are only €18,000. TCD only allocates 49 per cent of non-EU student fees to their medical school. Irish students who can afford foreign student fees should be allowed compete for places with these foreigners.

5

The Health Boards

The Health Act 1970 provided for the establishment of eight health boards which have been responsible for the administration of some of the health services in Ireland since 1971. Membership of the health boards consists of councillors, medical and paramedical representatives and three ministerial appointees. Each health board has a chief executive and boards divide up their work into three broad programmes, each run by a manager. These deal with community care, general hospital and special hospital services.

There are now 10 health boards plus the Eastern Regional Health Authority (ERHA) and the Department of Health. The health boards employ 96,000 people, of which 29,000 are nurses and 5,700 are doctors and dentists. Among the non-medical and nursing staff are ambulance crews and paramedical staff. In line with rising costs, the overall budget for the health boards will increase from €8.2 billion in 2002 to €8.9 billion in 2003. This is an average increase of 7 per cent with inflation running at 5 per cent and medical inflation at another 5–7 per cent. Services are likely to be reduced as pay accounts for at least 70 per cent of the budget and benchmarking will be implemented at the expense of patient services.

The most recent figure claims that 1 in 13 staff appointed to the health services is involved in direct clinical contact with patients. In the *Irish Independent* on 3 December 2002, Eilish O'Regan wrote a defence of the health boards and the criticism of the numbers of administrative staff hired. According to O'Regan, the number of administrative staff hired at the expense of more doctors and nurses in the system does not stand up to scrutiny when their job descriptions are analysed. Sixty per cent of the extra staff were in frontline service – working as social workers, community welfare officers or ambulance staff.

Throughout the country, the efficacy and efficiency of health boards have long been called into question, none more so than in the case of the

A Cure for the Crisis

ERHA. Its administration of health services, particularly in respect of buying treatments, is wholly unsatisfactory.

Eastern Regional Health Authority

The ERHA was established in March 2000 from the ashes of the Eastern Health Board (EHB) when three new health boards – the Northern Area, East Coast Area and South Western Area Health Authorities – were appointed with an overarching ERHA. The purpose of the ERHA was to remove the Department of Health from directly funding the Dublin Voluntary Teaching Hospitals and place a buffer between the providers and the paymasters. In practice, the proliferation of administration posts and transfers of junior administration staff from hospitals like Beaumont to the ERHA and Northern Area Health Board was witnessed.

On the basis of an annual service plan, the ERHA is given a block grant to fund services and buy them for public patients from the hospitals. With current spending, the Dublin hospitals were approximately €50 million overspent by the end of 2002.

In November 2002, the Government directed that the new chief executive of the ERHA should be appointed for two years only. This was to allow change in health service administration in response to the Prospectus Report, 2003. Days later on Wednesday, 13 November, perhaps by coincidence, a four-page commercial supplement appeared in *The Irish Times* with the banner headline "ERHA: Eastern Regional Health Authority – Buying and assuring best health for you". The self-serving tone of posturing condescension in the text was risible. Never was the key question put – would the overnight elimination of the ERHA superstructure have any deleterious effect on the level of services in the greater Dublin area? To give you a taste of the "administrator speak" and the type of paternalistic pomposity in vogue, a short quotation is needed:

> The ERHA is unique... in that it 'purchases' services, treatments and procedures for its clients from the three area health boards in the east ... and from 36 voluntary agencies in the region, including the major acute teaching hospitals and those who provide services for persons with physical and intellectual disabilities. The extent of the services that the authority buys is agreed annually with each of the provider agencies.
>
> The ERHA purchases the whole range of health and personal social services including primary care, community services, acute hospi-

The Health Boards

tal services, mental health services, services for persons with intellectual and physical disabilities, services for children and families, services for older persons, addiction services and services for the socially disadvantaged. In the current year the authority's budget is €2.8 billion.

What is worth noting here is that there is no mention at all of patient choice. Furthermore, so inefficacious is this administrative behemoth that each service goes on largely oblivious to the ERHA's "machinations". Tight control of the purse strings, while seeming to espouse advances in the medical treatment of patients, underpins the inherent contradiction in their philosophy. According to ERHA chief executive and veteran administrator, Donal O'Shea:

> There has been a major expansion of health and personal social services in the east in recent years but needs are always increasing and technology developing, so we face major challenges on an ongoing basis, which is as it should be.... We are committed to working with all our provider agencies to look for new answers and new solutions. And of course this must all be done in the context of a finite amount of resources. **Indeed the prudent fiscal management of the services is one of the major tasks facing each agency.** [my emphasis]

How then does a market take out a flabby, poorly performing agency? The answer is patently clear – through COMPETITION. However, that aspect of market forces is one strangely not applied to the governance of public hospitals, despite being run ever more increasingly along the lines of public limited companies. According to the supplement, the Authority uses two yardsticks in buying services – "scientific assessment of need and the view of clients and patients on the type of services which they themselves feel they require. Underpinning all this is value for money." The question of who undertakes these scientific assessments and how is strangely lacking. The same applies to patient choice.

Taking the credit

The ERHA takes credit for opening up minor injury units and specialist treatment units for chest pain, deep venous thrombosis and respiratory illnesses in acute hospitals as if the advent of the ERHA had accelerated these events. The reality is rather different. Indeed, the professional staff in hospitals have been driving this agenda for years. For example, the

A Cure for the Crisis

Chest Pain Evaluation and Treatment Unit for Beaumont Hospital was first discussed with the cardiologist Prof John H. Horgan back in 1994. Managerial inertia was the reason for the delay, however. The benefits of such units were well known to the profession for many years. Throughout the 1990s, formal evaluations were published in the *Annals of Emergency Medicine* in the US. Similarly, the distress of patients and the scrum at the Warfarin Clinic at Beaumont Hospital was a major driver of reform in that area. Raising such issues in a public forum can often act as a catalyst for change. The broadcaster Gay Byrne with his guests on radio and the *Late Late Show* was far more effective than any ERHA in making things happen. In fact, accountability in public is the key. That applies to all professionals, not least of all medical.

In elaborating on its functions, the article makes reference to the ERHA's role in evaluating and monitoring services: "Part of the authority's role is also to evaluate and monitor the services which it buys from each of the different agencies to ensure that they are effective, efficient, of high quality and delivered in an equitable and accountable manner." This seems to me to effectively supplant the remit of professional bodies. Where does it leave the efforts of the Medical Council with regard to continuing medical education, audits, reaccreditation, recertification and the efforts of the RCSI (Royal College of Surgeons in Ireland) and RCPI (Royal College of Physicians of Ireland) with regard to surgical and medical standards?

The hospital building and refurbishment programme in the region is yet another initiative seized as an ERHA success. According to the EHRA, they have been responsible for upgrading such hospitals as Naas General Hospital, James Connolly Memorial Hospital, the Mater Hospital, The Children's Hospital, Temple Street (to transfer to Eccles Street), St Vincent's University Hospital, St Columcille's Hospital, Loughlinstown and finally Our Lady's Hospital for Sick Children, Crumlin. Time was when the Fianna Fáil Government claimed that as a Department of Health success.

Next the ERHA claims credit for the reputed falls in the death rates for various cancers over the past decade. The Public Health Department of the ERHA reported that the death rate from cancer for the period 1992 to 1997 fell by 8 per cent in men and 9.7 per cent in women. A dramatic increase in the level of hospital treatments and early detection are cited as ERHA achievements. In reality, cancer treatment units should be

The Health Boards

present in every large teaching hospital and the results of international clinical trials drive investigation and treatment modalities.

A colour piece on a baby from Waterford who had a surgical procedure by Mr Martin Corbally, paediatric surgeon at Our Lady's Hospital for Sick Children, is also the focus of ERHA pride. Subliminally, are we supposed to be grateful to the ERHA for providing such a quality service in the Eastern region? Headlined as "Speedy diagnosis saves the day", it goes on to say that "at six-weeks of age, her check up showed a rare liver complaint... swift action and great co-operation led to a successful outcome for baby Aisling". There is nothing extraordinary about cross-referral and co-operation in medicine. In fact, it is the norm. In medicine, the common problem is not inappropriate non-referral but of trying to admit patients from other hospitals when all beds are full from routine medicine cases admitted through the A&E Department.

The ERHA procurement team also gets a splash. Part of the Eastern Health Shared Services, the team is designed to give volume weight and bargaining power to a central procurement agency and then to subsupply the three Dublin health boards. For example, it provided counselling and communications for Irish families affected by the events of 9/11 in New York, organised disinfection for foot-and-mouth disease protection in recent years, and helped the Ringsend, Dublin area residents after the River Dodder flooding. The director of procurement and materials management, Mr John Swords, purchased smallpox vaccines and ciprofloxacin antibiotics for anthrax as a contingency to counter biological terrorism, which was a sensible move. The iodine tablets distributed to each household to block radio-iodine cancers from nuclear fallout were also part of their remit. Although, how many households could put their hands on their supply six months later? A statistically valid random survey should be carried to find out the effectiveness of this strategy before self-congratulation is warranted. This procurement department also acts as agents for the Department of Health and Children and the various health boards in buying vaccines for all immunisation programmes. They also warehouse supplies for the Dublin area. In fact, this group would be better served as a section of the Department of Health and, if effective, it should bargain for therapeutics supplies for the whole country.

The hagiography continues apace on the next page of the supplement with human-interest stories. First up is a story about Mr Mark Redmond from Our Lady's Hospital for Sick Children, Crumlin who operated on an Ennistymon child with a cardiac lesion after transferring the 10-year-old

A Cure for the Crisis

boy to Johns Hopkins Hospital in Baltimore, Maryland. The final quote from the mother is telling: "It was simply brilliant for a medical card patient to be treated this way – all our expenses were paid." If you remember the ethical duty of the doctor to do whatever he can for each patient, then it is not surprising that Mark Redmond would wish to properly treat the boy in the best conditions possible. One other question remains, however. Let's assume that the boy is the patient of the ERHA rather than Mark Redmond. Did the ERHA look into a cheaper option in the European Union for this boy? An E112 form would have allowed the boy public health treatment in the EU, if available.

Next up is the cochlear implant service for deafness run by ENT surgeon Dr Laura Viani at Beaumont Hospital. This service started in 1994, which was some considerable time before it was procured by the ERHA. The hearing therapists do a fantastic job after the surgery and display great skill and patience.

The next vignette was on home-based treatment of chronic obstructive pulmonary disease (COPD) from Beaumont Hospital and headed "Economic medicine". The COPD Outreach team for home help has ensured that such patients spend an average of 2.6 days per admission to hospital for an acute exacerbation instead of a previous average of 8–10 days. On discharge, patients are visited daily at home by the COPD team. The team monitors the patient by phone also and provides education on the disease, lifestyle and medication. They also give advice on exercise, chest clearance, smoking cessation, coping mechanisms and self-management plans. In essence, this is a large infringement of the role of the GP and it is unclear how this practice will work into the future. The related issue of rewriting hospital prescriptions for GMS patients will annoy GPs and certainly needs reform.

Control of prescribing

Control of prescribing is one measure which the ERHA has decided to promote in order to curb spending and allow hospitals to stay within budget. In 2002, CEO of the Mater Hospital, Martin Cowley, presented a memo to his hospital board in which he claimed that all the main Dublin hospitals were in agreement on the need for a restriction on the traditional freedom of prescription by doctors: "It was agreed (at a September meeting) there is a requirement for national protocols on drug prescribing which would cap the range of drugs that can be prescribed in hospitals. The ERHA will be raising this with the Department of Health."

The memo got a front-page airing in *The Sunday Tribune* in November. The article drew attention to the fact that Minister for Health Micheál Martin had planned to establish a new agency, the Health Information Evaluation Agency, which was to assess new technologies and new drug treatments before they were introduced to State hospitals. Spin doctors at the Department of Health, however, intimated that the Minister would be opposed to the introduction of any capping of drug treatments for public patients. It is obvious that a version of the British National Institute for Clinical Excellence (NICE) is heading this way. *Plus ça change?*

Health board cull on the agenda

In an *Irish Examiner* editorial in November 2002, headlined "Health crisis bureaucratic excess must be eliminated", the case for rationalisation of the health boards was strongly put:

> It is astonishing that only one out of every 13 people recruited by the health service in recent times is engaged in direct clinical contact with patients ... administrative staff employed by the country's health boards are devouring 70 per cent of the health budget amid mounting calls for greater value for taxpayers' money.... If ever there was a compelling argument for rationalization of the health boards, Health Minister Michael Martin will find it in the unnecessary duplication of costly services spawned by a proliferation of officialdom. Apparently, the recruitment of additional nurses and doctors, urgently needed to work at the coalface, is being outstripped by the appointment of administrative personnel. As a result, nursing and medical staff are leaving the service in droves.... The conditions in local health centres in some parts of the country remain Dickensian while managers occupy state-of-the-art offices.... Incredibly, a value-for-money audit of the health service failed to include the government department at the centre of the crisis.... Arguably a hospital authority should be set up to make decisions currently made by health boards.... Ireland has a lower standard of health service than most other EU countries and still has Europe's lowest per capita number of hospital beds.... It would be a major step towards giving taxpayers more value for money if the government overhauled the country's lumbering health board system. It is time for Mr Martin to grasp the nettle.[1]

Clearly, reform of the health boards is long overdue. In the Prospectus Report released in June 2003, it was proposed that the 11 health boards

A Cure for the Crisis

and the ERHA should be abolished and replaced by a new Health Service Executive (HSE). Essentially, the HSE will take over many of the functions controlled by the Department of Finance and will control all hospitals through a National Hospitals Office, in addition to managing primary, community and long-term health services. In my view, any proposed changes to the health boards should bear the following solutions in mind.

Solutions

- Health boards should reflect regional health priorities. The mix of political and professional interests should be preserved on the management boards.
- The health board role in managing hospitals should be removed.
- Health boards should ensure that step-down facilities and community care are sufficient for the population.
- Health boards should be involved in public health; for example, vaccination programmes, home care, homelessness, care of disturbed children and the treatment of drug addictions.
- The boards should have a role in facilitating the development of general practice in association with the Irish College of General Practitioners (ICGP), the Irish Medical Organisation (IMO) and the independent GP organisations.
- Health boards should employ consultant geriatricians and psychogeriatricians in association with hospitals to care for the elderly.
- Health boards should have a co-ordinating role in ensuring full services for the mentally and physically handicapped. They should fill gaps where the current agencies are deficient.
- Health board payments to GPs should not be postponed in the fourth quarter to arrive in January, even when interest is paid under the Prompt Payment of Accounts Act 1997. This activity merely adds to GP cynicism regarding the administrative system.

6

The General Medical Services (GMS)

Since its inception in 1972, the Government-funded General Medical Services (GMS) scheme has provided free medical care to those on low incomes. The scheme can be improved and is certainly worth improving. Undeniably, it will always facilitate a two-tier system as long as there are "private patients". Nonetheless, it is relatively efficient and keeps the volume of paperwork bearable. Many patients with GMS cards are under the mistaken impression that the doctor is paid for their every visit. Indeed, some would be very surprised at the fee levels actually paid to the GP. However, additional payments towards pension contributions, holiday and locum allowances as well as nurse and secretary salaries make the true figures less parsimonious.

GMS entry

Entry to the scheme is restricted. It is based on capitation for primary care services with choice of doctor and choice of patient. A GP with relevant qualifications, who on 1 March 1999, was engaged in full-time general practice in one location for five consecutive years starting before 1 March 1999 is entitled to enter the GMS scheme at the end of the five years' wait. The GP can only take on patients who become eligible for a medical card for the first time. Three years later (after the first five-year wait), any GMS patient is able to transfer to the practice. Participating doctors who have a GMS panel of 500 patients or more would normally be entitled to apply for a partner/assistant with a view to up to five years before retirement.

In June 2001, a once-off entry arrangement was agreed in association with the new over-70s scheme. It gave the right of entry to any fully qualified and vocationally trained GP who was in practice on 1 July 2001, and who had been in that practice for one whole year or had bought or entered into partnership with an existing GP. This right of

A Cure for the Crisis

entry restricted the GP for five years to public patients in the new over-70s medical card scheme. In other words, the GP could hold on to older private patients. If the GP was in partnership on the date of limited entry, then the wait period was reduced to two years before unrestricted access was given.

Capitation

Capitation fees are based on the age, sex and distance from the practice and on whether the patient is entitled to a medical card at 69 years of age or not. Fees for means-tested over-70s in March 1999 are shown in Table 6.1.

Table 6.1 Fees for means-tested over-70s

Distance (miles)	<3	3–5	5–7	7–10	>10
Male (IR£)	62.67	70.32	81.70	92.88	106.77
Female (IR£)	69.90	77.57	88.95	100.13	114.03

Eighty per cent of the over-70s are paid at €100 per year rate. Capitation fees in November 2002 are shown in Table 6.2.

Table 6.2 Capitation fees (as of November 2002)

Age (yrs)	Male (€)	Female (€)
0–4	57.55	56.13
5–15	33.38	33.77
16–44	42.61	69.71
45–64	85.14	93.56
65–69	89.70	100.07
70+	92.62	103.30
New 70+	462.16	462.16

If private patients are paying more than €32 per visit, the GMS is obviously a cheap deal for the taxpayer. For years, private practice subsidised the GMS. Essentially, this is a hangover from the Poor Law and medical professionalism and the doctor's duty to society at large. I fully accept this duty, which is why some of the new American innovations of super GPs with high private capitation fees are ethically dubious as they exclude a whole swathe of society.

Value for money

In these cost-effective times we live in, the question of value for money inevitably arises. How then am I fairly certain that the taxpayers are getting cracking good value for the capitation fees? A British study of over 10,000 patients in two practices in inner-city Sheffield showed the frequency of attendances related to age and sex. The mean (average) attendance of women was between 5 and 6 times per year each decade from 15 to 75 years of age. The mean attendance for males was approximately 2.6 per year under 30 years old to approximately 4 times per year from 45 to 55, to peak at nearly 5 times per year at 65 and falls slightly after that.[1] Frequent attendees at those practices were defined as the top 3 per cent and their annual attendances are shown in Table 6.3 below.

Table 6.3 Annual attendances at GP practices (top 3 per cent)

Age (years)	Male (No.)	Female (No.)
15–25	11	17
26–35	12	18
36–45	14	19
46–55	18	20
56–65	18	20
66–75	16	22

In Ireland the GMS is likely to have similar attendance figures. The fee-per-visit confirms that the GMS is below the French GP strike threshold. How about the loss leaders who are the frequent attenders? That is why criticising GPs is unwise. Indeed, we should be grateful to them for their efforts.

Practice nurses and secretaries

There are tiered allowances for hiring practice nurses and secretaries. The 2001 maximum rates were IR£22,000 for a practice nurse with three years' experience and IR£14,000 for a secretary with three years' relevant experience. A weighting of 3:1 for any person aged 70 on a doctor's panel is used to calculate the panel size for the purpose of calculation of the allowance for a practice nurse and secretary. Certainly, these GMS payments have greatly facilitated an expansion in the numbers of practice nurses and secretaries. In addition, the GMS paid a once-off IR£100 per asylum seeker on a doctor's list. There was also a pro rata payment covering loss of income from discretionary medical cardholders.

Indicative drug budgeting

Schemes that reward doctors for staying within a drug budget are ethically inimical in my opinion. Under the Indicative Drug Budgeting Scheme introduced in 1993, doctors can use "savings" to fund practice developments. National averages of drug costs for age/gender bands are used. A grant equal to 50 per cent of the difference between their net costs and the net national age/gender-related average cost is paid. Consequently, if you are ahead of the posse and up to the latest trial evidence in your medical field, your drug costs are likely to be above the national figures. Practice development funding is an area that should be handled differently.

Drug costs

In 2002, the cost of the GMS was €1.4 billion. The cost of drugs to the scheme was €434 million in the same year. There has been a 65 per cent increase in the number of items prescribed over the 10 years to 2001. Compared to 1991, there has been a doubling of the number of six-item prescriptions and a threefold increase in the number with more than seven items. In Europe the value of healthcare consumed by the over-65s is about 2.3 times greater than for the under-65s. Thus, it clear that expenditure on drugs for the over-70s will escalate out of control. For example, selective serotonin reuptake inhibitors (SSRIs) accounted for 5 per cent of the GMS drug expenditure in 2001 and statins and proton pump inhibitors accounted for 20 per cent. The statin, atorvastatin (Lipitor), is the world's bestselling drug. This is not surprising given the prevalence of arterial disease in the western world.[2]

Warfarin and INR service

In recent years, the management of anticoagulation therapy has been extended to GP surgeries. However, GPs are not always prepared to run their own anticoagulation clinics due to a variety of reasons, namely lack of time, knowledge, training and facilities, in addition to the need for more finance. A possible solution to this problem is the following: Patients are given target INR (international normalised ratio) values from the hospitals and go to their GPs to have values measured and dose

The General Medical Services (GMS)

adjustments made. This is an obvious use of near-patient testing which is hugely cost-effective to the patient. In 2001, the GMS agreed a pilot study on the basis of a fixed budget, which had expired before the end of the year, resulting in some GPs not being paid. Technophiles should buy their own machines, check their performance in the local laboratory and avoid the continuous hassle of hospitals and GPs altogether.

"Ghosts"

Newspapers made much mileage out of the Comptroller and Auditor General's report in September 2002 that GPs could have been overpaid in the region of €12 million per annum for treating about 20,000 dead or ineligible patients. Apparently, out-of-date Central Statistics Office lists resulted in the inclusion of 20,000 doubly registered or dead patients on the national list. An investigation resulted in the removal of 14,100 medical cards from people who had died or had been duplicated.

Clearly, the problem is an administrative mess of farcical proportions. So much so that health board officials are being sent out to surgeries throughout the country in search of "ghost patients". In response, IMO GP chairman Dr James Reilly advised non-cooperation and requested an independent audit from Deloitte & Touche or its equivalent. That GPs have no control over which patients are covered by the GMS is clear from Dr Reilly's comments: "We don't apply for payment for patients we treat who have a medical card. The health board sends us a sum every month, and it is very rarely that my records would balance with their cheque." According to Dr Reilly, there are about 25,000 people who are unregistered on health board GMS lists, but who still have to be treated as they present a valid medical card. Where did this figure spring from? Dr Reilly explained the situation as follows: "They have a [medical] card but their names are not on any database. What are we supposed to do? Turn them away? We usually end up not getting paid for these patients. The system is in chaos and needs an urgent review."

Those not entitled to medical cards include single people living alone whose income is more than €132 per week; a single-working mother earning the minimum wage of €250; a married couple with two children, one of whom works 39 hours on minimum pay. This is outrageous when you consider that retired people with pensions in excess of €50,000 per year are entitled to free medical care.

The Department of Health will collect any overpayment made when data are available on individual doctors. Tackling the administrative chaos by the Department is clearly the most appropriate response, as evidenced in an *Irish Examiner* report: "The Department has also instructed health boards to put in place an effective management system for reviewing medical card eligibility in the future."[3]

In all likelihood GPs were not overpaid in the round, given that they are owed money from maternity and newborn child schemes and from vaccinations. For over 14 years GPs have been unable to state with certainty exactly who they have been paid for. There are problems for GPs in three areas. First, newborn infants where the parent has a medical card, but the infant is not yet registered with the health board. Second, a patient whose medical card has been withdrawn by the health board yet who still attends with a "valid" up-to-date card, but is not on the health board payment list. Third, expired medical cardholders who have not bothered to renew their card and are therefore not registered on the health board list, but who still attend the GP and expect not to be charged.

Medical cards for students

As it currently stands, students are not entitled to medical cards. By denying medical cards to them, the State is treating them as parental appendages and not as autonomous adults. The Union of Students in Ireland (USI) claims that up to 50,000 students cannot afford to visit their local GPs. A USI survey found that 20 per cent cannot afford medical care; 16 per cent changed GP due to poor service; 24 per cent had to wait one day to see a college doctor; 12 per cent had to wait three days and 17 per cent had to wait one week. In 2001, USI president Colm Jordan demanded a medical card for every student because they are low-income adults and not simply students. He is absolutely right.[4]

GPs on patients

The shift in emphasis to patients as consumers and their attendant rights has meant striving for an efficiency and best practice in GP surgeries which is often unattainable. A survey of GPs for *Reader's Digest* in 2002 found that doctors are frustrated by patients' lack of trust, untruthfulness (lies), and the assumption that GPs have unlimited time and can work miracles. The research group, NOP, interviewed 200 GPs for the poll and their findings include:

The General Medical Services (GMS)

- 71 per cent said that they would not turn away a patient who had failed to keep a previous appointment.
- 66 per cent would love to say "you're too fat" but don't.
- 50 per cent did not think that patients took the medication prescribed.
- 50 per cent believe that patients lie about what they eat.
- 50 per cent would love to say "please wash yourself before coming in here".
- 25 per cent would love to say "why should I see you, you did not keep your last appointment". Other comments that give a flavour of what many GPs would like to say but cannot include: "Please do not answer your mobile phone while I am giving you a smear test." "Don't treat me like a supermarket assistant." "There is nothing really wrong with you, you need a social worker."
- 66 per cent feel that patients are frustrated if they leave without a prescription. Indeed, public patients think that the doctors are just trying to save money.
- Most doctors would love to say "tell me what is really worrying you straightaway and not when you are leaving".

There is a considerable body of research on why some patients overattend GPs. Some but not all are a considerable source of stress and exasperation to their GPs. Clinically inexplicable frequent attenders (about 15 times per year) in Donegal were recently analysed and had high levels of kinship. The GPs often resorted to psychiatric medications, other prescriptions and referral to cope. These patients consume a disproportionate amount of medical time.[5,6] The issue of frequent attenders is a serious one. For that reason patients who are frequent attenders should probably move practices every five years to lessen the chance of a serious complaint being missed because of exasperation and the disinclination to treat them.

Medical cards for the over-70s

In 2001, the Government originally estimated that about 39,000 people over-70 would automatically become eligible for medical cards at a cost of €19 million. However, the true number turned out to be more than 77,000 at an extra cost of €55 million. By all accounts, the health boards

A Cure for the Crisis

miscalculated the number by 20,000 people. By 2003, the numbers had escalated to 80,000 and is set to rise.

Clearly, this was a naked vote-buying exercise by the Government which obviously worked, but had clear consequences for practising GPs. More than 80 per cent of the over-70s are still paid at the old €100 per annum rate, irrespective of the number of visits to their GP. In reality, some over-70s patients visit the GP surgery more than 12 times per year. These patients are uneconomic to treat; and are in fact a form of charity.

Extending the medical card to all over-70s has meant that retired doctors, lawyers and judges get free primary healthcare although they can well afford to pay. On those unable to pay, Dr Ronan Boland from the IMO is quoted as saying: "I am in no doubt that because of the cost of GP visits and medicine, there are people out there who can't afford this, and as a result have to delay or put off their visit to the doctor." Effectively, the over-70s scheme has led to huge inequality and increased rigidity in the healthcare system.

Meath GP, Dr Martin White believes that the extension of the GMS to the over-70s without a means test has contributed to rising costs for GP practices. "Doctors fees are increasing because of this scheme and this is obviously a problem for low earners. Even a single parent not working a full week could earn over the medical card limit quite easily. The marginalised are becoming more marginalised."[7] I do not believe he is correct about the rising GP practice costs. The fee paid for the wealthy medical cards is much higher than for others and the opposite is more likely the case. Furthermore, I believe that many GPs charge fees that are excessive, which will lead to political pressure and obviously impact on their independent practice.

The Department of Health in reply pointed out that there were discretionary medical cards and that community welfare officers are there to help people. Indeed, the Drug Repayment Scheme had also been set up for this purpose. An interesting question is whether health board officials issue relatively *more* discretionary medical cards to 69-year-olds now than prior to the over-70s extension of the scheme to reduce the capitation fees for GPs. Certainly, a study of the actions and attitudes of health board officials regarding this question would make compelling reading.

7

Nursing

What is exceptional in nursing is the nature of the work: the continuous and intimate association with pain and not infrequent contact with death.... Not every man or woman would feel themselves able to undertake the duties of a nurse. [1]

Brian Abel-Smith
A History of the Nursing Profession

Nurses are the traditional frontline carers in medicine – the Florence Nightingales with hearts of gold. Over the years my experience of nurses has been hugely positive, but now working mainly in the laboratory or directly seeing my own patients, I do not have as much interaction as previously with my nursing colleagues. Nonetheless, it is clear that nursing has changed. It is more assertive and much less calming and pleasant than formerly. Attitudes have hardened and the public discourse has coarsened. For an overwhelmingly female profession, nurses are spoken for in the public arena by male union officials. However, administrators and politicians, who failed to ensure that nurses' pay allowed them to have a decent standard of living and to house themselves near their hospitals or community care areas, are also responsible for these attitude changes. Patients are never best served by closed nurse-free wards. Lamentably, nursing has moved from being regarded as a vocation into the realm of being a "mere job".

Nurse shortages

The extent of true nurse shortages can only be known when nurses spend all their time nursing. Using highly trained nurses to clean rooms and remove food trays is a waste of a scarce resource and is demoralising for nurses. Worldwide, there is a wide-ranging personnel crisis in nursing. There are nurse shortages in the US, Australia, New Zealand, Ireland and Britain. Each country is trying to recruit from each other and from

43

the developing world. In Britain in 2001, the NHS lost one nurse to emigration while importing two others. Some 6,256 nurses emigrated from Britain that year alone.

The general secretary of the British Royal College of Nursing, Beverley Malone, regards overseas recruiting as a long-term measure, not merely a short-term solution. The College supports the activity once it is done ethically and once proper support is given to the new recruits when they arrive in Britain. I think this is a pious platitude. "We must work with our overseas colleagues and embrace them. There are just not enough home-grown nurses." Admittedly, the situation is acute in Britain. There are 400,000 nurses working in that country. There were 16,000 new foreign nurses employed in 2001, of which only 1,091 were from EU countries. The NHS plan published in July 2000 targets an extra 20,000 nurses by 2005. This target has already been achieved through overseas recruitment and the British government has set a new target of recruiting an extra 35,000 nurses by 2008.

There is global competition for skilled nurses and UK and Irish recruitment overseas will become more difficult. The US needs to recruit 1 million nurses over the next 10 years, and as the Western world population age profile gets older, increased demands for carers and caring services follow. The US is offering $5,000 to any nurse who brings a nurse friend to work in the US plus another $5,000 for the friend. Some overseas nurses are being exploited by British recruitment agencies who charge the nurses £2,000 to bring them to Britain. In the US in the 1990s, the number of students entering nursing school dropped by 25 per cent and the age of the average nurse increased from 37.7 to 45.2 years.

Nurses are discovering that they have economic power and organisations like the Irish nurses' unions will not be slow to exploit the opportunities that shortages present. Nurses are demanding a 35-hour working week, a Dublin weighting allowance (€4,000) and improved shift allowance. In addition, under the Benchmarking report nurses have been recommended to get an 8 per cent pay rise.

Impact of shortages

The Health Strategy promised an extra 3,000 beds by 2011, with the first 709 in place by the end of 2003. There are also plans to increase by 700 the number of elderly and step-down beds. If the public-sector freeze on new recruits hits nursing, then these beds will be merely aspirational.

Budget 2003 ordered a cut of 5,000 in the number of public sector workers in the next three years.

When the nursing establishment chooses to preserve the new status quo, what happens when we have no nurses and the Third World cops on? Or when a tribunal of inquiry is set up here about an as-yet unknown medical scandal, can we credibly say that we have examined all the avenues to redress the nursing shortage?

Nursing restructured

In an interview in *The Irish Times*, a colleague of mine at Beaumont Hospital, Mr David Hickey, was critical of the current nursing degree. He claimed that it laid too much emphasis on academic achievement and was flooding the healthcare system with unsuitable nurses. Many new nurses had no long-term interest in the job and only pursued it as a means to a career in other areas of healthcare, such as pharmaceutical sales representatives. This viewpoint is shared by many nurses and hospital consultants since the nursing education system was restructured. Admittedly, I agree with this general thesis. Certainly, it is quite common to find that drug reps from pharmaceutical companies are qualified nurses.

On the other hand, there is another medical view to which I only partly subscribe. This is where the specialist nurse augments the role of the doctor as a cost-cutting measure. In 2002, the Medical Division at Beaumont Hospital agreed to "support the development of clinical nurse specialist and practitioners". Other specialties within the hospital where this nursing role has been and is being developed include oncology, respiratory medicine and cardiology hypertension. Seeing that nurse practitioners are actively involved in clinical services, there is need for greater clarity in defining their role, responsibilities and line management. Undoubtedly, when these crucial points are clarified, there are many areas where the nurse specialist can significantly enhance patient services. For example, endocrinologist Dr Chris Thompson is requesting the appointment of a nurse specialist for diabetes at Beaumont Hospital.

My interpretation of these developments is that there is a shortage of doctors and a large number of patients. Therefore, the idea to "let's train nurses to perform a limited number of procedures which doctors usually do" has gained currency. Essentially, it means that there is no need to hire extra doctors. In addition, nurses' pay is lower so the operation is

A Cure for the Crisis

cheaper and the outcomes may be similar, if the focus is kept sufficiently narrow. This also facilitates the operation of a restrictive practice where the pressure for a specialist-led service is diluted and the specialists can retreat to seeing the more difficult and complicated patients, and of course "skip off" to the private clinic. At present, nurses are also less likely to be blamed for a poor outcome and sued for damages.

In reality, a great number of these patients could be looked after by GPs. However, this begs the question, why do we have so many primary care patients attending hospitals in the first place? What are primary care nurses supposed to do? Give vaccinations, check baby weights, speak to patients about their diets, exercise and weight, take blood pressures, give vitamin B_{12} injections, offer advice about diabetes, perform cervical smears and maybe prescribe? Where does that leave the GP? This is a key question because already 80 per cent of the proposed staff increases in primary healthcare in the greater Glasgow area in Scotland will be nurses.[2]

There are other technical areas where nurses are also employed. Because so many invasive procedures are now performed in Radiology Departments, nurses are employed in a supportive role to look after the many patients having these procedures. X-ray nurses also give gadolinium injections for MRI and CT scans and assist in cerebral and coronary angiography.

The advent of nurse specialists and practictioners inevitably comes with added costs. In many instances, it has led to recent disputes over parity in pay and conditions. For example, radiology nurses at St Vincent's University Hospital withdrew from out-of-hours work seeking parity in pay and conditions with the liver transplant nurses. Similarly, there was a five-month work-to-rule at Waterford Regional Hospital in pursuit of better pay for on-call. A local agreement was reached because an anomaly existed whereby a nurse involved in a six-hour operation was paid the same as a nurse called in for a one-hour operation. The INO statement from Tony FitzPatrick was evocative: "A skilled, highly trained nurse involved in life-saving surgery would have to pay more to her untrained babysitter than she would receive for a night on-call." Nurses in St John's Hospital, Sligo went on strike for one day in protest at practices which, they claimed, were unsafe. Public health nurses were incensed that the Benchmarking Body report should

Nursing

have them earn 3 per cent less than the clinical nurse specialists. In October 2002, 93 per cent voted to take industrial action over the issue.

Clearly, there is an increasing militancy across the caring professions. A trade-off of money for status has occurred.

Nurse selection

The Central Admissions Office (CAO) for third-level education is perhaps not the optimum method for selecting nurse trainees. Even with the nursing shortage, 2001 saw an increase of 21 per cent in applications for nurse training, while there are 1,500 nurse-training places up to 2003. In 2002, there were 8,822 applications to the CAO for the direct entry degree programme in nursing, which is an increase of 35 per cent on 2001. The new four-year degree course will put nursing education on a par with other healthcare professionals. This programme will include a continuous 12-month rostered clinical placement, inclusive of four weeks' holidays plus public holidays during the third and fourth years. For the other three years, the student will receive a combination of theoretical and clinical instruction.

Currently, general nursing course CAO points are in the range 325–395. Psychiatric nursing in DCU dropped to 280 points in round 2 in 2001, whereas in 2003 it was 245 in round 1 and 235 in round 2. Mental handicap nursing at Dundalk RTC dropped to 225 in round 2 in 2001. In 2003, it was 185 points in both rounds 1 and 2.

Admission points from the Irish Leaving Certificate requirements for UCD courses are shown in Table 7.1. The recent huge jump in the number of points for nursing confirms the success of the recruitment campaign which has greatly increased competition. How many will remain in nursing after graduation remains the unanswered question, however. Imagine the future frustration of these high-achieving women when reality hits home!

Table 7.1 CAO points requirements for medicine and nursing at UCD

Place	2000	2001	2002	2003
Medicine	550*	545*	555*	570*
General Nursing Mater		330	440*	
General Nursing St Vincents		325	470*	340*
General Nursing St Michaels			370*	
Psychiatric Nursing St John of Gods		310	425	

* Some but not all applicants with that number of points were offered places
Source: Central Applications Office (CAO)

With the establishment of degree courses for nurses, university-based nursing departments are not always associated with the respective medical school attached to the hospital. For example, it is extraordinary that Beaumont Hospital should be the Royal College of Surgeons' main teaching hospital with many joint medical appointments and much postgraduate medical education. However, the nursing school is part of Dublin City University, which has no medical school at all. Given that the RCSI Medical School is now largely onsite at Beaumont, it would have made better sense to affiliate the nursing school with that!

Nurse retention

Recent years have been marked by high wastage of nurses following graduation. Formerly, this was unusual. Up to the recent past, the Dublin Teaching Hospitals had nursing schools and trained their own nurses. Many students had to pay an entrance fee into the nursing schools and after basic training were introduced to patients in the hospital wards early. They gained an *espris de corps* and became part of the institution. In so doing, it was very good for morale and greatly helped patient care.

In 2000, the churning of nurses in the system could be seen by the Health Service Employers Agency figures. While they had recruited an extra 4,226 nurses by the end of March, 2,954 had resigned or retired over the same period, leaving a net increase of 1,272 in the system. The public hospitals in particular have a large turnover. In the Mater Hospital, 350 nurses resigned while 486 were recruited, whereas St Vincent's University Hospital saw 232 leave, while 160 were recruited. The Nursing Recruitment and Retention Report 2000 found that 60 per cent of nurses leaving the profession were aged between 20 and 29. To counteract the loss, they recommended nurse tracking, subsidised accommodation, flexitime, anti-bullying policies and overseas recruitment.

Ireland is not the only country experiencing retention problems. In Britain, data from the British Household Panel Survey found that 42.6 per cent of nurses left the profession between 1991 and 1996 and 14.5 per cent were not working. About 50 per cent of those still working were involved in social or child care. Thirty-three per cent of working nurses were not satisfied with their jobs. In England, 30 per cent of newly qualified nurses are reluctant to stay in the NHS.

Nursing

Nurse effectiveness

The relationship between hours of nursing care and better care for patients is a clear indicator of nurse effectiveness. A higher proportion of hours of nursing care provided by registered nurses and a greater number of hours of care by registered nurses per day are associated with better care for hospitalised patients.[3] Among medical patients, these outcomes included a shortened length of stay in hospital, fewer urinary infections and lower rates of upper gut bleeding. A similar relationship does not exist for care assistants and licensed practical nurses.[4]

Doctor substitutes

The concept of using nurses as doctor substitutes in certain instances, as discussed earlier, has been the subject of much debate and study. In 2002, Kinley *et al.* found favour with the practice at pre-registration level, i.e. intern level in Ireland.

> Appropriately trained nurses are no worse than pre-registration house officers in assessing patients before elective surgery. Reforms in postgraduate medical training and the introduction of reduced working hours have increased pressure to substitute non-medical staff for pre-registration house officers.[5]

Kinley *et al.* note that house officers will have to undertake some of the work to satisfy training requirements, however. In the study the patients included those for general, vascular, urological or breast surgery. In my view, this practice is questionable and is likely to curb the clinical experience of interns. How will the new generation of doctors recognise a normal or abnormal patient with clinical exposure which will be much less than the previous cohorts? The word "reform" implies improvement, but all change is not necessarily better, even when dubbed reform. That said, there is a role for clinical nurse specialists as "one disease doctors" (ODDs), particularly in endoscopy. Studies have found that nurses have been shown to be proficient at gastroscopy and can substitute for doctors.[6] Similarly, they have also been trained in sigmoidoscopy and colonoscopy.[7] However, I would caution doctors that skills are like rugby balls – if you don't use it, you lose it!

In primary care there are analyses which report that "nurse practitioners can provide care that leads to increased patient satisfaction and similar health outcomes when compared to care from a doctor. Nurse practitioners seemed to provide a quality of care that is at least as good,

49

A Cure for the Crisis

and in some ways better than doctors." Nurse practitioners seemed to identify physical abnormalities more often. A systematic review in the *British Medical Journal (BMJ)* in 2002[8] showed that in one study nurse practitioners gave more information to patients. Nurse practitioners made more complete records and scored better on communication than did doctors. They also offered more advice on self-care and management. Two studies in A&E suggested that nurse practitioners were as accurate as doctors at ordering and interpreting X-ray films, with small in-study variations depending on the relative experience of both providers. The response to such a crucial evaluation naturally evoked strong reaction. In reply to the *BMJ* review, Dr Richard Costello from the RCSI wrote:

> I am sorry to see that the *BMJ* continues its descent into the banal world of 'systematic reviews'. These are not projects of any research value, they diminish the value of reasonable trials and add confusion. Am I to conclude that there is no need to see a GP when a nurse is just as good?[9]

Another GP, Dr Adrian Midgeley, wrote that "when the length of a consultation is 3.6 minutes longer, patients will be more satisfied" but agreed that the conclusions were valid. Certainly, I agree with Dr Midgeley, but must indicate to the reader that there is yet another viewpoint. I can attest that experienced night superintendents in the A&E Department of Beaumont Hospital are excellent and proficient in dealing with emergencies. Therefore, it is not surprising that some nurses and doctors could have equivalent outcomes once the field is narrowed. Doctors also are increasingly specialising in the care of narrower areas and most forget the detail of what they do not use.

European Working Time Directive

The effect of the European Working Time Directive on junior doctors' working hours – which allows a maximum of 58 hours per week from August 2004 – has "forced" NHS Trusts to put nurses in charge of wards at night. The British government announced big cuts in night cover, which has raised doubts about patient safety. Currently, one-third of junior doctors work more than 72 hours per week and cover the wards at night. In January 2003, 19 pilot schemes to have nurses replace junior doctors at night were launched. In Birmingham Heartlands and Solihull NHS Trust, senior nurses replaced doctors from 5 pm to 9 am on weekdays and all day at weekends on acute medical wards. Advocating the

Nursing

scheme, an administrator told *The Independent* (London): "We are matching resources to the need. There will be doctors available if urgent help is needed." At Burton Hospitals NHS Trust, interns will not be on duty at night. At Northern Devon Hospital NHS Trust, a medical assessment unit will switch to 24-hour working and will be led by a nurse practitioner. At Nottingham City Hospital, five intensive care nurses specialising in heart patients "will ensure 24-hour comprehensive cover".[10]

Commenting on the scheme, a British Department of Health spokesperson said: "This is about giving staff extra responsibility, breaking down traditional barriers and encouraging people to take on new skills. Obviously patient safety is a primary concern." The reaction from both the Royal College of Physicians (RCP) London and the British Medical Association (BMA) is one of restrained wariness. The RCP is quoted as welcoming the "thoughtful and detailed guidance", but warned that "there are many emergencies where only immediate help from a skilled doctor is appropriate". Similarly, the BMA supported giving extra responsibility to nurses provided they were properly trained and available: "In principle we are in favour but whether it is practicable is questionable." On the other hand, Royal College of Nursing policy adviser, Helen Caulfield was enthusiastic about the scheme: "We may see really ambitious nurses wanting to develop specialist skills so they can run services out of hours. It is a tremendous vote of confidence in nursing."

Personally, I believe that this pilot scheme shows a contempt for and misunderstanding of the role of the doctor. It causes ethical problems for doctors and calls into question continuity of care, referral ethics and ultimately who controls patient care. Clearly, the Labour government have got it wrong, unlike the Tories. The Shadow Secretary of State for Health, Dr Liam Fox, pinpointed the crux of the problem: "I understand the need to reduce the hours.... but you can only do that when you have sufficient doctors. This will mean increasing the pressure on senior staff to provide cover for patients or the level of care will potentially diminish." The British medical establishment has "lost the plot".

Six months later an early evaluation of the scheme revealed some of the challenges associated with the implementation of the pilot. They included restrictions on doctors' training, an increased workload for consultants and specialist registrars, an impact on doctors' salaries, difficulties in recruiting new posts from existing staff, and professional antagonism particularly between doctors and nurses. Progress in many cases was impeded because of a failure or delay to recruit a dedicated project manager.

The issue of doctor substitutes has reached its nadir in the United States, with the advent of the interdisciplinary workforce in healthcare. This confirms my view of the likely progression of doctor substitutes. In an editorial in the *New England Journal of Medicine*, a nurse proponent of this interdisciplinary approach wrote:

> Large medical care organisations routinely circumvent state practice acts and reimbursement regulations that restrict the authority to prescribe drugs and require that licensed nonphysician clinicians be supervised by on-site physicians....Consolidation of services and the quest for cost savings appear to be forcing greater integration of services provided by different types of providers than has been achieved by other strategies.[11]

Noting the conflicting aims of medical and non-medical professionals, she writes:

> Nurses, social workers, occupational and physical therapists, and other nonphysician health professionals provide care that is more holistic than that provided by physicians. They have a demonstrated interest and expertise in helping the chronically ill, frail elderly, and their family caregivers manage the day-to-day aspects of their chronic conditions and treatments...

To infer that geriatricians are somehow inferior and superfluous in the overall care of the elderly is ludicrous. Certainly, doctors have no intention of becoming home helps – it would be an inappropriate use of their time! Here in Ireland, however, the question of maximising, not minimising, doctors' training is paramount. We are threatening to close A&E departments in county hospitals in the name of standards and training, while the Americans allow nurses to practise.

Solutions

- The Nursing Recruitment and Retention Report should be implemented. Nurses working in shortage areas should be given a loyalty bonus. This should be a flexible version of a "city weighting".
- A look at the comments from nurses on the *irishhealth.com* website will dispel any doubts about the need to ensure adequate nurse staffing levels to reduce stress and encourage staff to remain in nursing.

Nursing

- I believe that hospitals should retain their own nursing schools with consultant commitment to teaching.
- The above listed "hospital nurses" should have a registerable qualification in nursing.
- Those who wish to specialise in nursing care in a medical or surgical specialty should have the benefit of a postgraduate MSc or equivalent at the hospital's medical school. This would encourage many of the people who are not particularly academically inclined to enter nursing. Clearly, some imaginative solution is necessary or hospital wards will be unsupportable from a nursing standpoint.
- Hospitals should be able to come to their own pay arrangements with their nurses in the interests of patient care (a pseudonym for good nursing and unit morale).
- The CAO figures prove that there is no shortage of interest in nursing in this country.
- If the new clinical nurse specialists could be arguably redefined as "one disease doctors" (ODDs), then nursing could be reinvented as "medical assistants in caring" (MACs). The British have their SRNs (state registered nurses) and SENs (state enrolled nurses), the latter qualification unrecognised in Ireland. Advanced nurse practitioners have seemingly advanced beyond the ODDs to which terminus I'm not sure. (See consultants in Chapter 44, Action Plan for Ireland.) SENs from the NHS should be able to convert in Ireland to SRNs registerable by An Bord Altranais. At present, SENs can complete a conversion programme in Britain and convert to SRNs. There is a non-means-tested grant available from Ireland to do this.
- The law should be changed to allow the current NHS SENs to be registered with An Bord Altranais.
- Nurses do not need to be in operating theatres, but operating technicians can be specifically trained.
- A high complement of nurses does not need to be in outpatient departments (OPD). Instead, my friends the MACs could check blood pressures in OPD and also dipstick urines, if necessary. They could finger-prick for glucose checks and also be trained to take blood. They could weigh the patient and be considerate to stressed people.
- A cohort of nurses should be attached to wards and a separate group to individual medical and surgical teams. Theatre nurses could be

A Cure for the Crisis

reassigned to the intensive care units/high-dependency units, whereas OPD nurses could be transferred to the wards depending on their preferences. Then the impact of the absence of rigid core units in some hospital wards would be diminished; however, hospitals should, as far as possible, have their specialty patients on the same wards. It makes for more effective and safe medical and nursing management.

- The scheme to allow experienced care assistants to train as nurses, with their pay continuing, in exchange for an agreement to work for the health service for five years after graduation, should be extended to cover all candidates who reach an agreed entry standard.

- St Michael's House and other specialist bodies should be supported in extending their specialist nurse-training programmes.

- There should be a minimum of one nurse to five patients in a general medical or surgical ward. The ratio in psychiatry should be one nurse to every six patients. There should be a minimum of one nurse to every two patients in delivery units and intensive care units. These figures are *minima*.

- There should be a Dublin allowance to attract and retain staff due to the higher cost of living in the capital city.

8

Self-preservation for administrators

Role of administrators

Ongoing conflict between doctors and administrators is a common feature of hospital life. Nonetheless, there is a role for hospital administrators, especially in our increasingly secular society with the absence of the religious communities running hospitals. However, their lack of ideology sets them apart from their predecessors. In years gone by, the medical and nursing professions and religious orders were united in a common goal; providing the ultimate care for the sick. Every means at their disposal whether state aid, private finances or fundraising was utilised to ensure patients benefited from the latest advances in medicine and technology. In contrast, hospital administrators, in the absence of ideology, have one primary goal in sight – keeping within budgets regardless of patient welfare. Therefore, on the issue of resources, conflict between doctors and administrators is inevitable.

When there is a clamour for change in the media among commentators, columnists and economists and with leaking from political sources that downsizing of health boards is necessary, then you can expect a reaction from the nomenclatura. Cue the chairman of the Health Boards CEO Group Michael Lyons, who in late November 2002 indicated that, while they supported change, they believed that some regional management units would be needed.[1] In their view, integrated regional management should oversee the various strands of healthcare, including hospitals, community care and continuing care. In essence, the CEOs want the Department of Health and Children to remain responsible for policy matters and devolve greater control over personnel and capital projects to agencies on the ground.

A Cure for the Crisis

Integrated regional management

The health board CEOs argue that merging health boards will not of itself develop a more effective health service. This is largely true. However, they deny that they are top heavy with administrators and claim that 73 per cent of new staff employed since 1999 are frontline personnel dealing directly with patients and the public. Essentially, the CEOs want a National Hospitals Plan that would agree which medical and surgical services should be sited at which institutions. To this end, they hope to persuade the public that every hospital in every region cannot deal with every specialty and also remove local politicians from having a say in what happens in local hospitals. Personally, I reject this disregard for the public's representatives.

There is a residual problem for local hospitals, which has recently become apparent. The RCSI announced that Louth County Hospital in Dundalk would not be recognised as a training hospital for some surgical staff because of inadequate consultant cover. Clearly, some of these hospitals will need the appointment of journeymen consultants – good midfielders who will keep the show on the road, have a good quality of life and provide a service which the local people want. The obvious solution is to keep A&E units open by appointing appropriate consultant staff that could also look after basic medical inpatients with appropriate training. Certainly, Ireland is a wealthy country and can safely indulge the public's appetite for local hospitals.

CEOs & medics

In the healthcare scenario envisaged by CEOs hospital consultants would act as managers within their hospitals controlling their own budgets. My experience forces me to guffaw at that pious aspiration. Administrators usually show a *de facto* disregard for consultants and often seem to miss the central point of a hospital's mission.

In an attempt to curtail investment, CEOs also want new national protocols for assessing new technology or drug treatments. Currently, there are standard professional protocols for such activities in buying new machines and reagents for laboratories, etc., and these should be preserved, not supplanted. New drugs are introduced into large hospitals nearly always as a result of published evidence and trial reports in major journals such as *The Lancet, New England Journal of Medicine, Circula-*

Self-preservation for administrators

tion, *British Medical Journal, Journal of the American Medical Association (JAMA)* and many others.

The issue of renegotiating GP public contracts also falls within their sights. They want performance-related pay with regard to immunization and screening programmes. GPs should immunize all their relevant patients as part of their professional mission as doctors. However, GPs are already paid a fee-per-item, which somehow seems to have escaped officialdom. In practice, some mothers refuse to have their children immunized. Remember the furore over the MMR vaccine and autism. Demands for single vaccines at high cost became commonplace, despite the absence of corroborating safety data, resulting in the Irish Medicines Board having to publicly state that some of these vaccines did not have a national product licence.

Numbers game

Mr Michael Lyons – who in addition to being chairman of the Health Boards Chief Executive Officers' Group is also CEO of the East Coast Area Health Board – wrote a substantial article in the op-ed page of *The Irish Times* on 25 November 2002, headed "Reducing number of health boards is not the real issue in reform of service". However, reduction is certainly one! In the piece, he complains about the pressure being put on hospital administration by recent commentaries in the media and claims that "administration" is used to define anyone outside of medicine or nursing. This is not the case. We know that ambulance workers, community welfare officers, social workers, environmental health officers are not administrators in the pejorative sense. Equally, he rejects the assertion by an ESRI official that one in 13 new staff appointed in recent years was a service provider. On the contrary, he claims that 73 per cent were involved in frontline service delivery, as shown in Table 8.1.

Table 8.1 Staff increases, 1999–2001

Staff	Percentage (%)
Health & social care professionals	13.00
Medical/dental	5.23
Nursing	16.18
Other patient/client care	24.00
Management/admin dealing with patient care	15.06
Total	73.47

Source: Health Boards Chief Executive Officers' Group

Interestingly, numbers are not put on these figures. Not surprisingly, Mr Lyons slides over the question of value for money commensurate with the growth of staff numbers. Instead he claims credit for the 89 per cent satisfaction rating of a patient/client survey published by the ERHA in August 2002.

Organisational structure

That no health administration has come up with the ideal organisational structure is a point rightly made by Mr Lyons. By and large there is no consensus on the ideal number of health boards. He cites New Zealand with 21 district health boards up from four. Scotland has 14 health authorities (Scotland is socialised beyond belief and for decades has a bigger health budget per head than England, which obviously would make a difference). The Canadian province of Saskatchewan has 10, whereas Greater Manchester, England has one. Mr Lyons states that "we [health boards] have been centrally involved in, and have supported, all of the organisational changes in the health system throughout the years and are fully supportive of the present audit of structures being carried out by the Department of Health and Children". On that point, he is correct. Health board officials have taken to themselves a mass of power over many years and this has lead to ineffective, sluggish and relatively unaccountable decision-making on their part. Change has strengthened the hands of administrators and left medical cynicism to fester and undermine morale. Like turkeys voting for Christmas, health boards are unlikely to support downsizing.

The subtitle to his article implies as much: "Reducing the issue of providing better health services to the simple question 'do we need 11 health boards?' misses the point altogether." Michael Lyons calls for the removal of unnecessary overlaps and duplication and wants clear governance and accountability arrangements put in place. I think he'll find medics would agree with that sentiment entirely. In identifying what the goal of health-care should be, he is correct about the means to achieving it:

> It is also about how people, within and between health service organisations, co-operate and collaborate with each other in the interests of patient care. It is also crucial that other obstacles to the achievement of a high-quality, fair and equitable health service are addressed so that any new organisational structures put in place can contribute effectively to the ideal that we all continue to strive

Self-preservation for administrators

for – the care of our patients and clients. Structural change in itself will not be sufficient.[2]

The question of co-operation and collaboration among medics is central to their code of practice. The *Guide to Ethical Conduct and Behaviour* from the Medical Council addresses the responsibilities of doctors with regard to appropriate referral and treatments. The patients are the doctors' patients not the administrators'. There is no recognition of the conflict of interest between the legal obligation of these CEOs to balance their budgets and the duty of the doctor as advocates of continuous improving patient care.

External and internal audits

Independent review group

An independent three-person committee report on the health services for the Minister for Finance, published in conjunction with Budget 2003, stated that "there were serious doubts about the efficacy of the existing health board structures," as reported in *The Irish Times* of 5 December 2002. It called for the control of health service staffing to be returned to the Department of Health after it had been devolved to the health boards only two years earlier. Michael Lyons rejected the report's conclusion that recent investment in the health service had not brought significant improvements. On that point, he is correct; nonetheless his special pleading can be judged from what he is reported to have said:

> However, the report's emphasis on structural reform alone is a narrow and simplistic solution for the wider reforms that are necessary in the health system.... Structural reforms, accepted by the health boards, are not enough, and there are other equal, if not greater, obstacles to a better and more equitable health service. These include, for example, the consultants' common contract, GP contracts, and current pay rates for health service staff – issues that are decided at national level and not at health board level. Indeed the current difficulties experienced by the National Treatment Purchase Fund, concerning the treatment of patients abroad, provide ample evidence of some of the non-structural obstacles the health services face when trying to imaginatively deal with the problems of capacity.

A Cure for the Crisis

CEO Group of the Health Boards Audit

Prior to Christmas 2002, *The Irish Times* obtained a draft report by the CEO Group of the Health Boards for the audit of health service structures by the Department of Health.[3] Not surprisingly, the CEOs wanted the number of boards to remain the same. In fact, they wanted the boards to be smaller with fewer political representatives and to include a broader representation from specialists, such as health economists, policy analysts and business experts. They called for a dilution of local public representatives whose remit, they say, is to protect existing services at all costs, because that is what is expected of them by the local community and by their peers. Furthermore, the CEOs claim that local representatives do not even have a regional vision and prevent the development of regionalisation or subspecialisation. The lack of a National Hospitals Plan was cited as a major impediment to the delivery of acute care within the country. By their reckoning, funding and planning of hospitals should be given over to a national agency which should continue to run hospitals at local level. In addition, the CEOs want a reduction of the 50 statutory health agencies in the State. On this matter, I certainly agree.

They suggest that consultants should be rostered to work 24 hours (not the way they want) and that administrative and support systems across the whole of the health service be unified. These proposals find little favour among consultants. As it stands, consultants are already on-call out-of-hours and come in for difficult cases. In Beaumont Hospital, consultants regularly operate upon and see patients out-of-hours. I have often received phone calls from consultants about patients at night or at weekends from all the Dublin general and children's hospitals. This is not beyond the call of duty; we are paid to look after our patients. Instituting a regime where consultants are rostered to work 24 hours will impact on training for junior doctors. Registrars get experience like we did in our turn at the coalface. Problems can arise in the event of consultants not being available or contactable; however, the law has had much to say on that subject.

Pressure on the Minister for Health is such that he is sure to cut a few health boards and introduce a Hospitals Agency of some description. He might be better off beefing up the people in the Department of Health, who might surprise him by their ability if given the chance. The obvious solution is to remove health board management from hospitals.

Self-preservation for administrators

Leaks of health board culls by the Government are not ignored. Again CEO Michael Lyons wrote to *The Irish Times* in May 2003 to say that all the extra money spent by the ERHA went on frontline services.[4] Noting that the population of the area had increased by 106,000 in the past six years, he claimed the ERHA has a staff of 136 people administering a budget of €2.9 billion. Despite the obvious crisis in the acute Dublin hospitals with more than 100 bed closures and more to come, Mr Lyons claimed that there are sufficient funds to buy the same level of services as 2002. Experience in the hospitals would suggest otherwise.

Prospectus Report

In June 2003, Prospectus Management Consultants detailed an audit of the health services. In their report they recommended reducing health boards to four regional executive bodies and the creation of a National Hospitals Office within a Health Service Executive.[5] In effect, there would be more professional and executive functions and less say for local political interests. This is not wise because it patronises the people being served and will create remote and bureaucratic structures.

Brennan Report

Also in June 2003, the Commission on Financial Management and Control Systems in the Health Service (also known as the Brennan Report) reported to considerable controversy. The recommended centralised command and control of hospital medicine by a new group of administrators in a Health Service Executive with various subservient health boards and hospital agencies is a recipe for unrest and administrative treacle. Monitoring the activities of GPs and consultants in detail will be unenforceable without a massive collapse of professional morale. In the Report, there is a mad determination that medics must be controlled by administrators. Moreover, there is a heavy assumption of malfeasance and bad faith on the part of consultants, as outlined in the comments on page 73:

> The provisions of Consultants' existing common contract should be enforced to ensure that the following is undertaken: (i) The setting of core times when a Consultant must be available to patients in the public hospital; and (ii) formal active monitoring of work commitment in respect of public patients.[6]

61

A Cure for the Crisis

In my experience in North Dublin hospitals, I am unaware of doctors not attending public patients in any systematic way. If it were the case, corridor whispers would point the finger at any such behaviour. However, no evidence was offered by the members of the Commission for such innuendoes, which I consider to verge on the defamatory.

The Commission defines the key question as: "How can the health services contract with individual clinical consultants in ways that make it possible to negotiate with them, in a systematic way, the resources they need for their practices without interfering in any way with their clinical independence in the treatment of their patients?" I would suggest that the true question is that posed by the primary role of the doctor. How does the doctor make sure that the welfare of each patient is put first despite a limitation in resources? When a patient can pay for care that is rationed to publicly funded patients, what is the public advocacy role of the doctor? As I have indicated, conflict between doctors and administrators is inevitable on the issue of resources.

9

Waiting lists and treatment plans

Hospital waiting lists

For successive governments, the issue of hospital waiting lists has become the bugbear of the health services. On 6 May 2002, Bertie Ahern told a press conference that Fianna Fáil would "permanently end hospital waiting lists within two years if returned to power". By June 2002, there were 24,850 adults on hospital waiting lists. This was 1,809 down on the previous year. Waiting lists for cardiac surgery, ENT, ophthalmology and orthopaedic surgery decreased but the lists for general surgery and gynaecology increased. There were 7,890 adults waiting for more than one year, yet the National Health Strategy promised that such a wait would be eliminated by the end of 2002. The target for adults is one year maximum and six months for children.

In the late autumn, the SRSV (winter vomiting bug, Norwalk virus) infection caused the cancellation of over 1,000 surgical procedures in Beaumont Hospital. In turn, this affected the Mater Hospital through patient transfer. There were also serious problems in the Waterford and Wexford areas from the same pathogen. By the end of September 2002, there were 22,718 people on waiting lists, a drop of 3,627 or 14 per cent in one year. Of these, 19,236 were waiting for treatment that involved one overnight stay. The total number of adults waiting more than one year for admission to hospital fell from 7,407 to 6,273 from June to September – a drop of 15 per cent but well off the intended policy figure. There were 9,938 people waiting for day case admission in September.[1] The number of children waiting for more than six months was 1,201 by September 2002, down from 1,576 in three months. (See Table 9.1 for waiting lists, June–December 2002; note that figures for lists and procedures published in the press relating to specific times often conflict.)

A Cure for the Crisis

Figure 9.1 Waiting lists, June–December 2002

Waiting lists	June 2002	Sept 2002	Dec 2002
Total adults	24,850	22,718	29,017
Overnight		19,236	18,390
Day case		9,938	10,627
>1 year	7,408*	6,276	5,209
<1 year	7,890		
>6 months (children)	1,576	1,201	1,081

* Figures published in press may be contradictory
Source: Department of Health & Children, 2002

Just when you pretend to believe the figures stated above, the *Irish Independent* on the very next day, 5 December, pointed out that the total adult figure on the waiting list was not the 22,718, but the sum of the 9,938 day cases plus the 19,236 for overnight admission. Thus the true figure was 29,174. By way of explanation, Eilish O'Regan wrote: "A new method of calculating public hospital waiting list figures has uncovered 9,938 people previously undocumented, it emerged yesterday. They bring the total number waiting to nearly 30,000."[2] Besides, that cannot be the entire story because how many of the 9,938 day case patients have been waiting for more than one year? The Minister for Health in defending himself claimed that figures from the South Eastern Health Board showed that of 600 people supposedly on the list for 12 months or more, 279 had been operated on. The fact of the matter is that it proves official figures needed to be carefully scrutinised.[3]

An *Irish Examiner* editorial sums up the waiting list debacle. "In fact, hospital waiting lists have grown longer. The combined statistics total 29,174, a rise of 4,300 in the numbers awaiting treatment. The inescapable conclusion is that there are lies, damned lies and official waiting lists."[4] In addition, when the year-end figures were finally released in May 2003, *The Irish Times* noted that the "list adds up to a broken promise". Some hospitals were not even included on the waiting list figures, according to health correspondent Eithne Donnellan.[5] In May, five of the Dublin Academic Teaching Hospitals (DATH) announced bed closures totalling 250, which will result in 14,000 fewer patients being treated in 2003 compared to the previous year. The Fianna Fáil strategy is in tatters.

Waiting lists and treatment plans

Bed pressures

In 1987, 3,000 beds were taken out of the hospital system and it is costing €118 million to return 709 new beds. On 28 October 2002, the *Irish Examiner* reported that there were 26,350 people on inpatient waiting lists, 100,000 waiting for an OPD appointment, 450–600 beds occupied unnecessarily every day and finally that only 258 of the promised quota of 709 beds from the National Health Strategy were on-stream for 2002. The Department of Health promised that 600 extra beds would be in service by the end of the year and the rest would follow in 2003.

IHCA secretary general, Finbarr Fitzpatrick noted that the majority of patients occupying acute beds unnecessarily are elderly and incapable of independent living, but could be discharged if they had a home help, nursing home or rehabilitation facilities. Many of them are in hospital for several months to one year, without needing to be there. In October 2002, there were 105 patients in the Mater Hospital who were passed fit for medical discharge. Similarly, Beaumont Hospital had about 45 at the same time. The inability to discharge patients is costing the State approximately €75 to €100 million per year. Blocked beds are an obvious cause of patients for admission languishing on trolleys in A&E departments, sometimes for days.

The National Treatment Purchase Fund

The National Treatment Purchase Fund (NTPF) was set up to offer patients, who have been on hospital waiting lists for more than one year, an overseas alternative in a bid to eliminate hospital waiting lists. The scheme was allocated €30 million in Budget 2001 but only became operational in July 2001. By October 2002, about €10 million had been spent and 1,037 people had been sent abroad. However, €3 million remained unspent in 2002. Nonetheless, *The Irish Times* reported that the Fund achieved its 2002 target of treating 1,900 patients on waiting lists.[6] The Government's target was to clear 8,305 patients from the waiting list by November 2003.

The Fund has the capacity to pay for 600 patients per month in 2003, 400 in Ireland and 200 in Britain. The organisers have contracted four private hospitals in Britain at an average cost of €3,658 per surgical procedure at an average two nights' stay. They claim to have full co-operation from GPs but not from consultants, according to a report in the *Irish Independent*: "It is understood there is a reluctance among medics to

65

A Cure for the Crisis

send the patients to the UK."[7] In response, the IHCA declared that consultants will and have facilitated the patients who wished to be treated in the UK. "This co-operation does not preclude the IHCA from criticising the fact that we should have sufficient capacity in our public hospital services to treat patients with uncomplicated routine health problems within a medically acceptable timeframe." Minister Martin claims that the lack of capacity in Irish hospitals has forced the Department to look abroad.

The National Treatment Purchase Fund ran an information meeting for doctors, nurses and healthcare professionals in the Imperial Hotel in Cork in December 2002. The questions advertised included: "Are your patients sick waiting for treatment?" "How quickly can they be treated?" "Where will they be treated?" "How do you refer patients?" On the issue of referral, my personal practice is to refer patients to individual doctors within different institutions. Personally, I rarely refer patients to "whoever it happens to be" except when sending them into A&E departments.

Private care in Britain is more expensive than the equivalent here. For example, tonsillectomies in Britain cost between €2,600 and €2,700, whereas in Ireland the same procedure costs €1,900 to €2,500. Varicose veins vary from €1,800 to €2,300 in Ireland, whereas the cost is €1,900 to €2,800 in Britain. BUPA hospitals in Liverpool and Manchester are being used in the scheme.

However, utilising public surgical beds in the State for their express purpose should be done, before any money is spent on the scheme. As economist Moore McDowell pointed out, the Minister of Finance should insist that "the Minister [of Health] pay for private operations on public patients if and only if all the public surgical beds provided are being used for surgical purposes."[8]

The Norwegians have provided a similar scheme for 5,000 patients who were treated in Sweden, Austria and Germany. Similarly, Germany has also used other European countries.

Outside of the NTPF scheme, other patients have been sent for procedures not available in this country. For example, patients are sent to England for lung transplants to the Freeman Hospital in Newcastle, usually for cystic fibrosis and fibrosing alveolitis. Others have been sent for specialised neurosurgery to England.

The Commission on Health Funding Report 1989 claimed that some doctors did not discharge their public hospital responsibilities because of the economic incentive to pursue private practice. The claim sprang

Waiting lists and treatment plans

from the belief that long waiting lists would suit some doctors because it encouraged patients who could pay to attend the same doctors in the private sector. The charge was rejected by the IHCA. Nonetheless, could the charge have a tincture of truth? Obviously, it could. Over a decade ago, the population was much smaller and what could be done medically for people was much less. Therefore, demand was less. Indeed, some doctors might have underperformed in their attendance at public outpatients. Nowadays, inspections for training of NCHDs and a culture change make this much less likely. Consider that the public and private waiting lists for neurologists, rheumatologists, dermatologists, orthopaedic surgeons are now similar and are often up to one year. Demand greatly exceeds supply, therefore, there clearly is no economic incentive for these doctors to divert patients to the private sector.

Predictable consequences of the NTPF can occur. Patients may be admitted to ring-fenced beds in a public hospital for routine hernias and varicose veins, while dangerously ill patients remain in A&E units due to lack of beds. Some cost comparison figures are shown in Table 9.2.[9] This study was conducted by the School of Health and Related Research at the University of Sheffield and commissioned by *HospitalHealthcare.com*. The Irish costs came from the Department of Health.

Table 9.2 Cost comparisons of surgical treatments carried out in EU

Country	Hip* (€)	Knee* (€)	Thyroidec- tomy (€)	Aortic valve replacement (€)	Cataract† (€)	Hernia‡ (€)
UK	6,355	7,156	2,383	11,287	1,430	1,319
Germany	8,819–15,126	19,031	4,270	22,837–37,113	3,212	3,775–5,055
Austria	4,979–6,806	7,994	2,570	12,460	2,585	1,685
Netherlands	6,862	6,776	2,633	14,472	1,527	1,902
Denmark	6,943	6,943	3,369	18,663	813–1,008	2,334
France	7,283	7,283	3,063	18,629–21,622	1,850	1,745–2,964
Ireland	7,013	7,013	3,263	22,720	1,830	2,028

*Hip/knee replacements
†Cataracts removed
‡Inguinal hernias repaired
Source: School of Health and Related Research, University of Sheffield. Irish costs courtesy of Department of Health and Children

EU transnational borders opened for treatment

Cross-border medical care is available to people where services are unavailable in their home state "within a time limit that is justifiable".

A Cure for the Crisis

Patients will be able to travel to other EU countries for treatment, if local hospitals cannot provide urgent care again within a reasonable period of time. Public health authorities will be obliged to cover the cost of treatment. How each individual case will be judged has yet to be finalised. EU officials declare that decisions will be based on doctor's advice and that health authorities will have the right to seek a second medical opinion. Whether the patients will have to pay upfront and then recoup the cost is as yet undecided. National health authorities will have to sanction the treatment before it can be provided but will not be able to refuse valid cases.[10] This opens the way for some interesting manoeuvres by dissatisfied impatient people.

Solutions

1. Use all available public and private operating theatres from Monday to Friday.
2. The public sector should buy theatre and bed spaces in the private sector, where appropriate facilities are available.
3. Divert city waiting lists to peripheral hospitals for basic surgical procedures, such as for hernias, varicose veins, ENT, etc.
4. Money from any NTPF should follow such patients.
5. Use surgical beds for surgery only.
6. Purchase nursing home spaces for discharged "bed block" patients in hospitals.
7. Fund nursing home placements by means testing.
8. Equip hospitals properly with scanners and endoscopes.

10

Pay and expenditure vs cutbacks

Pay and public health expenditure

Nearly 70 per cent of the huge increase in health spending in Ireland since 1997 has gone on pay. The health sector pay bill has increased by €2.4 billion over the past 5 years. Only €1 billion of the €3.4 billion increase in health spending since 1997 has been non-pay related. When asked by Damian Kiberd in *The Sunday Times* where all the money had gone, a senior civil servant answered "hiring suits". Obviously, there are many cynics. Nonetheless in 2002, the numbers employed in the public health sector were about 93,850 compared to 69,726 in 1998.

The per capita health spending in Ireland is now above the EU average, whereas in 1996 it was 74 per cent of the comparative figure. Overall Exchequer spending on health is almost double that of 1997 with current spending rising by 78 per cent and capital spending nearly doubled in five years. Spending on pay and pensions has risen by 77 per cent or €5 billion in five years and €2.6 billion is due to higher pay rates.

Benchmarking

Benchmarking – otherwise known as pseudo-comparison of jobs in the public and private sector – was dreamed up during the height of the boom in the Celtic Tiger in what seemed like an attempt to placate schoolteachers. But when it comes to public sector pay, lawyers seem outstanding in that field. Given the spate of tribunals of inquiry in Ireland in the last decade, the exorbitant fees charged by senior counsels have been well documented.

Are consultants working for the public any less valuable to the community than such august senior counsel? Maybe I have a grossly exaggerated sense of the value and importance of senior doctors but if, for the sake of argument, such doctors are at least as valuable as these elite lawyers, then that has implications for formal pay assessments such as that carried out by the Review Body on Higher Remuneration in the Public

Sector (Buckley Review), which is the mechanism used to quantify consultant's pay along with senior civil servants and politicians.

If consultants work at the coalface for four days per week, 42 weeks of the year, then pay for senior consultants at Morris Tribunal rates would be €378,000 per annum for full-time geographic wholetime appointees. At Moriarty Tribunal rates this would rise to €420,000 per annum. This, on the assumption that there are no signing-on fees (like brief fees or hospital retainers), no pay for time spent in continuing medical education and no holiday pay. Could you imagine the media uproar? Why then is current pay only a fraction of this? Or is it the case that lawyers are overvalued by the Government or that doctors are undervalued? Or are both professions guilty of the George Bernard Shaw crime of being conspiracies against the public? The geographic wholetime contract without private fees was abolished in 1996 by the Buckley Review on the recommendation of the Department of Health. Therefore, all consultants have an entitlement to private practice. I would guess that a large number of consultants would opt for a full-time public job at lawyer-equivalent pay rates.

Foolish and unwise cuts proposals

In light of reduced Exchequer funds, cutbacks are now the order of the day in Irish hospitals. Certainly, the proposed cutbacks at Beaumont Hospital in 2003 reached absurd proportions. When Mr Pat Rabbitte TD questioned An Taoiseach, Bertie Ahern, in the Dáil on 26 February 2003 on the proposals from the senior management of Beaumont Hospital concerning the details of the cuts possible in 2003, a minor quake erupted. Amusingly, Mr Ahern seemed to think that the hospital management had deliberately publicised their financial difficulties. Any hospital management that considers taking actions that would directly lead to patient deaths, however, will be determinedly exposed and opposed by consultants, who have an overriding ethical duty to be advocates for their patients.

Despite an announcement by Minister McCreevy that there would be no cuts prior to the 2002 General Election, Beaumont Hospital was about to face savage cutbacks. The 10 February cuts list included the possibility of closing night-shift dialysis (i.e. precipitating the deaths of 60 to 70 patients), eliminating the use of drug-eluting stents for coronary patients (i.e. increasing the death rate), eliminating neurosurgical coils

Pay and expenditure vs cutbacks

(i.e. increasing the death rate from intracerebral aneurysms), capping activity in cancer treatments, returning nursing home patients to Beaumont Hospital (i.e. blocking beds), capping GP laboratory referrals and many other administrative contract-breaking manoeuvres.

Nephrologist Dr Peter Conlon felt obliged to leave a management meeting due to the offensiveness of the proposals. On reading the list of options, one is struck by the madness of the strategy. The dilemma it poses for doctors is an ethical one. Doctors are obliged to let the public know, so that there is clarity on the actions of hospitals.

When the details became public in the Dáil, the Medical Board of Beaumont issued a statement stating that doctors would not tolerate cuts that directly hit patients' lives. Prof Shane O'Neill and Dr Peter Conlon appeared on TV and radio and underlined that the doctors would not lie down or be quiet in the face of pressure from any source. The retired health board official and new chairman of Beaumont Hospital Board, Donal O'Shea, had a cold-water immersion baptism as to the attitude and professionalism of Dublin consultants. Contrary to popular opinion, this issue had no personal financial stake for consultants. In fact, the proposal of management to maximise the usage of private beds was also opposed, if the usage was clinically inappropriate.

An *Irish Examiner* editorial on 28 February 2003 highlighted the conflicting aims of Government:

> ...the Taoiseach's implicit Dáil threat, that Beaumont Hospital could suffer over what he termed the 'cheap stunt' of leaking a document outlining its shortfall of €21 million, was particularly unhelpful. Any Taoiseach who goes down the road of berating specialists for focusing attention on the acute problems confronting one of the country's leading hospitals, inevitably opens himself to a charge of being more concerned about the government's political embarrassment than the real issues involved. If, as consultants say, dialysis patients are facing a life or death situation, then it is surely in the general interest to bring the matter into the public domain.

The obvious strategy of issuing protective notices to IMPACT and SIPTU members in the hospital as a means of reducing the wage bill, which accounts for 75 per cent of expenditure, was not listed. It seems obvious that these powerful bodies should be enlisted to fight for adequate resources as part of their partnership negotiations. Beaumont Hospital is obliged at present to cut expenditure by 10 per cent and 100 beds when demand is rising. Other examples include James Connolly Memorial

A Cure for the Crisis

Hospital, Blanchardstown where 32 beds are to close, Tralee General Hospital 30 beds and Cork University Hospital 24 beds. So what gives? Certainly, not medical ethics in this instance.

The Sunday Tribune reported Minister Martin as saying that the proposal to axe dialysis services "was never a runner and was not feasible in any shape or form". Minister Martin was also critical that the management proposal contained no costings. He was certainly correct, but will he change anything as a consequence? The Beaumont Hospital car park fiasco revealed by the Comptroller and Auditor General's report in November 2002, where the State may have lost between €9 and €13 million, should have alerted the Minister to the problem of hidden deals from inexperienced administrators. The brief glance at the penalty conditions attached to the deal for "improperly" parked cars should have been obvious to anyone with common sense. It certainly begs the question why the hospital did not go to the banks and do the deal themselves.

However, Beaumont Hospital is not alone in dealing with cutbacks and budget deficits. All the large general hospitals in Dublin have a similar story to tell. The Mater Hospital may be forced to close 175 beds and treat 11,000 fewer patients due to a 20 per cent shortfall projected in February for 2003. Tallaght Hospital is 15 per cent underfunded, while St James's Hospital has a shortfall of approximately €20 million.

Solutions

1. Reduce administrative waste.
2. Cut numbers through natural wastage.
3. Ensure that service department consultants have the authority to respond to changes in service plans.
4. Allocate budgets to professional functions and allow market rigour to vary pay levels, e.g. pay more to nurses in A&E and ITUs (intensive therapy units).

11

Private health insurance

There are a number of players in the health insurance market in Ireland. Chief among them is the Voluntary Health Insurance (VHI), the British United Provident Association (BUPA) and small occupational schemes like St Paul's Medical Aid for the Garda, ESB medical aid and the prison officers' medical fund. Some small numbers are in other schemes. In general, there are three principles that apply to health insurance in Ireland.

1. *Open enrolment.* At present health insurance companies must accept everyone under 65 regardless of age, sex or health status.

2. *Lifetime cover.* Once you pay the premium the company must continue cover.

3. *Community rating.* The companies must charge the same rate regardless of age, sex or health status. Your record and past medical history are not reflected in the premium. There are restrictions and waiting times when the person enrols to avoid people joining at the time that an illness is discovered. Pre-existing illness may not be covered for a set period but any new condition is unaffected by this condition. The exact rules are usually set out by the companies in their literature.

VHI

The VHI was set up under the Voluntary Health Insurance Act 1957. The company has arrangements that they pay hospitals directly and the doctors are also paid directly net of retention tax deducted. The VHI has lists of so-called participating doctors who accept that their fee will be that agreed with the VHI in central negotiations. Thus, these doctors do not extra bill and are paid more per procedure or code number for a particular service than non-participating doctors. The vast bulk of consultants (80 per cent plus) are participating and, therefore, VHI members know that they are covered for services from any doctor listed as "participating". There is a gap of 25 to 35 per cent in the fees paid to each category.

73

A Cure for the Crisis

This has the effect of fee-fixing and creating a non-competitive environment. It also allows anomalies to arise between the fee paid for various procedures.

The VHI also assesses the suitability of the institutional hotel accommodation for private patients and agrees charges. BUPA has followed the same system. In broad terms, the VHI has been an excellent vehicle for financing the Irish medical profession, and certainly, VHI-tis is an Irish endemic disease worth acquiring.

Health rationer

The VHI behaves like a health rationer just like an American health maintenance organisation (HMO). For example, if you want to open a new private hospital or diagnostic clinic, the VHI may or may not agree to cover the costs of its members using the facility. Thus, the patient is not really insured, it is the institution that is covered and such cover includes those doctors working there. BUPA has a controlling interest in the Blackrock Clinic and Hospital and is largely able to fix its costs there.

The VHI refused to cover its subscribers for MRI scans using mobile units supplied by MRI Ireland Limited. This company offered radiologist-interpreted scans at €412 provided more than 1,000 were performed per year. The VHI will only pay for fixed scans subject to their general rules. In response, MRI Ireland complained to the Competition Authority.

In 2000, a Government White Paper on health insurance provided for the establishment of the VHI as a company under the Companies Act with full commercial autonomy and in the ownership of the Minister for Finance. It also allowed for third-party investment or for the eventual full-sale of the State's interest. A full privatisation would merely replace a state oligopoly (controlling about 85 per cent of the market) with a private one. Part privatisation is still on the Government agenda.

Claims and premiums

In 2001, the VHI took in €482 million in premiums and paid out 350,000 claims at a cost of €419 million, leaving it with a clear profit. The VHI made a profit of €14.7 million in 2002, which was a 48 per cent decline. For 2003, public hospitals are expected to take an extra €15 million from VHI and BUPA. Consequently, Minister Martin announced that "in the major teaching hospitals... it is estimated that the income from private

74

Private health insurance

beds represents less than half the costs of treating private patients. In the interests of equity, it is government policy to gradually eliminate the subsidy." The Government again raised the charges on private beds in public hospitals by 5 per cent in December 2002. This constitutes a 25 per cent total increase since August 2002.

VHI claims that the cost of providing healthcare for a 70-year-old is on average eight times that of a 20-year-old. It has over 1.5 million members and its subscription rates have been rising quickly. However, the VHI claims that a disproportionate number of younger people have joined its competitor, BUPA. Community rating, i.e. levelling the market through risk equalisation, has remained Government policy. Therefore, the VHI expects BUPA to compensate the VHI for the latter's heavy burden of expensive older patients. The VHI made a 42-page submission to the EU in which it claimed that the health insurance market in Ireland needs to be protected from predatory picking of low-risk clients. It claimed that "health insurance premiums have already started to spiral out of control", which is the case. BUPA has 15 per cent of the market for health insurance in Ireland (Republic) but has 3 per cent of the claims. VHI has most of the rest and attracts 97 per cent of claims, a situation which is clearly untenable in the intermediate term. The VHI believes that the client age disparity is adding about 30 per cent to its premiums.

The VHI warns that "death spirals", where an insurance company is forced to constantly increase premiums because of the high-risk profile of its clientele, may be forced on it, unless community rating is truly enforced. This would force BUPA to transfer about €20 million to the VHI. Clearly, BUPA would be none too happy about that. VHI premiums increased by 18 per cent in 2002, 4 per cent of which was attributed to the lack of risk equalisation. Not surprisingly, BUPA raised their prices by 14 per cent in March 2003.

Risk equalisation

The Minister for Health told the *Sunday Business Post* in November 2002 that he plans to introduce a risk equalisation scheme as soon as the necessary legislation is passed in the Dáil. The Government's 48-page reply to complaints made by BUPA Ireland to the EU Commission about the introduction of risk equalisation, which would force BUPA to compensate rivals as BUPA's clientele is significantly younger, is firm in tone and content. The Government claims that BUPA was trying to engineer a position where it could make exorbitant profits and was price shadowing the VHI, thus creating a competitive advantage.

To maintain community rating in Ireland, there is no alternative to risk equalisation. The Health Insurance Authority (HIA) makes the recommendations to the Minister about risk equalisation payments. The Authority does not view the issue as straightforward. A HIA report concluded that "the authority will need to be mindful of the likely effectiveness of risk equalisation in addressing any problems existing in the market and any potential harm that the commencement of risk equalisation may cause to the best overall interests of consumers".

Anti-competitive practices

BUPA complained to the EU Commission that the Government's policy was anti-competitive and would result in 260,000 BUPA members having to transfer €114 million over the next five years to the VHI, which has more than 1.5 million subscribers. BUPA also claimed that this would make their Irish business non-viable. The Government argued that the BUPA position was merely a stalling tactic to delay the implementation of risk equalisation, which has been part of Irish Statute law since 1994 and was not *bona fide*.

The Government document indicated that there were signs in the Irish market that the VHI was "paying most of the claims, is losing profitability and is facing the scenario of a diminishing reserve ratio and is leading the market in terms of premium increases necessary to keep pace with claims". Furthermore, the Government also claimed that BUPA Ireland had the benefit of a fully capitalised parent insurer and had benefited from the size and expertise of that parent, including the impact of advertising and sponsorship undertaken in the UK.[1]

The HIA intends to take into consideration the relative size of the insurers, the rate of premium inflation, the number of competitors and new entrants into the market, the effect of premium transfers on consumers, the overall size of the market and the commercial status of the insurers, before it comes to a decision on payment transfer.

A 1992 EU Directive allows Member States to operate specific legal provisions to protect the general good. The EU's Competition Directorate examined a BUPA complaint in 1999 and did not have a particular concern about risk equalisation and state aid.[2] Moreover, the Government sent a copy of the Health Insurance (Amendment) Bill 2000, which paved

Private health insurance

the way for risk equilisation, to the EU where Brussels officials did not query the details.

In 2002, Bank of Ireland planned to enter the health insurance market but did not intend to underwrite the insurance risk themselves, which would be passed on to an established health insurance underwriter. For its part, Bank of Ireland would earn fees from the sale, placing and administration of the business. However, having decided that the returns were unlikely to exceed €10 million per annum and together with the risk of collateral damage from the loss of banking from VHI and BUPA, Bank of Ireland backed out. This is a great pity, as it will limit competition. Finally in May 2003, the EU agreed to allow risk equalisation in Ireland.[3]

Solutions

1. Insist on risk equalisation.
2. Preserve the VHI in the public sector.
3. In the event of the introduction of universal health insurance, the VHI is the obvious vehicle to cover the GMS patient segment (excluding the over-70s).
4. Insist that the VHI becomes an insurance company, not in reality a health maintenance organisation (HMO). This will immediately result in the provision of more private sector beds.
5. Again money should follow the patient and every patient should be private.

12

Medical indemnity

More and more people feel that they somehow have a right to compensation for every vicissitude of life. There is a widespread "compo" culture to which at last some judges are giving short shrift. Legal costs are a problem. Some solicitors have been ambulance chasing, inviting people to sue when they feel in any way aggrieved. Court awards in medical negligence cases in Ireland are four times higher than comparable cases in Britain.

For decades Irish doctors have been indemnified against malpractice suits by the UK-based Medical Protection Society (MPS) and the Medical Defence Union (MDU). The MDU has been loaded with a heavy obstetrical burden of recent years which has become unsustainable. Fees have skyrocketed into the €400,000 area. The State repays 90 or 80 per cent of the premium to category 1 or 2 common contract holders. Yet the figures net of that are substantial. The cost of cover for consultants has risen from IR£120 in 1980 to average €40,000 in 2002. In 2001, the MDU added an insurance contract with Eagle Star to their cover without the prior knowledge of their members. Thus, Eagle Star is legally obliged to defend the insured member for claims made during the life of the insurance policy.

There is clearly a crisis in insurance cover for malpractice. This is most acute in obstetrics. The Rotunda Hospital currently spends 20 per cent of its annual budget on insurance compared to 3 per cent in 1995. The malpractice insurance bill in the Rotunda was €5.1 million in 2001. This is greater than the €5 million paid to consultants, including obstetricians, paediatricians and anaesthetists. Most obstetricians now pay €78,622 net.

Enterprise liability

Enterprise liability now operates in the UK and is most likely to be introduced in Ireland. If introduced without a deal with the Department of Health on historic liabilities (which may be as high as €200 million to

Medical indemnity

€500 million), private practice in Ireland will become almost unsustainable. This would effectively close the 2,500 beds in the private hospital sector. Enterprise indemnity has already been forced on junior doctors who must take out extra cover for out-of-hospital prescriptions. The medical indemnity organisations set their subscription levels every year to take account of current claims and to fund past claims. At the time of these past incidents, MDU/MPS subscriptions were much lower as were court awards. There is usually a five- to ten-year interval between the incident being pursued and the time of litigation or settlement. Obstetric cases may occur decades later.

A recent MDU case is a pointer. In January 1969, a right oophorectomy (removal of right ovary) for a cyst was performed. In 1983, the left ovary was found to be absent when the patient was 13-years-old. The case was notified to the MDU in 1985 and was settled in 1997 for IR£150,000. The subscription fee in 1969 was £8. That is the reason for the guesstimate above on the extent of current historic liabilities. Allowance cannot be made for cases that are unknown at present but are "out there". The MDU may have huge obstetrical liabilities that have yet to start coming to court, but the MPS has no apparent problem at present. That is no guarantee into the future.

In 2001, the MDU had assets of £211 million and liabilities that matched. Their accounts in 2001 read: "The level of indemnity provision in the accounts has been restricted to £81.7 million because of the reduction in the total assets mentioned earlier. This sum is covered by our re-insurance programme and *capital funding* if required." Capital funding is a call on members to pay up. In 1990 by contrast, the MDU had a £15 million asset cushion ahead of liabilities and the MPS was £9 million to the good. You could say that things have worsened. There appears to be some obfuscation of the MDU's true position. Mr Brian Lenihan TD, Minister of State at the Department of Health, raised the issue in the Seanad:

> ...only one of the defence bodies, the MDU, is suggesting that this is a problem, but its recently published annual report and accounts for 2001 do not highlight it. The notes to the accounts suggest that liabilities not backed by assets in the balance sheet are backed by reinsurance arrangements and access to capital. If this is the case, there is no reason to suggest that taxpayers should take on liabilities properly accounted for.

Minister Lenihan is entirely correct, but he probably does not realise (at least in public) that "access to capital" is a whip-round in the consultants' staff rooms.

Clearly, if the State takes up new cases from 2003 only, then someone will have to pay for historic case awards or settlements. The remaining MDU members or former members will have to pay up. In all likelihood, the MDU/MPS would have to collapse and the doctors would find themselves as a group individually liable. Doctors are only too well aware of the gravity of the situation; the key points of this issue were set out in an MDU circular to members in November 2002.

State Claims Agency

The Government intends to give the State Claims Agency (SCA), part of the National Treasury Management Agency, the responsibility for handling medical negligence cases in the public health system, covering public and private patients on a public hospital site. The proposed Clinical Indemnity Scheme will take responsibility for the acts and omissions of health board, hospital and other health service employees in respect of personal injury arising as a result of clinical negligence or malpractice.

Mr Adrian Kearns, director of the SCA, claims that significant savings will be made by having only one defendant and one set of lawyers, instead of a separate legal team for each person as at present.[1] However, the State scheme may increase rather than reduce the frequency of claims. Without doubt, it will not reduce the level of awards but may lead to earlier settlement.

As well as private practice considerations, there are other material concerns of consultants. There will be a loss of a personal indemnifier with a separate and distinct contract. The MDU/MPS also provide an advisory service to members who go before a tribunal or an inquest. Who will now provide this service and who pays? The defence organisations have a century of experience and expertise in the area. Clearly, this issue fits in well with the extension of the control agenda of the Department of Health.

If the State goes ahead with the scheme as outlined at present, consultants in private practice everywhere will have to make their own extraneous insurance arrangements. There are 150 consultants in full-time private practice in the State. Historic liabilities would have to be covered by MDU/MPS residual members and bankruptcy would loom

Medical indemnity

large. There is also the question of members' responsibility for liabilities, if they occurred while members. Then there is the problem of the State agreeing liability with complainants where the consultant feels the case is justifiably defendable. Does that mean that the hospital employer will suspend or dismiss the consultant under the terms of the common contract? Undoubtedly, there will be a loss of contractual security. Over 100 consultants are under suspension at present in the NHS often for very questionable reasons.

Litigation

The frequency of accidents in Ireland is the same as in the rest of Europe but litigation rates are much higher. The growth in subscription rates in Ireland for obstetrics is shown in Table 12.1.

Table 12.1 Subscription rates; MDU and MPS

Year	MDU (£)	MPS (£)
1989	4,380	4,380
1992	16,186	16,500
1993	21,554	19,000
1994	16,381	20,425
1995	23,950	24,409
1998	36,525	34,240
1999	68,665	35,950
2000	68,665	43,000
2001	393,000	51,600
2002	499,007	78,622

In June 2002, 35 obstetricians left the MDU and joined the MPS in a deal with the Department of Health. The malpractice insurance fees in obstetrics had soared to €2,000 per working day. The value of obstetrics settlements has increased by 26.5 per cent per year – i.e. they doubled every three years. It is impossible for any investment policy to keep up with that rate of claim settlement inflation. The deal covers obstetrics in the Bons Secours Hospital in Cork – a subsidy for private industry not much different to industrial or farming grants or subsidies! The obstetricians who left the MDU did not get a guarantee that the traditional occurrence-based system would still operate. Each case would be considered on its merits – i.e. a "get-out" clause. Current general subscriptions are shown in Table 12.2.

A Cure for the Crisis

Table 12.2 General subscriptions rates, 2001–2002

	2002		2001	
	MDU (€)	MPS (€)	MDU (€)	MPS (€)
Obstetrics	499,007	78,622	499,007	65,518
Surgery	48,665*	60,338†	41,774	47,500 60,338†
High risk	35,635	37,394	31,534	37,394
Medium risk	25,355	30,118	22,538	30,118
Low risk	14,260	10,894	12,240	10,984

*The MDU has set neurosurgery at €83,000
† Two cosmetic surgeons only

The MDU is involved in the private sector in Britain and in both the public and private sectors in Ireland. The MPS is involved in Britain and Ireland, Hong Kong, Singapore and New Zealand. Now the MDU must defend the member and is in reality only slightly different to an insurance broker, but the rules of the MPS mean that all benefits are discretionary. Legal advice and indemnity are discretionary and given by the decision of each organisation's governing body. Both organisations have the final decision on handling all aspects of claims. Both can call on members for extra funds. Indeed, this has happened in Australia where another mutual malpractice organisation called up AUS$19 million due to a cerebral palsy case being awarded a much greater sum than anticipated. Consequently, the local defence organisation shut up shop. The doctors stopped carrying out procedures and within 24 hours, the government stepped in to make another arrangement, having earlier denied any involvement or responsibility. The Australian Federal Government has introduced a form of enterprise liability.

Therefore, Irish doctors are a bit like Lloyd's names – they have unlimited liability, but do not share in any profits. It is possible that future cases could impact hugely on members of both bodies, if historic liabilities are not carried by the State. The defence organisations can settle cases without the doctor's agreement. There are circumstances where this could lead to disciplinary action and referral to the Medical Council. Two cases, involving a paediatrician and an obstetrician, were settled out of court with an admission of liability by the defence organisations made without the doctors' consent. The claimants then sought enquiries with either the employing health boards or the Medical Council. To date we have seen obstetrics and gynaecology take the brunt of malpractice

Medical indemnity

claims, however in the future, cosmetic and orthopaedic surgery indemnity rates will escalate.

State indemnity

When Crown Indemnity was introduced into the NHS in 1989, the UK Exchequer bought off historic liabilities for a £50–£56 million contribution, with both MDU and MPS paying about £28 million each. All consultants with public appointments were insured by the state. Private practice insurance is still provided by the MPS/MDU. Representation before the General Medical Council (GMC) is still provided by both organisations.

The Bons Secours Hospital, Cork/MPS obstetrics deal with the Department of Health and Children (DOHC) is only another step along the way to the development of state indemnity. The agreement includes:

(a) "MPS shall exercise its discretion to provide assistance and indemnity to any transferring members or residual obstetrician members in accordance with its prevailing practices and policies but will not confirm or refuse indemnity without prior consultation with the DOHC."

(b) "MPS undertakes to use its best endeavours to ensure that relevant civil claims are managed in an efficient and cost effective manner in accordance with best practice. DOHC shall have the right at any time to take over the conduct of any relevant claim in which event MPS undertakes to deliver its files and relevant data to DOHC at the earliest opportunity and DOHC shall be responsible for the costs of management and conduct thereof."

The MPS has also agreed to hand over a special fund for private and non-private work. For its part, the DOHC has agreed to indemnify the MPS for costs incurred in excess of the amount in either the special fund (private) or special fund (non-private). Subscription increases will only take place following consultation with the DOHC.

Clearly, the MDU wants enterprise liability. Dr Michael Saunders of the MDU said on 14 June 2001:

> It is anomalous that obstetricians in Ireland, members of a profession which has amongst the best rates of mortality and morbidity in Western Europe, find themselves funding such a high level of

A Cure for the Crisis

claims. We believe that this could be resolved by the introduction of Enterprise Liability now.

There is widespread agreement among doctors that enterprise liability is the way forward. Certainly, the professional academic body, the Institute of Obstetricians and Gynaecologists at the RCPI, is also calling for enterprise liability.

Risk management, more bureaucracy

The independence of the MPS/MDU is now a mirage. The Department of Health is in reality the guarantor of last resort. It is only a matter of time before state indemnity spreads widely throughout the high- and medium-risk specialties because the alternative is unaffordable. Inevitably, risk managers will be employed across the health system to try to limit risk. This will have the effect of slowing patient throughput and holding up care when the facilities are inadequate or less than ideal. In the past, doctors often fudged and muddled through, doing their best for the patients in the face of severe cutbacks and lack of adequate development funding. However, no more! At the very least consultants must have security of tenure, clinical autonomy, a reliable defence (consultants are at risk when liability is inappropriately admitted), advisory services and, lastly, affordable services.

Litigation – the American way of life

Litigation is at world record levels in the US. Doctors have not escaped and the cost consequences are hurting. In 2003 in the US, doctor strikes have taken place, to protest over crippling malpractice insurance premiums. In West Virginia, several hospitals had to transfer patients across state lines because of a strike by about 30 surgeons. In that state, spiralling lawsuits have forced numerous doctors to move or retire. Juries in West Virginia have seemed incapable of understanding the concept of genetic birth defects. A striking doctor described his job as "a hostile work environment. The problem just grows every day. Physicians no longer want to come to work".[2]

A similar strike was just averted in Pennsylvania when the state promised a new malpractice insurance plan. In May 2002, Las Vegas obstetricians placed a ban on new patients, citing insurance premiums equivalent to €60,000 per year. The American College of Obstetricians

Medical indemnity

and Gynaecologists reports that average medical liability awards jumped 43 per cent in a single year from £451,000 in 1999 to £650,000 in 2000.

There has been a huge rise in allegations that "neurologically impaired" children suffered brain trauma during birth. The average award in such cases is £645,000, but one jury in Philadelphia recently awarded a child £64.5 million. Similarly, radiologists are being sued for failing to see early signs of breast cancer on mammograms. Mississippi recently drafted laws to cap damages for emotional distress at £322,000.

Solutions

1. Risk reduction must be given a higher priority within the whole health service.
2. Enterprise liability.
3. The State must pick up historic liabilities. The MDU no longer has any obstetrical members, yet may face huge liabilities with no obstetrical income to cover it.
4. Academic contracts must be fully state-covered. In the case of RCSI, the College should make a contribution to the state scheme covering undergraduate activities only.
5. State indemnity should be available for GPs covering all their patients. It will cover health board clinics.
6. GPs on the Specialist Register or eligible for inclusion should be covered by a state scheme administered by the MPS or MDU or commercial insurer.
7. Doctors should be allowed state cover through the defence organisations for sports events and acts of charity whether remunerated or not.
8. Locums should be covered through the state system in line with the arrangements of the practitioner, whose practice is being covered.
9. Category 2 consultants working offsite should have a state arrangement operating through the MPS/MDU/commercial insurer as well as their onsite hospital or clinic cover.
10. Cork has a citywide rota of all obstetricians in public or private hospitals. Private hospital consultants can cover all patients in public and private hospitals at weekends. This arrangement should be continued and extended to other services where appropriate.

A Cure for the Crisis

11. Consultants working in teaching hospitals with private hospitals attached, such as St Vincent's University Hospital and St Vincent's Private Hospital or the Mater public and private hospitals, should be treated as integrated from the standpoint of medical indemnity.

12. Private clinics on a public hospital site should be included in the overall hospital scheme.

13. Private hospitals should be able to buy into the state scheme at a subsidised rate otherwise they may face closure.

14. Public patients treated in private hospitals under the National Treatment Purchase Fund or similar plans should be covered in full by the state scheme.

15. Ethical clinical trials in public hospitals should be covered by enterprise liability.

16. For an advisory service the MPS is likely to charge €400 to €1,000 per annum related to income. Alternatively, the IMO/IHCA should initiate such a service for members.

17. Tort reform. A Constitutional referendum is needed for real changes to tort law but it may not be passed. The Constitution is very strong on individual rights. Awards cannot be capped and there is no statute of limitations.

18. Vigorous defence of spurious claims must be made, including the pursuit of costs.

19. A public information campaign must be launched to inform the public that all intrauterine growth retardation and cerebral palsy is not due to medical intervention.

20. A no-fault scheme should be agreed for cerebral palsy cases.

21. Whatever arrangements are agreed for private practice, retired consultants who continue to do medico-legal or medical work must have the right to participate. MPS members who earn life membership can continue to practise free, but MDU must pay a subscription related to their income.

13

Prescription medicines

In Ireland in the private sector, all citizens can avail of the Drug Payment Scheme (DPS). The scheme was set up initially to help the long-term ill on chronic medication. Des Byrne set out the interesting – reverse Robin Hood – recent history of the scheme.[1] Up to 1998, those who spent more than IR£32 per month on medication and at least IR£96 in three months could apply to a health board for a refund over this figure. This meant that once-off expensive drug bills were not covered but chronic illnesses were. Then the scheme was computerised and the three-month IR£96 requirement was scrapped. However, the threshold was increased to IR£42 per month. The chronically ill then had to pay an extra IR£120 per year, whereas those with once-off illness had their costs reduced to IR£42, if the condition was, as many are, circumscribed – a redistribution towards those without chronic disease.

In January 2002, the threshold converted to €53.33 and was shortly after increased to €65, while the Budget that year raised it to €75. (In fact, the Minister assumed the figure was €70, but the effect is unchanged but reduced by 6.6 per cent.) That was the second rise within six months. In comparison to four years ago, those on long-term illness will be paying an additional €363.12 per annum. This is an 85 per cent increase in the threshold in four years and is unfair on asthmatics, people in cardiac failure, renal failure and so on, who need continuous medication. For 2004, the threshold will be €78 per month.

Switch to generic drugs

Minister for Health, Micheál Martin wants to reduce the cost of the DPS by €20 million in 2003. He claims that it is possible to introduce generic drugs in about 18 per cent of prescriptions and such substitution will reduce costs by €2 million. Seamus Feely of the Irish Pharmaceutical Union advised: "We're suggesting that pharmacists themselves do a review of a person's medication, which would help secure value for money and improve patient outcomes."[2] However, no individual or family is required to pay more than €70 per month on prescription medicines. The soaring cost is the reason for raising the threshold. Evidence-based drug treatments for the major cardiovascular diseases of high blood pressure, cardiac failure and coronary artery disease are advancing rapidly and are costly.

Essentially, generic drugs are agents whose patent has expired. They are copies of the original compound manufactured by a separate company. In Ireland, each drug must have a product licence from the Irish Medicines Board, which sets standards and safeguards the public against therapeutic misadventure and fraud. The biological activity of the generic drug must be identical to the original. Generics are usually considerably cheaper than the parent.

Under the proposal presented to the Minister, if a generic drug is not available to an individual, then the next-cheapest drug would be prescribed. If a patient insists on a more expensive option or a GP chooses to prescribe a more costly drug, then the patient would have to pay for it themself. Dr Muiris Houston in *The Irish Times* (28 November 2002) highlights the unsatisfactory nature of this proposal: "Some doctors will object citing the principle of autonomy and object to state interference in the doctor–patient relationship."

The economic point is that the DPS offers no economic incentive to economise once the €65 threshold is exceeded. All additional medication is free to the consumer but paid for in taxes. The DPS cost €177.6 million in 2001 and was used by 1.156 million people, 30.13 per cent of the population. Thus, it is important to a huge number of families. This was 24 per cent of the total costs of the state drug schemes and the cost in 2001 was 26 per cent greater than in 2000. The Labour Party Spokesperson on Health, Liz McManus TD, accurately summed up the effect of the rising DPS threshold: "A single person earning €132 per week is still not entitled to a medical card and will now have to pay up to €70 per month for prescription drugs."

Worldwide increase in prescription costs

In the US, drug prescription costs grew by 17.3 per cent from 1999 to 2000. In 1990, drugs accounted for 6 per cent of total healthcare spending, whereas by 2000 this had risen to 9 per cent and it is projected to rise

Prescription medicines

to 14 per cent by 2010. Pharmaceutical expenditure in Ireland will grow to approach €1 billion within the next one to two years.

In Canada, Can$12.3 billion (US$7.8 billion) was spent on prescription drugs in 2001, a 10.6 per cent increase over 2000 and a huge 46.4 per cent increase over 1997 when the bill was Can$8.4 billion. Canadians also spent an additional Can$3.3 billion on over-the-counter drugs. The total drug cost is 15.2 per cent of the Can$105 billion spent on healthcare in 2001. The Canadian Institute for Health Information reported that an ageing population and the growing prevalence of cardiovascular, respiratory and gastroenterology diseases, AIDS and hepatitis were factors. The comprehensive and universal nature of the drug subsidy programme also played a major role in rising utilisation rates.

Since February 2002, pharmacists in Germany have been told to dispense medicines from the cheapest third of the price range of drugs, unless the doctor specifies no change to the prescribed drug on the prescription. Dr Zollner of the NAV-Virchow-Bund, a regional doctors' union, has protested that the law change is unnecessary. "In over 70 per cent of all possible types of medicines we have already changed over to generics," he explains. Dr Zollner protested at the interference in the doctor's freedom to prescribe. "We have had a clear division of powers in healthcare since about the second century or thereabouts – the chemist has the task of making up a written prescription and the doctor has the responsibility for prescribing." The German Health Department noted however that there is a long-standing practice at night and in emergencies for pharmacists to replace prescribed drugs when unavailable.[3] There is an expectation that 4.6 per cent can be saved from the drug budget over the year. In Germany, prescribed drugs are paid for by statutory health insurance companies. Most health insurance is administered by non-profit sickness funds to which 90 per cent of Germans make statutory contributions.

Concerns have been expressed about possible allergic effects of generic drugs and the lack of records in case of adverse reactions. It may also confuse the patient because a different-looking drug may be dispensed every time. Unlike doctors, chemists do not have to keep records of drugs they dispense. Doctors can still prescribe brand names but must specifically say so on the prescription.

Pharmacoeconomic evaluations are being carried out in Britain, the Netherlands, Italy, Portugal, Greece, Norway, Sweden and Finland in an attempt to ensure value for money, i.e. cost-effectiveness. The economic argument for the fire-and-forget method of treatment is put very well by Dr J Shepherd in the *Lancet*.[4] Most of the clinical benefit from statin therapy is achieved by reduction of the initial high or high normal cholesterol by 25 per cent. A doubling of the dose of a statin only reduces the cholesterol by a further 5–6 per cent but at great cost. Two-thirds of the maximum lipid-lowering benefit of a statin are achieved at the starting dose.[5]

The assumption that price competition is pristine with generics has been holed. Indeed, the British Department of Health has sued three pharmaceutical companies for £180 million compensation for price fixing and anti-competitive cartel arrangements in dealing with NHS purchasers.

Monitoring pharmaceutical companies

Any industry making huge profits will use its muscle to protect their interests. The pharmaceutical industry is no exception. This industry is the single largest sponsor of medical research. In the US, Canada and the UK, it plays a huge role, and in some countries is the only source of research support. Industry-funded research is overwhelmingly drug orientated. Ninety per cent of the world's health problems attract only 10 per cent of global health resources. In fact, multinationals have traditionally ignored work on tropical diseases because of the low potential return.

Evidence capture

Health policies often blindly follow published evidence irrespective of whether the information provided is reliable or appropriate to the needs of society at large. As Joe Collier and Ike Iheanacho, editors of *Drug and Therapeutics Bulletin* put it: "The sheer weight of industry sponsored new evidence rather than its quality might lead to inappropriate shifts in therapeutic practice away from the tried familiar and usually cheaper approach to novel unfamiliar and generally more expensive alternatives that offer no real clinical advantage."[6]

Regulatory agencies

Pharmaceutical companies try to exert influence over state regulatory agencies. There is often a revolving-door system with state agencies hiring staff from the industry and later these people return to industry at a

Prescription medicines

higher level. The US Food and Drugs Administration (FDA) and the British Committee on the Safety of Medicines (CSM) are both affected. Regulatory capture is important because the risk–benefit assessment of drugs has a high degree of technical uncertainty, which is inherent in toxicology, clinical trials and epidemiology. In the *Lancet*, Prof Abraham of the University of Sussex wrote about the alarming bias found in a regulatory agency such as the FDA:

> In 2002, an internal inquiry into the views of regulatory staff at the FDA's Centre for Drug Evaluation and Review reported that a third of respondents did not feel comfortable expressing their scientific opinions, with some reporting pressure to favour the wishes of manufacturers over the interests of science and public health, and receiving requests from senior agency officials to alter their opinions... in the late 1990s, when some FDA scientists released documents to congress because of their concerns about the risks of troglitazone while it was on the US market, they received threats of disciplinary action from agency management.[7]

Conflicts of interests

In 1996, data showed that only 25 per cent of expert advisers to the CSM had no financial interests in the industry. Of 23 members of the CSM with financial interests in 1996, 3 had interests in at least 20 companies, 7 had interests in at least 10 and 20 had interests in at least 5. In the FDA, up to 90 per cent of the members of advisory committees could have conflicts of interest.

Tricks

The medicalisation of female sexual problems in a concerted and co-ordinated manner by multinational pharmaceutical companies is their latest wheeze to find lifestyle fashions that can be lucratively treated with patented drugs. For the past six years, there has been a concerted effort to have female sexual dysfunction defined as a medical condition requiring treatment. This predated the launch of Viagra which earned Pfizer $1.5 billion in sales in 2001. The emerging competitors, Bayer's vardenafil and Lilly-ICOS's tadalafil, are expected to have sales of $1 billion each annually. Extensive efforts were funded by the industry to define a new concept of female sexual dysfunction outside that normally seen such as vaginismus, dyspareunia and postmenopausal dryness and irritation. This was necessary to run clinical trials to get licences for the female

A Cure for the Crisis

market before patents expire. Ray Moynihan in the *British Medical Journal* described the making of a disease:

> In a ground breaking gathering in May 1997, clinicians, researchers, and drug company representatives met for two days at a Cape Cod Hotel to discuss the future direction of clinical trials in this area, against a backdrop of widespread lack of agreement about the definition of female sexual dysfunction.[8]

Eighteen of the 19 authors had financial or other relationships with a total of 22 drug companies. There were nine drug companies involved in sponsoring the meeting.

In 1999, a report in the *Journal of the American Medical Association (JAMA)* claimed that 43 per cent of women aged from 18 to 59 suffered from some sexual dysfunction.[9] About 1,500 women were surveyed as to whether they had experienced any of seven sexual problems for two months or more during the previous year. The problems included anxiety about sexual performance, difficulties with vaginal lubrication and a lack of desire for sex. A "yes" to any counted in the 43 per cent. However, the *JAMA* article stated that its data were "not equivalent to clinical diagnosis". Two of the authors belatedly disclosed links to Pfizer. Sexual dysfunction has complex social, personal and physical causes and using Viagra to treat these is unlikely to offer a solution. There is a likelihood that women will be made to feel that they have a physical malfunction when they do not. The unfortunate consequence is that doctors may feel that drugs are an appropriate intervention when the problems are elsewhere. The price of Viagra in MIMS is €34.87 for four 100 mg tablets or €24.62 for four 25 mg tablets. Good for the industry – a lucrectomy for the patient or the victim!

The new disorder of ill-defined female sexual disorder is the invention of pharmaceutical companies at a corporate-sponsored meeting in 1998. Dr John Bancroft of the Kinsey Institute at Indiana University believes that the term dysfunction is highly misleading. Dr Bancroft argues that "an inhibition of sexual desire is in many situations a healthy and functional response for women faced with stress, tiredness, or threatening patterns of behaviour from their partners". The original author concedes that many of the women in the 43 per cent are "perfectly normal" where a lot of their problems "arise out of perfectly reasonable responses of the human organism to challenges and stress".

Prescription medicines

The disgraceful piece in this saga is the admission in 1999 by Dr Jennifer Berman, assistant professor of urology at the University of California at Los Angeles that "normative data are being gathered for comparison to determine what normal physiological responses are for women in particular age groups".[10] In other words, there is a disease or a disorder but the propagators of the new paradigm do not know the reference range of normals without the disease.

The late D. Brian Morgan, professor of chemical pathology at Leeds University, offered the following definition of a disease as "a difference from the normal which is a biological disadvantage to the holder", during the course of his inaugural address at Leeds in 1979. This definition is truer, more accurate and perceptive than that found in the *Concise Oxford Dictionary* – "an unhealthy condition of body or part of, or of the mind; illness, sickness. A particular kind of disease with special symptoms of location." George Bernard Shaw would have loved the latter – a disease is a disease! However, there has to be rigorous scrutiny of the definitions of disease when there is substantial money to made in treating newly defined entities – for example, myalgic encephalomyelitis (ME).

Drugs and equipment advertising

Medics' trips on the Orient Express to discuss the merits of a particular drug seem to have gone out of fashion. In the US, direct-to-consumer marketing of drugs is allowed and is big business. In the UK, most drugs are available only on prescription and therefore advertising to GPs and consultants is important for pharmaceutical companies.

Misleading advertising is a serious issue. Recently, Dr Joe Collier, editor of *Drugs and Therapeutics Bulletin*, called for an inquiry into how the Medicines Control Agency (MCA) in Britain let an advertisement for a new oral contraceptive Yasmin go through in June 2002, which claims that this pill avoids weight gain and gives the taker a sense of well-being. The manufacturer Schering Health Care also claimed that Yasmin had a "demonstrable positive effect" on premenstrual symptoms and skin conditions. The Prescriptions Medicines Code of Practice Authority looked at the advertisement in September and found that it breached the code of practice on 10 counts. The weight gain and skin claims could not be substantiated. The MCA then found there were grounds for concern. Nonetheless, Schering still hold that the claims are true and are appealing the MCA ruling.[11]

Solutions

1. Drug costs should be covered for a flagship therapeutic agent in each group for each condition, and drugs that cost more than that should be subsidised up to the base cost of the index agent. This would allow freedom of medical practice, contain costs and allow any therapeutic advantage that may be published about newer drugs to be available to the public at a cheaper cost. The doctor will also have to explain to the patient the advantage of one drug over the other. There could be a number of base agents per disease which would be fully covered under the GMS. These should be named and ranked by a new National Therapeutics Agency. The German scheme on generic substitution, noted above, is worth considering with modifications.

   Therapeutics often has an element of belief included in the clinical effect. Witness the power of placebo in many trials. It is not unusual for a patient to state categorically that drug X does something specific for them therapeutically or to them in the case of undesirable side-effects, whereas drug Y does not. Yet the two drugs may be identical. So undoubtedly some patients will be upset by changing from a black Ford Model T to a dark blue one. Patients could be asked to pay the difference from the base index price, if they insist on a proprietary drug. This should apply to all prescriptions, whether funded wholly by the GMS or in part by the DPS.

2. Package inserts should include more than one language in the EU to allow parallel drug importing and thus price competition in proprietary drugs. The prices of statins and antihypertensives are still much lower in Spain than in Dublin.

3. The EU should proceed with the proposal for a directive to ensure that large print labelling and braille form part of package inserts. Apparently, about 21 per cent of adults have difficulty reading labels and 73 per cent have sight problems. Telephone helplines and websites should also be set up as a source of product information.

4. New agents, such as antibodies like infliximab or etanercept, which are shown internationally to be effective, should bypass the system via direct interaction between the prescribing consultant and the National Therapeutics Agency.

5. Competition should be introduced into dispensing. At present, there is a 50 per cent mark-up on drugs dispensed. This is part of the DPS and is an anti-competitive fixed cost on the taxpayer. It should be

Prescription medicines

replaced by a dispensing charge and a stock payment for holding medicines with short expiry times based on each pharmacy's record. There is a same-day delivery service from drug wholesalers in Dublin, so the costs must be readily containable at least in the larger urban areas.

6. The National Centre for Pharmacoeconomics at St James's Hospital should be commissioned to evaluate the cost-effectiveness of drug interventions in the major clinical areas. Their findings could be incorporated into a national indicative formulary, updated yearly and used with co-payments as a gesture in drug cost control.

7. Drug prices should be monitored to combat anti-competitive practices at all levels.

8. The Competition Authority should prevent large pharmacy chains monopolising the market. Since the Pharmacy Act 1875, a chemist shop must be operated and personally supervised by a pharmacist. All registered EU pharmacists should satisfy the legal requirements. The derogation from EU law which prevents Irish pharmacists, trained in the UK, to independently operate a pharmacy in Ireland must be dropped. The Pharmacy Review Group wants to limit to 8 per cent the number of GMS pharmacy contracts which any pharmacy group may hold in any health board area. This might not survive a legal challenge.

9. Drug regulatory systems are needed which act uncompromisingly in the interests of public health. Expert advisers to regulatory agencies should be required to divest themselves of all conflicts of interest during their period of appointment.

10. Regulatory systems should have the ability to check key tests independently.

11. The State should ensure that regulatory agencies are funded entirely independently of industry.

12. Disease definitions in licence applications must be expertly scrutinised for accuracy.

14

Impact of advances in technology

Technology deficiencies in Irish hospitals render them inefficient, unsafe and unaccreditable. The current administrative structures fail the public because they refuse to respond to technology advances in anything like a timely or appropriate fashion. Innovation is always suppressed by "procedure".

Technology changes happen very quickly in medicine and some simple conventional practices of 20 years ago would now be considered dangerous. For example, it is now standard practice to do a CT brain scan on patients before a spinal tap for meningitis, to ensure that the vital brain centres are not squeezed into the spinal cord exit at the lower end of the brain. This is all very well in Beaumont Hospital, but where does that leave you in Portlaoise General Hospital, where there is no CT scanner and someone presents with possible or probable meningitis?

Other surgical specialties may change. In 1990 in neurosurgery, a detachable platinum coil was first introduced into clinical use in the US and in 1992 it was first used in Europe. It is called the Guglielmi detachable coil and was approved by the FDA in 1995. The device allowed the development of endovascular techniques for the occlusion of intracranial aneurysms, which offered the prospect of reducing the risk of further rupture without the need for craniotomy. Since 1995, this technique has become widely used in patients with ruptured and unruptured intracranial aneurysms.

In 2002, a trial of surgical clipping versus endovascular coiling in a selected subgroup of patients with subarachnoid haemorrhage reported an absolute reduction of 6.9 per cent in dependency and death at one year in favour of coiling over surgery, representing a relative risk reduction of 22.6 per cent.[1,2] The consequences for the demand for neurosurgeons and interventionist neuroradiologists are obvious.

Specialties develop into a myriad of linked subspecialties. In cardiology, subdivisions have developed where general cardiologists do

Impact of advances in technology

echocardiograms (ECHOs) and diagnostic angiograms and refer to superspecialists for stenting or surgery. Other cardiologists are electophysiologists who look after arrhythmias and map the sites of the rhythm disturbances. They then burn therapeutic lesions often around the pulmonary veins.

Endoscopy

In Ireland, efforts are being made at present to carry out screening of over 50-year-olds for colon cancer. In 2000, 47 per cent of people over 50 in the US were not being screened. The US National Colorectal Cancer Awareness Month in March 2000 set out to educate over 50-year-olds and their doctors about the importance of large bowel cancer screening. Nurses are being trained in the skills necessary because of the huge logistic requirement. Refinements in CT virtual colonoscopy will aid this effort and imaging centres will proliferate, generating many new patients who will need therapeutic polyp snaring.

Open access endoscopy is important as a service to clinicians in the hospitals and in primary care. Endoscopy, *Helicobacter pylori* eradication and anti-gastric acid drugs have massively reduced the demand and indications for gastric surgery. Trained nurses are being used in some hospitals to provide much of this service as an effective cheaper alternative.

Laboratory science

Laboratory science is in constant evolution. Scientists have been very flexible in their work changes. Modular systems like Roche can be used to analyse the overwhelming volume of the daily workload with a saving in staff numbers. This allows redeployment and facilitates change in the laboratory menu and service for patients, which is a very welcome development. Blinkered management could regard these developments as an excuse for redundancies, but that is the path of instant stagnation for the services. New tests, new methods and new demands are constantly being introduced, which requires constant staff retraining. Laboratory scientists will increasingly be responsible for the quality assurance of near-patient testing equipment in the hospitals, health centres and GPs surgeries.

Current equipment, smaller than a kitchen microwave oven, allows GPs to safely do 70 per cent of their routine blood testing in the surgery. The machine does its own quality control (QC) automatically and will refuse to give a test result if the QC is wrong (i.e. it is safe for patients).

The equipment can be monitored by qualified laboratory staff. This is what the Department of Health should be encouraging as it is cost-effective in the round – it saves on laboratory staff, repeat visits, transport, communications, phlebotomy costs, hospital administration costs, etc. Home INR testing for warfarin treatment has also been shown to improve the anticoagulation control and is cost-effective and convenient for the patient.

Scanning equipment

PET scanners

Positron emission tomography (PET) with 18-fluorodeoxyglucose (FDG) has been used for staging cancers since the early 1990s. In July 2001, Medicare in the US started covering PET scanning for staging non-small cell lung cancers. These public sector insurers considered the data sufficiently strong to cover its appropriate use. FDG-PET is more accurate than CT and radionuclide scans in staging lung cancer. Furthermore, PET is accurate in 83 per cent of patients, whereas conventional imaging is accurate in 65 per cent. A study from the Netherlands reported that the addition of PET scanning to conventional work-up prevented unnecessary surgery in one in five patients with suspected non-small cell lung cancer.[3]

The Irish National Cancer Registry (1994–98) reported five-year survival with lung cancer in Ireland at 10 per cent in females and 8.5 per cent in males. At Beaumont Hospital, there are about 250 cases of lung cancer per year with median age 64, that is, a new one every working day.

Research in the US has shown that the availability of PET saves between €1,000 and €20,000 per patient and results in more appropriate management and treatment in almost 40 per cent of cancer cases. A small number of public patients are scanned using the PET scanner in the Blackrock Clinic at €2,600 per patient. There is also a PET scanner in Belfast which has also been used for some patients from the Republic. European recommendations suggest a need for one PET scanner per million, whereas in Australia, the ratio recommended is one for three million. PET scanners also have a distinct role in neurological diagnosis.

The Department of Health is currently considering placing one machine in Dublin with a mobile machine for the rest of the country. A static machine will cost about €1 million, while another €1 million is needed to build a suitable facility.

Impact of advances in technology

CT and MRI scanners

Much is written and said about institution accreditation for Irish hospitals, but when CT scanners are not freely available as a basic tool, then scepticism is appropriate. Portlaoise General Hospital should get a CT scanner in 2003 at a cost €1.2 million for the machine, €300,000 in capital set-up costs and an annual revenue cost of €300,000.

The State should purchase a job lot of MRI scanners and place them in our general hospitals. The images generated should be downloaded to expert radiologists in this country or abroad by using broadband. This will make medical investigation more efficient and reduce the need for hospital bed stay in many specialities, including neurology.

New techniques

Scientists in Cambridge, England have harnessed a previously hidden spectrum of light, called terahertz, and used it to take precise images which can be used to identify cancers much earlier and assess their size and shape. The prototype is being tested at Addenbrooke's Hospital. Trials are also being set up at St Thomas' Hospital, London. The equipment costs between £200,000 and £300,000, which is cheaper than MRI and in the same price range as ultrasound. Science advances unpredictably and the public and the doctors demand the most effective and sensitive means of investigating and treating patients currently possible. Therefore, medical inflation will continue to outstrip general consumer price inflation.

Solutions

1. National technology deficiencies in CT/MRI/PET scanners should be corrected through a central purchase of a job lot.

2. Reporting of images by superspecialists should be made available to all imaging units by broadband.

3. Near-patient blood testing networks for GPs should be available and linked to the nearest large hospital pathology department.

4. There should also be open access to hospital service departments for all medical providers.

15

Life expectancy in Europe and beyond

One of the oldest and most widely used measures of the health of a population is life expectancy at birth. It is an indicator based entirely on mortality data. As an indicator, life expectancy is important because it is often used in comparative analysis regarding health and quality of life at national level. In the last four decades, there have been phenomenal gains in life expectancy in almost all OECD countries, although for certain sections of Irish society those gains have not been significant.

In 2000, 37 per cent of the EU population lived as part of a nuclear family. By 2005, this will decrease to 34 per cent, or 133 million people. Between 2000 and 2005, the number of children between three and nine years will fall by 2.6 million; the number of under-18s will fall by 3.5 million, while the number of retired people will rise by six million. Table 15.1 shows the life expectancy in delegate EU Member States in terms of population and GDP.

Table 15.1 Life expectancy in delegate EU Member States

Country	Population (millions)	GDP per head (£)	Life expectancy males (yrs)	Life expectancy females (yrs)
Czech Rep.	10.3	3,963	71.7	78.4
Cyprus	0.8	9,346	75.3	80.4
Estonia	1.4	2,897	64.7	76.2
Hungary	10.2	3,642	67.1	75.7
Latvia	2.4	2,319	65.2	76.6
Lithuania	3.5	2,460	65.9	77.4
Malta	0.4	6,629	76.1	80.8
Poland	38.6	3,269	70.2	78.4
Slovakia	5.4	2,730	69.1	77.2
Slovenia	2.0	6,757	72.1	79.6

Figures relate to 2001
Source: Eurostat

Life expectancy in Europe and beyond

Irish scenario

Between 1991 and 1996, life expectancy in Ireland improved by 0.7 years for males and 0.6 years for females. In 1926, an Irish male infant was expected to live 57.4 years and a female 57.9 years. Life expectancy of Irish males aged 65 improved by 1 year or 8 per cent over the last 70 years, while Irish females improved by 4 years or 30 per cent. The improvement in life expectancy is a direct result of decreasing mortality over the last 70 years, particularly infant mortality. Much of this occurred between 1946 and 1961.

In 1960, Irish male life expectancy at birth was above the EU average, ranked in fourth position. In the same year, Irish female life expectancy at birth ranked second last of 15 EU Member States. In 1996, the gap between the sexes was 5.5 years and the EU average gap was 6.4 years (see Tables 15.2–15.4).

Table 15.2 Life expectancy at birth and at age 65 (1960–1996)

Life expectancy	1960		1996	
	Males	Females	Males	Females
At birth				
Ireland	68.1	71.9	73.0	78.5
EU average	67.4	72.9	74.2	80.6
At age 65				
Ireland	12.6	14.4	13.8	17.4
EU average	12.7	15.1	15.4	19.2

Source: Central Statistics Office

Table 15.3 Life expectancy at birth in selected non-EU countries

Country	Males		Females	
	1980	2001	1980	2001
Russia	61.5	59.0	73.1	72.2
Belarus	65.9	63.4	75.5	74.0
San Marino	73.2	77.4	79.1	84.0
Switzerland	72.8	77.2	79.6	82.8
United States	70.0	74.4	77.4	80.0
Japan	73.3	77.6	78.8	84.2
India	52.9	62.2	52.1	63.5
China	66.7	69.8	68.9	73.6
Turkey	59.2	66.4	64.8	71.0

Source: OECD, 2002

A Cure for the Crisis

Table 15.4 Life expectancy at birth in EU countries

Country	Males		Females	
	1980	2001	1980	2001
EU	70.5	75.3	77.2	81.4
Belgium	70.0	74.4	76.8	80.8
Denmark	71.2	74.3	77.3	79.0
Germany	69.6	74.4	76.1	80.6
Greece	72.2	75.4	76.8	80.7
Spain	72.5	75.6	78.6	82.9
France	70.2	75.5	78.4	83.0
Ireland	70.1	73.0	75.6	78.5
Italy	70.6	76.7	77.4	82.9
Luxembourg	69.1	74.9	75.9	81.3
Netherlands	72.7	75.7	79.3	80.6
Austria	69.0	75.4	76.1	81.2
Portugal	67.7	73.5	75.2	80.3
Finland	69.2	74.6	77.6	81.5
Sweden	72.8	77.5	78.8	82.1
Britain	70.2	75.7	76.2	80.4

Source: Eurostat, 2001

In 2001, the average life expectancy for EU women was 81.4 years, but was 78.5 for Irish women. For men the average EU figure was 75.3 years and 73 for Irish men. French women live longest at 83 years, while Swedish men outlive other Europeans at 77.5 years. Infant mortality rate in the EU in 2001 is 4.6 per 1,000 livebirths, whereas the Irish figure is 5.8. Possibly abortion might have a bearing on this issue as would community health problems in the Irish Traveller population.

Clearly, our national vital statistics leave much to be achieved. It is also worth noting that our performance appears to have worsened in the late 1990s. Specifically, life expectancy slipped from 73.2 to 73 for males and 78.7 to 78.6 for females over 1994 to 1995.

Industrial earnings and literacy

Average weekly industrial earnings over all industries for June 2002 in Ireland were €497.45, up 6.3 per cent on the previous year, and the average number of hours worked per week was 39.4. The hourly rate was €12.63. The average gross earnings for male industrial workers was €534.61 (€13.28 per hour) and for females it was €360.44 (€9.84 per hour).

Life expectancy in Europe and beyond

In 1999, 23 per cent of Irish people were found to be functionally illiterate. This meant that they had difficulty in reading a bill or following instructions on a medicine bottle.

In the late 1990s, the US topped the poverty list with 16.5 per cent, Ireland was next on 15.3 per cent, Britain 15.1 per cent, while Sweden had 7 per cent.

Indigenous peoples

Alcohol, drug abuse and homicides, including domestic violence, are epidemic in the aboriginal community in Australia and lifespan statistics are shown in Table 15.5. Similarly, the longevity gap between Native Americans and the rest of Americans is about 3 years, while in New Zealand the gap between Maori and non-Maori is about 5 years.

Table 15.5 Life expectancy rates in Australia (1981–2002)

Australian	1981	2002
Aboriginal males	56	64
Aboriginal females	56	63
Other males		77
Other females		82

Source: The Lancet, 2002

In Ireland, life expectancy is shockingly poor for Travellers. The Census of Ireland, 1996 showed the age structure of Irish society and contrasted the Travellers with the rest of the population. The statistics from the Central Statistics Office speak for themselves. Despite a very high birth rate, the mortality is also stark.

Table 15.6 Age distibution of Travellers and others in Ireland

Age	Travellers		Total population	
	No.	Percentage (%)	No.	Percentage (%)
0–14	5,454	50.1	859,424	23.7
15–64	5,290	48.6	2,352,781	64.9
65+	147	1.3	413,882	11.4
Total	10,891	100	3,626,087	100

Source: 1996 Census of Ireland, Central Statistics Office

A Cure for the Crisis

These figures are an underestimate because only Travellers living on halting sites were counted and not Travellers in housing. Local authorities found 4,898 Traveller families with average 4.9 people, suggesting a real population of 24,000. In 40 years, the number has grown fourfold. Traveller families have 3.5 children per family on average compared to 1.8 in the general population.

Traveller men and women live an average 10 and 12 years less, respectively, than the general population, i.e. 62 years for men and 65 years for women. At all ages Traveller mortality is higher than the general population. Traveller infant mortality is 18.1 per 1,000 livebirths compared to a national figure of 7.4. These figures are worse for men than those for Australian Aborigines and nearly as bad for women.

Shameful treatment

Solutions and resources should be targeted at minority communities to prevent long-term ill health and disadvantage. There exists a Traveller Health National Strategy 2002–2005 that must be implemented. It is a comprehensive and worthy programme involving service, commitment and research, which includes child health, maternity care and adult care. The Strategy is in response to the key recommendations of the Report of the Task Force on the Travelling Community 1995. Sudden infant death syndrome is 12 times greater amongst Traveller families (8.8 v 0.7 per 1,000 livebirths) than for the rest of the population. The policy announces that:

> The focus of the new approach to Travellers' health needs must be on equality of outcome as well as equality of access to, and participation in, services beginning from the position that there is a greater need for healthcare for Travellers at present given their poor current health status.

In fact, I would add that there is need for recognition of the distinct Traveller culture.

The choices the Irish Government makes regarding public spending relative to other countries is apparent in the OECD data from 2001 in Table 15.7. From the data, it is clear that Ireland's social spending is low with obvious consequences.

Life expectancy in Europe and beyond

Table 15.7 Social spending (% GDP) in selected EU and non-EU states, 2001

Country	Total (minus interest)	Education	Health	Other social services	Total income transfers
Ireland GNP	33.6	4.9	5.2	0.6	12.1
Ireland GDP	29.5	4.3	4.6	0.5	10.6
Austria	46.0	6.0	5.8	2.0	19.0
Belgium	40.4	5.0	6.1	0.3	18.1
Denmark	47.8	6.8	6.8	5.2	17.8
Finland	44.0	5.7	5.3	3.0	18.3
France	48.4	5.9	7.3	1.9	19.7
Germany	42.7	4.4	7.8	1.6	18.0
Italy	39.8	4.8	5.5	0.5	19.1
Japan	32.7	3.6	5.6	0.6	8.4
Netherlands	38.8	4.5	5.9	1.7	16.1
Norway	43.9	6.8	7.1	4.7	15.2
Spain	36.1	4.4	5.3	0.4	13.9
Sweden	49.9	6.6	6.6	5.4	18.9
UK	34.3	4.6	5.6	1.3	8.2
US	26.4	4.8	5.8	0.3	17.8
OECD average	38.6	5.1	5.8	1.4	14.4

The figures are % GDP, except for the extra Irish GNP figure which shows the effect of multinational transfer pricing.
Source: OECD, 2001

16

National Health Service (NHS)

The National Health Service (NHS) was set up on 5 July 1948 by Aneurin Bevan, the son of a miner from Tredegar in Wales. Beyond doubt, it was the most magnificent social achievement in Britain after the Second World War. It followed the National Insurance Act 1946 which put in place the recommendations of the Beveridge Report. Bevan had fought to end inequality through the intervention of the state. Initially in January 1948, the British Medical Association (BMA) questioned doctors and found that 88 per cent were opposed to the idea of the NHS. They were frightened that they would lose their independence and be forced to take orders from the government. Hospital consultants were promised a salary and allowed to treat private patients in NHS hospitals. By July 1948, 90 per cent of doctors had joined the NHS, which took over responsibility for 1,143 voluntary hospitals and 1,545 municipal hospitals in Britain. Family doctors were provided free. However, Bevan (along with John Freeman and Harold Wilson, the future prime minister) resigned from government in 1951 in protest against the introduction of charges for dental care, spectacles and prescription charges. Already cost had intruded into Utopia.

To 2002 and the Wanless Report which claimed that the cumulative underinvestment in the NHS over 25 years, compared with the European average health spending over the period, was £267 billion by 1998. At present, the British government intends to increase health spending in Britain from £65.4 billion in 2002 to £105.6 billion by 2007/8 or from 7.7 per cent to 9.4 per cent of gross domestic product in the same five-year period. By 2008, an extra 42 major hospital schemes will be operating with 13 more under construction. This is expected to increase treatment capacity by 10,000 beds. Maximum waiting times are planned to be three months in 2008 and two weeks in the longer term.

However by 2 January 2003, *The Guardian* noted that 600,000 minor operations were carried out in GPs surgeries in 2002 and 1.1 million in

National Health Service (NHS)

outpatient departments. Since 1997, hip replacements have increased by 15 per cent, heart operations are up 40 per cent and cataract removals up 50 per cent. For quality, 73 per cent of heart-attack patients get clot-busters within 30 minutes in 2002 compared to 39 per cent in 2001 – a great achievement – and 40 per cent of CT scanners have been replaced in the last two years. There were 600,000 minor operations carried out in primary care in 2002 and a further 1.1 million in hospital outpatients.

NHS medical manpower

In 2000, the then Health Secretary Alan Milburn MP announced that he wanted 7,500 more consultants and 2,000 more GPs in the NHS by 2004. Furthermore, he stated that the government wanted an increase of 2,000 GPs, 550 extra GP trainees and 9,200 consultants between 2001 and 2008. In 2002, Milburn then announced a new target of an extra 15,000 more doctors in the NHS by 2008, an increase of 4,000 on the earlier target. By 2008, the government also intends to hire 30,000 more therapists and scientists and 35,000 more nurses and health visitors.

If only one-third of GPs in the UK who are currently eligible to retire did so immediately, then more than 17 million people would lose their GP. More than 16 per cent of NHS consultants are due to retire by 2008. The European Working Time Directive due for enforcement by 2004 will mean that 13,000 extra consultants will be needed, according to the Royal College of Physicians. Between 1991 and 2001, the number of GPs in the NHS increased from 26,249 to 28,802 (about 10 per cent). In March 2002, there were 30,860 GPs in the NHS. With this level of manpower, the British government targets are unlikely to be met even by 2008.

Recruitment from overseas was pursued, however, by July 2002, only 100 extra doctors had been recruited. The number of GPs in training has increased to 1,883, which is a record high, and this was done with golden "hello money" and greater worktime flexibility, especially for those with children.

General practice

General practice is declining in popularity among medical graduates. In 1983, 45 per cent chose GP training but by 1996, this figure had fallen to 20 per cent. Thus the level of growth in GP numbers is unsustainable on the present figures. A survey in 1998 found that 14 per cent of GPs wanted to quit within the next five years. This rose to 22 per cent in 2001.

A Cure for the Crisis

The main reason is plummeting job satisfaction. That which is causing most dissatisfaction, however, is the government's reforms and pace of change.

There is also a growing feeling that this rising dissatisfaction may be part of a more global discontent of doctors upset with their changing role in society. Long working hours are a factor and men working in deprived urban areas are more likely to be dissatisfied. Ethnic doctors in particular are unhappy. The proportion of under 35-year-olds planning to leave medicine rose from 4 per cent to 6 per cent in the three years to 2001. Commenting on the trend, Dr John Chisholm, chairman of the BMA's GP committee stated that the GP workload is increasing and so too the complexity of their work as the borderlines between GP surgeries and hospitals become blurred. GPs are increasingly being asked to take on semi-specialist clinics and minor operations. To help them cope, some of their traditional tasks are being shifted towards nurses and pharmacists.

Negotiations started in February 2003 for a new NHS GP contract. Dr Chisholm's objective is to "allow GPs to control and manage their workload better than they can at the moment and that does include more time with individual patients, rewarding practices for the quality of the care that they deliver and allocating resources according to the needs of the practice population". An editorial in the *British Journal of General Practice* noted how the new NHS GP contract would radically transform the nature of general practice:

> ...[the new NHS GP] contract proposals have the potential to save lives but also to sideline some of the core values of general practice.... The old adage that GPs treat 'the patient rather than the disease' may no longer be true, and 'general' practitioners may start to feel more like 'partial' practitioners.[1]

There is a provision to categorise chronic disease care as a non-essential service in general practice. In the face of such developments, it doesn't take a cynic to predict that sell-out and medical absurdity are only around the corner in the NHS. Currently, about 75 per cent of the 34,500 GPs in the UK operate as independent contractors. The government is trying to subdivide GPs into those providing the traditional services and those providing enhanced services, such as minor surgery and the management of complex diseases such as Parkinsonism. Income will be linked to about 80 measures of activity, including the standard of care and facilities. Clearly, control is the objective.

National Health Service (NHS)

Consultants

Consultant numbers in the NHS have grown by 4 per cent per year since 1994. This was made possible by reducing the duration of consultant training in 1993. However, this rate of growth is too low to hit the government's manpower target. If the current growth rates in GP and consultant numbers continue, there will be about 12,000 more GPs and consultants by 2008 – 3,000 short of the government's targets. Currently, it takes five years to complete undergraduate medical training. After a further compulsory pre-registration year, it takes at least three further years to become a GP and at least seven to become a consultant.

Solutions

Dr Diane Gray and Belinda Finlayson at the King's Fund Consultancy have made some suggestions on a way forward, which were published in *The Guardian* on 8 October 2002.

To meet the target for consultants, a number of steps have to be taken:

1. Current training post numbers will be hardly sufficient to replace retirements.
2. An increase in the number of training posts to allow more doctors to achieve specialist accreditation.
3. A reduction in the duration of specialist training.
4. A move away from the system of time served to a system of competence appraisal and immediate certification. A one-year reduction in the apprenticeship period would create another 5,000 consultants over five years.

Any move to shorten training periods will raise the questions of quality and of medical regulation through the General Medical Council and the Royal Colleges.

For more GPs to be recruited:

1. There would have to be more GP training posts and more GP trainers recruited and, I presume, trained. The attractiveness of general practice as a career would have to be sold. For example, more opportunity for flexible working time and family-friendly hours.

A Cure for the Crisis

2. Raising the profile of general practice will require more than just a new contract.

At basecamp, the British government hopes to provide 2,100 more places at medical schools by 2005, but the effects of this will take a long time to feed through to increase the cohort of GPs and consultants. Another problem for the British is that a greater number of medical graduates are opting out of medicine altogether, or are opting out of traditional training patterns or are pursuing careers outside the NHS or abroad. The reasons why are obvious.

St George's Hospital Medical School in South London runs a four-year graduate entry course for older students. For its 2003 entry course, there were 1,350 applicants for 70 places. Twenty per cent of the student intake of a new medical school at the University of East Anglia is over 30-years-old and five students are over 40. Graduates from engineering, financial services, bank managers and housewives are among the new medical students. This may be another means of rapidly increasing the number of doctors in some areas.

"Physician's assistants" may also be introduced.[2] In the USA, after a two-year intensive medical school programme, these practitioners are licensed to treat patients on a one-to-one basis without reference to a doctor. In the NHS, the "physician's assistant" will work under the direction of a GP and perform most of the normal duties of a family doctor, including diagnosis and making house calls. In the US, they can prescribe a wider range of drugs than any nurse, but in the NHS their prescriptions will have to be approved by a GP. In addition, they will be able to deal with low-risk pregnancies, child health surveillance, and a range of mental health problems. However, they are not allowed to perform any surgery or pose as fully qualified doctors.

Consultant contract in NHS – 2002 ballot

The deprofessionalisation of medicine in Britain continued with the Labour government offering consultants a 19 per cent pay rise in exchange for increased productivity at an annual cost of £300 million. Each consultant would have to work 10 four-hour sessions per week. This is an increase of three hours per week from the present 37-hour contract. Overtime would now be paid from 6 pm to 10 pm weekdays and Saturday and Sunday mornings at a standard rate. The current basic working day is 8 am–6 pm Monday to Friday. Overtime is subject to

National Health Service (NHS)

negotiation. Those who choose to forgo one-eleventh of their salary can do as much private work as they like, provided they devote substantially the whole of their professional time to the NHS. In the proposed new contract, every consultant would have to negotiate a job plan with hospital administrators. Evening shifts and weekend work would be counted as part of the normal working week. New consultants would have to do the first eight-hours' overtime for the NHS. After seven years, consultants wanting to do private work would be obliged to do four hours overtime for the NHS first. The maximum salary for most senior consultants would have risen to £85,250 from £68,599.

In a ballot of 33,000 hospital consultants and 12,000 specialist registrars in 2002, there was a two to one majority against the new contract. The deal was rejected by 66 per cent in England but supported by 59 per cent in Scotland and 54 per cent in Northern Ireland. Senior registrars opposed the deal, 84 per cent against to 16 per cent in favour. In response, the British Medical Association leaders said that consultants did not object to the money issue, but feared that the new contract would put too much power in the hands of hospital managers, forcing them to work unsocial weekend and evening hours.

In defending the new proposals, the then Health Secretary Alan Milburn was quoted in *The Guardian* as saying: "It's a 24/7 world in which we live and the NHS has become part of that world."[3] Moreover, he declared: "There can be no renegotiation. There can be no more resources. There can be no more veto on reform." Such comments highlight the bullying tactics at the heart of government, undermining the principles of democracy. In effect, Milburn wants to own doctors and strip them of all autonomy. Ironically, no allowance is made for the Working Time Directive with the maximum 48-hour working week as part of the EU Social Chapter which the Blair government had signed.

Once again, the issue of remuneration is not at stake. Chairman of the BMA, Dr Ian Bogle, said that consultants were not asking for more money, but wanted clearer undertakings that working unsocial hours would be voluntary. *The Guardian* editorial "Doctors in distress – No more national deals for consultants" attributes the rejection of the contract to private practice. In Scotland and Northern Ireland, there is little private practice, whereas in England about one-third of consultants have some private practice. Consultants already see patients in the evenings and at weekends when there is a serious clinical problem. Certainly in my experience, this has always been the case.

A Cure for the Crisis

To demonstrate the arrogance and unsophistication of the mindset of command bureaucracy, the *Guardian* editorial on 1 November 2002 is worth quoting:

> For the 54 years of the current contract's lifetime, going back to the start of the NHS, consultants have claimed autonomy. But that era is over. It is not Labour which is imposing this but international trends. Public services – medical services included – must now be publicly accountable. Independent autonomy is no longer acceptable. Ironically, the consultants who now plan to set up chambers, similar to barristers, would find themselves subject to more managerial control, not less. A fee-for-service would not allow doctors to be advocates for patients.

The reality is different, however. Doctors have always been accountable for their actions and the climate of litigation is a direct reflection of this fact. Training schemes, accreditation, specialist registration and continuous medical education are now part of the profession. Indeed, it is arguable that the profession is becoming over-regulated to the point of absurdity. A chambers system, which is slammed by *The Guardian,* would fulfill one of Arnold Relman's ethical imperatives and a fee-per-item is more likely to ensure patient advocacy than a threatening administrator or politician-run bullying dictatorship. It is also interesting that no mention is made of the effects of increasing the length of the official working week when international trends have been in the other direction for over a century. Dr Bob Bury from Leeds writing in *The Sunday Times* on 10 November 2002 pointed out that the average consultant already spends 48 hours per week on NHS work. Therefore, increasing the formal working week to 40 hours will have zero effect on output. Admittedly, this is not necessarily true if operating theatres and OPD departments are opened after 5 pm when they might otherwise be shut.

Ironically, at the same time, the 19 October edition of the *British Medical Journal* included a paper which confirmed that job strain where there are high demands, low job control and effort–reward imbalance elicit stress at work. Workers with high job stress had a doubling of the risk of cardiovascular death. High job strain and effort–reward imbalance also predicted adverse changes in biological factors such as plasma cholesterol and body weight.[4] I believe that the dead hand of bureaucracy is having a deleterious effect on doctors' health and medics know this only too well.

National Health Service (NHS)

Writing in *The Daily Telegraph* on 5 November 2002, Prof Norman Browse held out against managerial interference and erosion of medical autonomy.

> ...Doctors enter the medical profession to prevent, diagnose and treat disease, not to have their mouths stuffed with gold..... regulation of juniors' pay and working hours in the 1970s opened the door to greater interference by administrators in clinical care. This interference was boosted in the last years of the Conservative government by the introduction of Waiting List Initiatives, then vigorously encouraged by the Labour government's unachievable political promises, financial rewards for managers who achieved the politicians' targets and the setting of initiatives to treat some diseases before others, for political – not clinical – purposes.
>
> Consultants have clearly declared that managerial interference must stop. We, as an independent profession, must be the prime source of advice on medical care, not managers or politicians. The administrator's task is to provide the doctor with the best possible working facilities, not to direct when and whom the doctor should treat.... all clinicians will now stand firm against the progressive reduction of their independence by politicians.[5]

Prior to the vote on the new contract, the fear that this new document was an administrator/politician subterfuge to increase managerial control and strip doctors of professional and practice freedom was heightened by a leaked NHS document to hospital managers from Andrew Foster, head of human resources for the NHS. The memo urged managers to implement evening and weekend work and recommended that only "the deserving few who do the most" would receive significant extra pay.

League tables

In late November 2002, cardiac surgeons in the UK announced that it was no longer wise to treat high-risk patients because if they subsequently died, the surgeon's spot on the league table heads south. Despite 12 per cent of the UK population having private insurance and often using private hospitals, no league tables of private hospital's performance are published, while anecdotes about NHS bailouts of clinical emergencies from private hospitals are commonplace.[6]

A Cure for the Crisis

Undue pressure on hospital managers

On BBC Radio 4's *World at One*, Junior Health Minister David Lammy said that the government was doing well on the journey to get 75 per cent of A&E patients processed and out of hospital in four hours by December 2004. Officially, the British government claimed in October 2002 that nobody waits more than 24 hours in an A&E department. Ministers claimed that 77 per cent of A&E patients were treated, admitted or discharged within four hours. The Minister did not seem to notice, however, that the target had been met more than one year early.

On 28 October 2002, the BMA published a survey of 160 A&E departments which covered about 40 per cent of the British total, showing that 20 per cent of patients had waited more than 24 hours during the previous week and the longest reported wait was three and a half days. Half of the consultants surveyed did not accept the government's claim that most patients were cleared during that time. Official returns disguised the problem by not systematically measuring the time between the decision to admit and the delay in finding a bed in a ward.

To meet political targets, there is a managerial incentive to insist that quick and easy cases are dealt with before the more seriously ill and difficult. Managers are rewarded for fulfilling goals laid down by government. Consequently, the bottom line for managers is that if they don't shape up, in some cases they will ship out. Doctors' loyalties should first be to their patients, with secondary loyalties to colleagues and institutions. Dr Theodore Dalrymple has written of a colleague who complained of overwork to management only to be told that one solution to his problem was to lower his standards. His thesis is that consultants would rather have freedom to operate than gold.[7] This is a play on Bevan's famous reference on his handling of the consultants during the inception of the NHS: "I stuffed their mouths with gold."[8]

It is clear that the government's attitude towards the medical profession is bullying and contemptuous. They appear to act on the assumption that NHS managers from a non-clinical background have the insight and experience to dictate the course of modern medical practice. This is despite the presence of audit and revalidation. Practical examples appear constantly. Dr John Wales, a diabetologist at Leeds General Infirmary, provided the following in *The Times:*

> The present provision of care is lamentably thin in the NHS with little or no support or planning. For example, when we were

National Health Service (NHS)

directed to reduce waiting times for new patients to 26 weeks in our own medical obesity clinic the only response the Trust could make, other than outright closure, was to close our waiting list to new referrals.[9]

Poor auld Wales – a decent guy – the waiting list is too long so the administration and Dr Tony Blair just pretend that the disease is non-existent!

The managerial manpower juggernaut rolls along in Britain and in the past two years, health spending has risen by 21.5 per cent. There were 3,000 new managers recruited, yet the number of hospital admissions has fallen. There is evidence that the government is bullying and intimidating managers to meet waiting list targets. An Audit Commission report found that one-third of NHS Trusts are distorting waiting list figures. The inaccuracies were found by an unannounced spot check on 45 of 186 acute and specialist Trusts in England. Directors of some Trusts, found to have manipulated their figures, have been suspended or fired.

The Labour government in their 1997 manifesto promised to cut waiting lists by 100,000 within four years. The government's NHS plan stipulated that no one should wait more than 18 months for an operation, with the target time falling to 15, 12 and 6 months by 2005. Trusts that fail to meet their targets face severe financial penalties. In an anonymous survey of 400 NHS managers, 10 per cent admitted deliberately filing inaccurate reports on waiting lists and more than half said that they were afraid to raise concerns with senior colleagues for fear of reprisals.[10]

Foundation hospitals

Foundation hospitals free from government control are the new dispensation. These flagships would be semi-privatised and run as non-profit organisations. They will be able to raise funds on the private market for new developments, use funds released from land sales and pay extra to staff, and change terms and conditions of work. They will be held locally responsible to primary healthcare trusts, a local regulator, the Commission for Health Improvement and a new Stakeholder Council of locally elected people. Their primary purpose is to treat NHS patients but they can treat private patients, the income from which is limited by licence. Addenbrooke's Hospital in Cambridge, Kings College in London and hospitals in Sunderland and Sheffield are likely to be the first to come

A Cure for the Crisis

fully on-stream in 2004. On balance, I do not believe that the plan will work because the remit is too vague and the control too centralised.

The Lancet described the deal in a commentary in December 2002.[11] Failing hospitals such as United Bristol Healthcare NHS Trust and the Royal United Hospital Bath NHS Trust and Good Hope Hospital in Birmingham are to be taken over by outside management. The least well-run hospitals were poor at managing risk to patients, and staff were afraid to speak out. Management companies can bid for the jobs. They can be private like BUPA or can be other NHS Trusts. There are 62 three-star NHS Trusts eligible to bid and there are seven private companies, which include BUPA, BMI Health Care Limited and German and Canadian companies.

These moves have been bitterly opposed by many Labour MPs. Former Health Secretary Frank Dobson said that none of the private hospital organisations had appropriate experience. "The best known, BUPA, has 31 hospitals with a total of 1,700 beds. The average BUPA hospital has 55 beds and its biggest has 92. The Bristol Trust has 900 beds, making it 10 times as big as BUPA's biggest hospital." Similarly, the Conservative Party has declared its opposition to the move. Tory Shadow Health Secretary Dr Liam Fox said: "With hospitals financed by the private finance initiative being run by private sector companies and ultimately becoming foundation opt-out hospitals, Labour will never again be able to claim with any credibility that the Conservatives want to privatize the running of the NHS."

Diagnostic and treatment centres

We have the National Treatment Purchase Fund in Ireland. Not to be outdone, Alan Milburn introduced Diagnostic and Treatment Centres (DTCs) to deal with waiting list cases in Britain. Working alone or in joint ventures with the local NHS, these are designed to provide fast-track treatment free of the threat that operations will be cancelled in busy general hospitals to cater for emergency cases. Contracts for 11 new centres have gone to tender with the objective of providing 39,500 operations by 2005. Ten NHS DCTs are already running and are treating 39,000 patients per year. A further 12 NHS-run DTCs will cost £100 million and carry out surgery which has the highest waiting times, such as knee and hip replacements and cataract removals. These will allow an extra 37,000 non-urgent operations to be carried out each year by 2005.

National Health Service (NHS)

Championing the initiative, Milburn declared: "By changing working practices, by introducing new services and by using spare capacity inside and outside the NHS we can treat more NHS patients more quickly for free. I am determined to ease the dilemma for people, particularly older people, between being forced to wait in pain for NHS care or being forced to pay for private care."

In December 2002, there were 1.5 million on NHS hospital waiting lists, a rise of 18,000 in one year. The number waiting more than one year had fallen to 15,500, which was 60 per cent lower than one year earlier. A study of 1,200 people in Britain by *Which?* magazine in Autumn 2002 found that just over half who tell a receptionist that their condition is urgent or an emergency are seen the same day, but one-third must wait for two days to see their GP. One in eight patients wait for about five days. For routine appointments, 20 per cent waited for five days with about 10 per cent waiting for more than one week. Patients were usually happy with their GPs but concerned with the delays in being seen and with the lack of evening or Saturday surgeries.

17

Best healthcare system: France

The Organisation for Economic Co-operation and Development (OECD) rates the French health system as the best in the world, with no queues, ample beds and equal treatment for all. Ten per cent of their gross domestic product (GDP) is spent on health.[1] Employers contribute 13 per cent of what they pay to workers in a health contribution, while the employee pays 7 per cent. As well as this, almost 90 per cent take out medical insurance which costs an average of 2.5 per cent of their pay, and they also pay an additional amount to doctors and hospitals.

Each worker pays about 20 per cent of their gross income towards health expenses. This may seem a lot but the percentage GDP is lower in France than in the UK, Germany or Switzerland; nonetheless, the World Health Organization (WHO) rate France above these in outcome terms. Ireland came 19th in a WHO survey spending $1,200 per person on healthcare in 1997, whereas the French spent $2,125.

In France there is a free choice of doctor for general practice and consultants. Patients may go directly to consultants if they choose. All hospitals are the same. Patients pay doctors directly and then claim back 75 per cent of the cost from the national health agency. They can claim most of the balance from their private insurance company, however, the insurance system is in crisis with debts rising to €10 billion by 2003.

There are 30 serious illnesses where the treatment is completely free. These include cancer, heart disease and diabetes. All health contributions go into an independent fund overseen by a board of em oyers and trade unions.

WHO tried to relate health outcomes to spending and Sweden, Luxembourg and France came in the top three countries surveyed. Ireland was 14th followed by Portugal. For life expectancy, France was first at 73+ years, Ireland was third last at 69.6 years, followed by Denmark and Portugal. Ireland was third in the EU in fairness of health contributions, while France was tenth.

Best healthcare system: France

Seventy-five per cent of the French have used complementary medicine at least once. Budgets are allocated to each hospital by government who then pay staff. Doctors in hospitals often earn about €50,000 after a few years and also see private patients. Doctors have been campaigning for pay increases and there is much dissatisfaction of late. Currently, there are waiting lists for hospital admission, often with a waiting time of several weeks for surgery.

Recently, there has been a refocus of policy to try to help the elderly stay at home and to improve funding for their institutional care. The cost of caring for the elderly is covered by local government who reclaim the money from the estates of the elderly after they die. This is now capped at €50,000 but formerly had no limit. Such an initiative is unlikely to find favour here in Ireland.

The OECD found that good-quality care, freedom of choice and equality of access are the strengths in France, but the downside is that extensive health cover may lead to overconsumption of services by patients and overprescription of medicines. Regional hospital agencies decide on the size and number of hospitals and on the distribution of specialties. They also allocate scanners and high-tech equipment to correspond with clinical needs.

Trouble in paradise

There is a gathering crisis in French medicine. A prolonged strike by GPs over low pay, which started in November 2001, only ended in June 2002 when the government, health insurance companies and medical trade unions agreed a deal. During the strike, GPs refused to treat patients outside of office hours, forcing patients to call public emergency services or go to hospitals during the night, at weekends and public holidays. GPs had sought an increase in their consultation fee from €17.50 to €20 to resume their normal work. The deal negotiated is €20 per consultation and €30 for a home visit, which must be medically justified where there is an emergency or where the patient is unable to attend the surgery. The cost will be about €260 million per year. In terms of prescription costs, doctors have agreed to replace at least 25 per cent of all branded drug prescriptions with generics and reduce antibiotic prescriptions.

These measures could save €300 to €400 million per year but are unlikely to be met because French doctors only prescribe 3–4 per cent of generic drugs, a very low proportion by European standards. Primary care is underserved in many areas because of the high dropout rate from general practice as a result of economic problems related to inadequate reimbursement. And the situation is getting worse. Many French GPs earn about €51,000 net.

Paediatricians in France also went on strike in June 2002 over fees and, indeed, medical strikes have been common over the past five years. Consultants often earn about €70,000 per year and there is much dissatisfaction. The French government has said that €6,500 million will be needed by 2007 to tackle the shortage of doctors and nurses by creating thousands of new jobs and to fund modernisation programmes.[2] Furthermore, France is not yet compliant with the European Working Time Directive.[3] In October 2003, the French government increased the price of cigarettes by 20 per cent to fund €10 billion extra health service expenditure. The French health insurance system is €10 billion in debt and losses are mounting.

I have no doubt that the secret of the French healthcare success is their diet, weather, genes and the fact that they did not close hospital beds when that fetish was at its height.

18

Healthcare systems of selected countries

Looking around the world, there is no clear best solution to the provision of healthcare and countries develop various systems often based on a mix of direct government spending and insurance to fund services. Every country is struggling with the burgeoning costs. Here are a few examples.

Japan

Japan is in crisis and the welfare budget has been cut 2.4 per cent. Contributions from wage earners to health charges rose from 20 to 30 per cent in April 2003, while those older than 70 years are asked to pay 10 per cent of outpatient charges, or 20 per cent if they are in a high-income bracket. Employees covered by the state-run health insurance system will also have to pay 8.2 per cent of their incomes on premiums. The Japanese government has also lowered fees payable for blood and urine tests and for MRI scans. Alarmingly, Japan has an incipient demographic crisis with 25 per cent of the population older than 65 years by 2014.[1]

Germany

In Germany, there was a €1.5 billion hole in the 350 health insurance funds at the end of 2002, where overall health spending is €250 billion per year with €142 billion paid through the statutory health funds. The causes are attributed to the option of patients being allowed self-refer to many specialists for multiple expensive investigations, rising administrative costs and the use of health funds for pensions.

From January 2003, the Health Ministry has obliged drug companies, wholesalers and chemists to give rebates of 2.8–10 per cent for drugs sold to the statutory health insurance funds Gesetzliche Krankenversicherungen (GKVs). Rates paid to hospitals and doctors have been frozen. An income freeze is the equivalent of a pay cut and has irked the National Association of Insurance Physicians. There will be fewer staff in hospi-

A Cure for the Crisis

tals and the German Medical Association has warned that queues which are unknown at present, may develop. There is a continuing problem because the statutory health insurance scheme is under unbearable pressure from an ageing society with chronically high unemployment. Some insurance funds increased their charges which already take 14 per cent of basic salary. Admissions were stopped in the 885-bed Greifswald University Hospital in December 2002 due to scarcity of cash. The short-term cost savings amount to about €1.4 billion.

In July 2003, both the government and opposition parties agreed a reform package seen as a part solution to a system that is inefficient.

1. Overall cuts of €23 billion by 2007.
2. Health contributions to fall in 2004 to 13.6 from 14.4 per cent on gross wages with a target of 13 per cent by 2006.
3. Coverage of the statutory system is to be reduced with patients in future having to pay for dentures and sickness benefits.
4. Payments for newborn babies and funerals to be taken away from the statutory system and funded in future by a €1 increase in tobacco tax.
5. Patients to pay 10 per cent of each medical bill up to a maximum of 2 per cent of gross income.
6. Price controls for some patented drugs.
7. New limited scope for chains of chemists to operate.
8. Quality control institute to monitor drugs quality and health services.

The Netherlands

Health expenditure in the Netherlands rose from €28 billion in 1999 to €38 billion in 2002. Health cuts of €2.3 billion will be implemented in 2004. Patients will contribute €1.3 billion through charges for physiotherapy, dentistry, IVF treatment, contraceptive pill for over 21s, transport and a prescription charge of €1.70. Pharmacists' wages will be cut and there will be wages restraint, reduced sick leave and lower spending limits on home care. The Health Minister Hans Hoogervorst said: "We can only solve the problem of rising costs by increasing the own responsibility to patients, clients and healthcare professionals substantially."[2]

Hong Kong

Hong Kong (HK) began charging A&E fees of US$31 in November 2002 ending a century-old free treatment tradition. The charge covers all tests

Healthcare systems of selected countries

and medicines. Tourists or those without valid HK identity cards will be charged US$73. The unemployed are exempt. The objective is to encourage patients to attend primary care. Queues for A&E departments are usually about three hours. Last year, 75 per cent of A&E patients were classed as non-urgent. From April 2003, the charges rose by 26 per cent and prescription medicines will cost US$1.30 per item. This will bring in US$45 million per year. The government subsidy for public medical care will still be 96 per cent down from the previous 98 per cent. The HK Hospital Authority had a first-ever deficit of $29 million in 2001–2.

Canada

In Canada, there is a 40-year-old system of universally accessible publicly funded healthcare costing Can$100 billion (US$64 billion). The system is run by the provinces and territories under conditions laid down by the Federal Government, which shares the cost. These are the provision of all medically necessary medical and physician services; the public administration of the system; universal coverage of all residents; and the absence of user charges at the point of care delivery. Doctors practise mostly on a fee-per-service basis. There is a ban on the coverage of core services by private health insurers, which has prevented the emergence of a parallel private system. Thus, there is pressure on provinces to meet the expectations of the Canadian middle class. There is growing dissatisfaction with the system among the public and the doctors. Between 1986 and 1994, 27 per cent of acute hospital beds were closed, despite the increase in population numbers and age.

Healthcare expenditure reached Can$112.2 billion (US$71.7 billion) in 2002. This is a rise of 6.3 per cent on 2001 and a large 30 per cent increase in five years. The Canadian economy grew 20 per cent during the same period so health expenditure is soaring. Health now consumes 9.8 per cent of GDP, still less than the 13 per cent in the US. Drug costs amount to 16.2 per cent of the total, hospitals 32.1 per cent and doctors 13.4 per cent. Canadians spent an average of Can$3,572 per person on health in 2002. The provincial governments want the Federal Government to spend an unconditional Can$25 billion extra over three years on the present system.

Roy Romanow, who headed the Royal Commission on the Future of Health Care, issued a blueprint in November 2002. He argued that the Federal Government must invest $28 billion every five years just to ward off the advent of private for-profit medical services. This will cost the

123

taxpayers an extra Can$0.50 to $4 per day depending on their incomes. Senator Michael Kirby has claimed that, in exchange, Canadians will gain efficiencies within the system and guarantees of medical services when needed. There are 47 recommendations including expansion of one-stop-shop health clinics with capitation payments for doctors. It will also involve the creation of much cost-sharing programmes.

The core idea is to provide more competition in service delivery by devolving authority for managing healthcare to regional health authorities. This will include funding for doctors, hospitals and possibly prescription drugs. Money would follow the patient (as I have suggested for Ireland). Doctors could contract with the regional health authorities for their services on a capitation basis or work entirely outside the system. There is an intention to create a comprehensive system of clinics staffed around the clock by teams of doctors and healthcare professionals. Medicare should be expanded to cover home care and drugs. Also, there is a recommendation to establish a new agency to manage the approval and pricing of new prescription drugs.

At present, the system in Canada is creaking. The waiting time between being referred from a GP and undergoing treatment is 16.5 weeks, an increase of 77 per cent since 1993. However, life expectancy has increased from 74.9 in 1979 to 79 years in 1999. Worryingly, the diabetic population burden has increased from 4.7 per cent to 6.2 per cent during that time. Heart disease and stroke now account for 20.4 per cent of male and 11.4 per cent of female admissions to hospital. The number of prescriptions for antidepressants has risen spectacularly from 3.2 million to 14.5 million over 20 years. It must be the power of advertising!

European Union

EU systems of healthcare are diverse in terms of funding system, hospital type, costs per person and status. They are well summed up in an Irish Labour Party document in Table 18.1.

Healthcare systems of selected countries

Table 18.1 EU healthcare systems

Country	Funding system	Hospitals	Costs per person	Health status
Austria	Mandatory insurance	Mainly public	Average	Normal
Belgium	Mandatory insurance	Mainly private or non-profit	Average	Problems
Denmark	Mainly tax funded	Mainly public	Low	Problems
Finland	Mainly tax & some insurance	Mainly public or non-profit	Low	Problems
Germany	Mix of public & private insurance	Mainly private or non-profit	High	Normal
Greece	Mandatory insurance	Mainly private	Low	Mixed
Ireland	Mix of tax & insurance	Mainly public or non-profit	Low	Problems
Italy	Mandatory insurance	Mainly public & some private	Average	Good
Luxembourg	Mandatory insurance	Mainly public & non-profit	High	Problems
Netherlands	Mix of public & private insurance	Mostly private non-profit	Average	Good
Portugal	Mandatory insurance	Mainly public	Low	Poor
Spain	Mix of tax & insurance	Mainly private non-profit	Low	Good
Sweden	Tax funded	Public	Average	Good
UK	Tax funded	Public	Low	Problems
France	Mandatory insurance	Mainly public, some private	High	Good

Sources: European Parliament, OECD and WHO

19

Ireland:
medical incomes and party policies

Medical incomes

Background: patient category and health insurance

There are now two categories of patients in Ireland. Category 1 patients are means tested and are entitled to free investigation and treatment all the way. As there is no such thing as a free lunch, the taxpayer pays via many intermediaries. Visits to primary care, hospitals and drug costs are all covered. The over-70s medical card patients are not means tested and are entitled to all services free.

Category 2 includes everyone else. All, irrespective of category, are entitled to free care in a public hospital bed. However, access is the problem. The cost of a public bed in a hospital is about €3,500 per week. Category 2 patients must pay a €45 per day charge for the first 10 days only. The maximum charge is €450 per year. Self-referral to A&E costs €45. This is not levied on those admitted as a result of self-referral, on those with medical cards, on those with infectious diseases, on children up to six-weeks-old, children with some prescribed diseases or children referred from school medicals or from child health clinics. Furthermore, EU citizens with E111 and women receiving maternity benefit are also exempt. Return visits for the same illness are free. If you have a GP referral letter, then you are also exempt, except from inpatient charges, if admitted.

Hospital charges may be imposed on long-stay patients who do not have a medical card, have no dependents, have been an inpatient for more than 30 days or for more than 30 days in the previous 12 months. The charge is means tested and there is no set charge. Legally, €3.17 per week must be left to the patient after rent, insurance and other bills are met. All maternity costs are covered by the State and exempt from the day charge. Children under six weeks of age are also exempt, as are children referred from a health clinic or school examinations, anyone with a

126

Ireland: medical incomes and party policies

prescribed infectious disease, long-term patients, children with disabilities, including mental handicaps, cystic fibrosis, spina bifida and cerebral palsy.

As previously noted, there is massive demand and poorly monitored funding with continuing waiting lists. There are about 3,000 beds too few in the service. This was exacerbated in the 1980s by the mistaken official belief that there were sufficient beds, when a reduced turnaround time and increasing efficiency were factored in.

There are private beds in public hospitals and about 20 per cent of the beds and 23 per cent of admissions to public hospitals are designated private. In excess of 48 per cent of the population have private health insurance. Currently, there are 1.56 million subscribers to the VHI and 280,000 in BUPA. The VHI Plan B and the Essential Plus from BUPA account for 75 to 80 per cent of the total. Thus, a minority have the higher plans. For €7 to €8 per week, an adult can buy BUPA Essential Plus or VHI Plan B and can further upgrade to Health Manager and Health Steps for a further €2.50 to €3 per week. These costs are net of the 20 per cent standard rate of tax deductions.

The number buying health insurance has been rising for two reasons. First, there is a belief that to get necessary service at an appropriate time, you must have private insurance otherwise you join the well-publicised long queue for the public sector. Second, as the economy strengthened, more people could afford the cost of private insurance and more companies gave health cover as part of the remuneration package to their employees. It is likely that the sudden increase in premium charges combined with an economic slowdown will reduce the numbers who can afford insurance.

VHI PAYOUTS AND PREMIUMS

Table 19.1 shows the maximum amounts paid out by the VHI in private or semi-private wards in private hospitals up to February 2002. The annual cost of VHI Plan B for an individual is €429.78 or €1,172.40 for a family of two adults and two children.

A Cure for the Crisis

Table 19.1 VHI payout for selected procedures

Procedure	VHI payouts (€)
Coronary artery bypass	16,342.00
Knee replacement	10,545.00
Hip replacement	8,438.91
Hysterectomy	4,838.00
Prostatectomy	4,348.00
Partial mastectomy	4,145.00
Cardiac ultrasound	3,516.55

Source: VHI, 2002

BUPA PAYOUTS AND PREMIUMS

The Essential Plus plan costs €366.19 for an individual and €987.64 for a family of two adults and two children. The BUPA maternity grant under the Essential Plus scheme is up to €1,745 for a normal delivery. This consists of up to three nights in a private or semi-private room at a maximum of €1,080. The €1,200–1,500 in premiums that a family of four pays in Ireland costs an American family €12,000.

Table 19.2 BUPA payouts for selected specialists

Specialist services	BUPA payouts (€)
Gynaecologist	236.55
Paediatrician	76.76
Pathologist	65.16
Anaesthetist (for epidural)	230.00
Outpatient	385.00

Source: BUPA, 2002

Current medical incomes

GPs charge private fees varying from €30 to €50 per consultation and appear to act as a cartel. Most have add-ons for electrocardiograms (ECGs) and other procedures. These costs are forcing some poorer patients to stay away or to head for the nearest A&E to join the queue of trivial complaints which often means an eight-hour wait. The A&E self-referral charge of €40, recently increased to €45, appears to be a poor disincentive. In practice many avoid this charge by giving false home addresses and refusing to "cough up" in the end. GPs should take note of charges in the rest of the EU. GPs seeing 70 private patients each week

Ireland: medical incomes and party policies

for 46 weeks of the year earn in the region of €96,000 to €161,000 plus GMS, legal, insurance and other payments. The net figure depends on the costs of overheads which may be up to half the gross income.

If GPs allow themselves to be completely bought by the State, they will lose autonomy and become middle-grade civil servants controlled by administrators in the health boards. Practices would become overly structured, monitored and bureaucratic and morale would collapse. New innovations would be difficult to introduce and, if expensive, implementation would be patchy. Postcode therapeutics is well known in the NHS. The doctors would be almost totally at the mercy of health board finance. It is likely that GP public salaries would decline steadily over a period of time, with an attendant fall in morale, quality, service and effort leading to increasing inefficiency. Ultimately, the total costs would rise due to increasing inefficiency.

The consultation costs for French GPs are in the €20 range. They are as low as €10 in Spain where some consultant fees are only €15. By contrast, consultants are well paid in Ireland. There are approximately 1,731 consultants in public hospitals. There are two categories: category 1 consultants devote essentially the whole of their professional time, including private patients, to the public hospitals; category 2 consultants may engage in private practice onsite or offsite. About 20 per cent of public hospital beds are pay-beds.

Consultants in the Dublin region have their public salaries abated by 20 per cent in lieu of private practice. A wholetime contract without private fee rights is no longer offered. Consultant salaries from October 2002 are shown in Table 19.3 for a full-time 33-hour per week commitment. There are also call-out and on-call payments.

Table 19.3 Consultant salaries

Consultants (by region)	Wholetime (€)	Category 1 (€)	Category 2 (€)
All psychiatrists, geriatricians, palliative care, and those in Midlands, West and North West	149,184	142,406	134,760
Cork, Limerick, Clare and North East	149,184	135,241	120,715
Dublin region	149,184	128,465	114,718

Many procedure-based consultants earn another €150,000 plus from patients in the VHI and BUPA. However, about one-third earns little above the State salary. In 2002, the average payment from the VHI to a consultant was €98,569. In Canada in 2001, surgeons earned about €214,000 with physicians earning €162,000. In the US, specialists earned from €300,000 to €500,000. Salaries are much lower in many European countries, such as Denmark €100,000, Finland €45,000 and France €83,000.

Party polices: health service intentions

The foremost political parties in the State, Fianna Fáil, Fine Gael and Labour, were given an opportunity to make their cases in respect of the health service in the *Irish Examiner* on 13 December 2002.

Fianna Fáil

The Minister for Health and Children, Micheál Martin, whose goodwill and earnest intent is beyond doubt, batted for Fianna Fáil. He cited the National Health Strategy published in November 2001 as Government policy. According to him, work has begun on 70 per cent of the 121 actions in the Strategy:

> The Health Strategy had promised to provide 450 [extra] public beds during 2002. By the end of the year, we're on target to have 600 in place – all designated for public use only. More than 100 more will be in place early next year.... It's an oddity of the health service that significant increases, not just in capacity, but also in delivery, don't generate much recognition. The fact is that an enormous increase in throughput has been achieved, with enormous credit to those delivering services.

The Minister next cited a 7 per cent reduction in numbers on the "one year and over" waiting list compared to 2001. These figures on hospital waiting lists are discussed in detail in Chapter 9. The upshot of all this number crunching is that you can believe whatever figures you like, but their accuracy remains suspect.

The Minister also claimed progress on proper complaints procedures in hospitals which do not cost money. However, he made no comment on the ignored issue of vexatious complaints which do cost money.

The policy of primary care teams consisting of GPs, nurses/midwives, healthcare assistants, home helps, occupational therapist, physiothera-

Ireland: medical incomes and party policies

pist, social worker and administrative personnel is being implemented in 10 areas. This is going to change the nature of primary care delivery and deliver integrated services faster, more locally, in a more patient-friendly way.

In time, improvements will be obvious on a vast scale – big new purpose-built facilities. Others will see improvements on a small personal scale when they have a complaint, i.e. it will be dealt with properly. And the Minister finishes with this flourish: "But all of them will see the difference." Unfortunately, to date this Strategy is mere wishful thinking.

Fine Gael

Fine Gael spokesperson on Health, Olivia Mitchell TD, claimed that while there has been a more than doubling of healthcare spending in the past few years, there has been no perceptible pro rata increase in additional services or the quality of the healthcare system. By and large this statement is untrue. She also complained that:

> We cannot leave in place an administration so complex it struggles to plug the gaps in a system that is largely dysfunctional and which adds additional layers to itself simply to cope. [I agree.]

> We cannot expect patients to put up with a system characterised by delays, waiting lists, nursing shortages and duplication.... We need a seamless IT system across the health service. ... The provision of medical services cannot be left entirely to the vagaries of the market. However, there is no reason why governments should be involved in the running of hospitals. Instead the incentives and efficiencies which the market can bring must be captured in the interests of more cost effective and better patient-centred care. Similarly, government must stop controlling manpower supply and actually meet the need rather than shore up vested interests. [Does she mean the doctors?]

> There is a clear need to improve and rationalise the acute hospital structure to ensure patients in each region have ready access to the full range of specialities and the highest quality of care. Hospitals should become autonomous units with their own boards, responsible for their own manpower and financial management.

Focusing on the hospital bed crisis, she also claimed that much pressure could be taken off the acute hospital system if GPs were better resourced, supported and equipped. I am not so sure about that because patients will continue to self-refer, and seeing that it is a supply-side problem, the bed problem cannot be wished away.

A Cure for the Crisis

Also, Ms Mitchell believes in phasing in free GP services beginning with families with children. By her reckoning, GPs surgeries must be part of the essential state-of-the-art IT system. The creation of the post of Health Ombudsman would provide citizens with a free system of inquiry and redress for complaints concerning their treatment in any part of the healthcare system. Certainly, there is much merit in that proposal.

In the 2002 General Election, Fine Gael proposed in a 60-page document to provide free GP services to under-18s and over-65s. They also promised to double the income limit for medical card qualification, to introduce a universal insurance system which is tax funded, to back a loyalty bonus and a Dublin allowance to attract and retain nursing staff. Fine Gael costed these proposals at IR£990 million in one year.

The Labour Party

There is sense to much of the Labour Party policy on health. The Labour Spokesperson on Health, Liz McManus TD, identified the core issue:

> Our hospitals and specialists are encouraged to care for private patients because the money follows the patient. Public patients ... are burdens on budgets and there is no incentive for specialists in the public system. When the money follows the patient the system responds.

That truism is essentially why half the population takes out health insurance, even though we all have hospital cover as of right. The way forward is to extend insurance cover to all citizens by providing support for those on low incomes. The two tiers would then be integrated.

Ms McManus also made the point that our health outcomes show that the better off live longer. However, this is true right across the world. She noted the fact that doctors are paid more than four times the capitation fee for caring for a well-off over-70-year-old than a poor one who had a medical card before the age of 70. The unfairness of the medical card system is emphasised by the low-income eligibility limit of €132 per week. Fianna Fáil reneged on their promise to extend the medical card to 200,000 people on low incomes. The cost of this would have been €150 million only. However, I disagree with the costing, as GPs are not going to agree to State-funded fees at an uneconomic rate.

In relation to good health and sensible living, diet, exercise, living environment, family and social relationships and the avoidance of addictions are considered important by the Labour Party. Furthermore, the

132

Ireland: medical incomes and party policies

wider social issues such as housing, employment, anti-poverty strategies, education and sports facilities also make a difference to well-being and welfare. In effect, Labour proposes the following:

- A sustained programme of capacity building while reforms are introduced.
- Greater emphasis on health promotion and personal responsibility.
- Integration between primary care and the hospital system. Too many people end up in hospital who do not need to be there and who could be cared for at home or in the community with proper supports. A GP service free at the point of delivery, while maintaining the Drugs Payment Service, would ensure an appropriate level of care.
- An insurance-based system for everyone to cover healthcare, including GP services and hospital treatment that is based on a statutory Health Care Guarantee.

While much of the Labour policy is viable, I do not believe that a GP service free at the point of delivery yet sustaining the Drugs Payment Service is workable. Such a system would be unwieldy, incurring high administration costs.

20

Health inequalities

Research has shown that health inequalities are largely social class related. Greater societal investment is needed to strengthen prevention strategies. Some 11,407 of the approximately 18,000 1958 birth cohort of England, Scotland and Wales (born on March 3–9) were interviewed at 33 years of age. With few exceptions, there were strong significant trends of increasing disease risk from classes I and II to classes IV and V.[1] It was noted that social trends in adult disease risk factors accumulate over decades. The authors found that investment in education and emotional development is needed in all social groups to strengthen prevention strategies relating to health behaviour, workplace environment and income inequality.[2] Other studies found that sustained economic hardship leads to poorer physical, psychological and cognitive functioning.[3]

Poor growth *in utero* and in infancy may increase the risk of cardiovascular disease, obstructive lung disease and diabetes. Low weight at one year was a risk factor for type 2 diabetes. Obesity is also social class related. Short stature increases the risk of cardiorespiratory disease. Clearly, childhood experiences are important for psychological health. For depression, risk factors include parental divorce, premarital pregnancy, low social class, poor emotional support in adulthood, and high rates of adverse life events. Educational opportunity is also class related with obvious consequences. Thus, childhood deprivation may have long-term physical and mental consequences. For that reason, formal preschool programmes are a worthwhile societal investment.

Global burden of disease

The global burden of disease has recently been published both in attributable mortality and in disability adjusted life years (DALYs). The leading global risk factors for high mortality in descending order of importance for 26 selected risk factors are high blood pressure, tobacco,

Health inequalities

high cholesterol, underweight, unsafe sex, low fruit and vegetable intake, obesity, physical inactivity, alcohol, unsafe sanitation and hygiene, indoor smoke from solid fuels, iron deficiency, urban air pollution, zinc deficiency, vitamin A deficiency, and others. For DALYs, in descending order – underweight, unsafe sex, high blood pressure, tobacco, alcohol, water hygiene, high cholesterol, indoor smoke, iron deficiency, obesity, zinc deficiency and others.

In the developed world, tobacco (12.2 per cent), high blood pressure (10.9 per cent), alcohol (9.2 per cent), high cholesterol (7.6 per cent), obesity (7.4 per cent), low fruit and vegetable intake (3.8 per cent), physical inactivity (3.5 per cent), illicit drugs (1.8 per cent) and unsafe sex (1.0 per cent) are the leading causes of DALYs. The specific disease burden is ischaemic heart disease (9.1 per cent), unipolar depression (7.1 per cent), and cerebrovascular disease (6.2 per cent).[4] The vast burden of these diseases is best dealt with at a political level. Doctors can and should campaign to reduce all the known risk factors: tobacco control, reduced salt in food, moderate alcohol consumption, reduced calorie-dense food, improved diet, exercise promotion, heroin and cocaine avoidance, and condoms for all. The solutions are really quite simple. Confronting unhealthy choices is a stated objective of the WHO, whereby it forms the thrust of its 2002 World Health Report.[5]

Irish scenario

In Ireland, the Combat Poverty Agency found that in poor families (average income €124 per week for an adult and €50 for a child), one-third of children are in poor health; half of Dublin-based poor families lived in fear of local thuggery; lone mothers complained of being bullied; 25 per cent of children were bullied at school; 66 per cent of households had no money left at the end of an average week; parents generally put spending on their children first; 50 per cent considered their family the best thing in their lives; 75 per cent earned money babysitting; over 50 per cent wanted to stay at school to finish the Leaving Certificate.[6] Clearly, such inequalities cannot be overcome without the political will to enforce change. Ireland has a child poverty rate of 16.8 per cent and ranks sixth highest on a list of 23 OECD countries. Further details are available on the Combat Poverty Agency website.

A Cure for the Crisis

WHO: rights and responsibilities

The objectives of the World Health Organization (WHO) should be kept in mind as a yardstick to judge the actions of politicians and professional groups in terms of health inequalities. The WHO constitution states: "The enjoyment of the highest attainable standard of health is one of the fundamental rights of every human being without distinction of race, religion, political belief, economic or social condition."

More specifically, guiding principles were outlined by WHO at a meeting at Alma-Ata in 1978, where a long declaration on health and the necessity for primary healthcare throughout the world was issued. The declaration comprised 10 parts; parts I, II, IV and IV pertaining to rights and political responsibility are included below.

Part I

Health is a state of complete physical, mental and social wellbeing, and not merely the absence of disease or infirmity. It is a fundamental human right and the attainment of the highest possible level of health is a most important world-wide social goal whose realization requires the action of many other social and economic sectors in addition to the health sector.

Part II

The existing gross inequality in the health status of the people particularly between developed and developing countries as well as within countries is politically, socially and economically unacceptable and is, therefore, of common concern to all countries.

Part IV

The people have the right and duty to participate individually and collectively in the planning and implementation of their health care.

Part V

Governments have a responsibility for the health of their people which can be fulfilled only by the provision of adequate health and social measures. A main social target of governments, international organizations and the whole world community in the coming decades should be the attainment by all peoples of the world by the year 2000 of a level of health that will permit them to lead a socially and economically productive life. Primary health care is

Health inequalities

the key to attaining this target as part of development in the spirit of social justice.

It is clear that even in a wealthy country like Ireland inequality remains. According to the UN's 2002 World Development Report, the level of income inequality in Ireland is second only to the US among OECD countries.

21

Immigrants and the Irish

Immigration and racism

During the 1997 General Election campaign some local residents in the Phibsborough area of Dublin were fearful of the presence of Romanians and black people. In fact, racism and fear of immigrants were widespread. It is immaterial that there was no basis to such fears; the fear remained, nonetheless. Many objected to the fact that immigrants were in receipt of welfare cheques and rent allowances from the health board. This was compounded by the ridiculous restriction on the right to work for those seeking asylum. Fear of the unknown, the unfamiliar and the foreign are ubiquitous sentiments. Enoch Powell in 1964 observed: "The life of nations no less than that of men is lived largely in the imagination." The absence of any reform of the Aliens Act from the 1930s leaves the situation fraught for all concerned. Basically, unless you are a refugee, it is nearly impossible to get a work permit here. This also affects those from Canada, the United States, Australia and New Zealand.

It is the indigenous working class who generally feel threatened by immigrants. Immigrants often do jobs that the locals shun and are willing to work extremely hard in pursuit of a decent standard of living for themselves and, more especially, their families. For example, in Britain, the Pakistani corner shop became a symbol of dedication. Emigrants usually migrate socially upwards and are an addition to their host countries in economic terms. In Britain, a Home Office report called *Migration: An Economic and Social Analysis* found that migrants contribute £2.5 billion more in tax than they cost in benefits and other handouts.

Migrants are overrepresented at the top and bottom of the income scale. As regards the former, for example some 150,000 French entrepreneurs have moved to Britain since the mid-1990s. However, most migrants are concentrated in poorly paid jobs and live in certain areas, leading to tensions regarding schools and social housing. Of course, there

Immigrants and the Irish

are problems of culture and communication too. In Britain, there has been a net inflow of 1.2 million people in the last 20 years. The figures show that 33 per cent of doctors, 10 per cent of nurses, 13 per cent of university teachers and researchers and 70 per cent of catering workers are foreign.

Tolerance is important and it cuts both ways. I have no doubt that black people will and do suffer discrimination in Ireland. Certainly, the Boston Irish had a bad record over the issue of school busing in the late 1960s, opposing the Federal Government's attempts at racial integration. In Dublin in November 2002, non-EU workers took an action against their employers as they were on half the union rate of pay, not being paid overtime and claimed that they were bullied and harassed when they raised concerns about pay and conditions. At that time, they were working on the Dublin Port Tunnel. However, the company is no longer operating at the site.

There is a certain irony in the above situations. The American economic boom in the 1990s was fuelled by the highest number of immigrants in the country's history, greater even than the "great wave" of immigration at the turn of the 19th century. The Center for Labor Market Studies at Boston's Northeastern University estimated that more than 13.5 million people emigrated to the US in the 1990s and about 9 million were undocumented illegals.[1] They accounted for 40 per cent of the US population growth, but about 50 per cent of the growth in the labour market. The number of indigenous Americans in the 25–34-year age group declined by 4.5 million, but 2.8 million foreign workers in that age group joined the workforce at that time. Many of the poorly educated illegals worked in low-paid service jobs often pushing wages downwards. About 27 per cent had university degrees and worked in health, services, engineering and business. They are overrepresented in science, IT and engineering.

The study shows the need for the US to operate a selective immigration policy closely aligned to the needs of the labour market. Further immigration is needed to fuel economic growth, and security concerns should not be applied to limit the potential. Without such immigration, the US will stagnate economically with obvious global consequences for all. These issues also apply to the Irish economy.

Irish immigration

In the Irish Republic, there are 30,000 Chinese, 30,000 Africans, 20,000 Romanians, 18,000 Eastern Europeans and 6,000 Filipinos in residence. Approximately 35,000 work permits were issued to the end of November 2002. There were 38,678 asylum seekers up to that time. In addition, 3,000 to 4,000 children were born here in recent years to newly arrived immigrants. Two thousand of the 7,000 births in the Rotunda Hospital in 2002 were to foreign non-EU nationals, mostly from Nigeria and Eastern Europe. The figure in the National Maternity Hospital, Holles Street was 14 per cent. In January 2003, the Supreme Court delivered a five to two majority decision that a baby born to a non-EU national does not automatically confer residency on the parents. This affects more than 10,000 parents with a further 10,200 cases pending. Hitherto, Ireland was the only EU state with relatively unrestricted citizenship laws. Certainly, this ruling will have implications for social welfare payments and for asylum seekers. However, the *jus sanguinis* still applies to great grandparents and grandmothers. Nonetheless, it leaves the interesting anomaly that parents of a baby citizen cannot use that relationship to stay here, but grandsons of the man from Ballyporeen can get an Irish passport. There is more than a tincture of contradiction and racism about this ruling, and like many commentators, I am less than impressed.[2]

Dr Peter McKenna, a former Master of the Rotunda Hospital, is correct when he says that politicians have hidden behind the judiciary. He opined that "racism is inevitable if change happens so dramatically in society without any decision-making by its leaders".[3] He supported the legal decision because of the experiences in the Rotunda Hospital and its impact on staff morale. Ideally, this question should have been addressed by legislation and/or referendum, if necessary.

Solutions

1. Encourage immigration and target-selected skills to boost the Irish economy.
2. Redefine Irish citizenship in an objective manner.

Health screening

Immigration inevitably raises issues of public health. The question of screening immigrants for infectious diseases such as AIDS/HIV, tuberculosis, syphilis and hepatitis is a highly charged one, not least because of its perceived threat to civil liberties. However, the matter of public health cannot be underestimated.

AIDS/HIV

There are 42 million people infected with the HIV virus worldwide and 30 million of these live in Africa. Most of the 29.5 million with HIV in sub-Saharan Africa will die as only 300,000 are receiving treatment. In the first six months of 2002, the National Disease Surveillance Centre reported 157 new cases in Ireland. Twelve per cent were born in Ireland and 73 per cent were born in sub-Saharan Africa and many were found through screening during pregnancy. The total number of known HIV infections in Ireland at the end of 2002 is 2,802. The UN price tag placed on combating AIDS is $10 billion per year. Only $3 billion was spent in 2002.

In Britain, 41,000 people have HIV and about 15,000 have died since the early 1980s. The Public Health Laboratory Service in England reported that the number of new HIV diagnoses is running at twice the level of the late 1990s. There are about 1,500 new diagnoses in homosexual men per year and there were 1,437 new heterosexual cases in the first nine months of 2002 – up 17 per cent on 2001. Some 892 of these were acquired in Africa.

South Africa has about 4.7 million HIV sufferers, the highest of any country in the world. HIV is causing devastation across Africa on such a scale that it is reducing the life expectancy of whole populations. Rates of HIV adult prevalence are 38.8 per cent in Botswana, 31 per cent in Lesotho, 33.4 per cent in Swaziland and 33.7 per cent in Zimbabwe. The adult populations of Zambia, Zimbabwe, Lesotho, Mozambique, Malawi and Swaziland total 26 million, of whom more than 5 million are HIV positive.

In China, 1 million are now affected and this is expected to reach 10 million by 2010. In Indonesia, there are now 196,000 intravenous drug abusers and they have a HIV rate of about 50 per cent. Most are male and 66 per cent are sexually active. In addition, 9,000 women caught HIV after sex with a drug user. Ten years ago in Jakarta, intravenous drug abuse was reportedly very rare.

India has 1.2 million orphaned through AIDS, more than any other country. There were 3.97 million with HIV in India in 2001, where the total is projected to surge to 25 million by 2010.

A Cure for the Crisis

In the Russian Federation there has been a sudden epidemic of HIV with total infections rising from 10,993 only four years ago to 2 million by mid-2002. Ukraine is the worst-affected country in Europe with HIV at 1 per cent of the population. There were 250,000 cases at the end of 2001 and 11,000 had died. The epidemic started with young intravenous drug users but is now mainly spread by heterosexual sex.

Worldwide, 4.2 million adults were infected with HIV in 2002 and 2.5 million adults died in the same period. About 19.2 million women are infected, as are 3.2 million children under the age of 15. Some 610,000 children have died as a result of the infection. In sub-Saharan Africa 60 per cent of those infected are women.

Other diseases

Tuberculosis is also widespread in Africa. Often, political revolution can lead to immunisation failures. Witness the outbreak of diphtheria in St Petersburg after the fall of communism. In Russia, Ukraine and Moldova, life expectancy has fallen. In Russia only 50 per cent of 18-year-olds will reach retiring age. There are high rates of cardiovascular disease, cancers, injuries and alcoholism. In fact, there is a dual pandemic of HIV and tuberculosis. By 2001, there were 2.3–4.0 million intravenous drug users in the former Soviet Union. Currently, in Russia, 30,000 people die from tuberculosis per annum.

To screen or not to screen

Should Ireland screen immigrants for HIV, syphilis, tuberculosis and hepatitis B and C? Undoubtedly, the rise of syphilis is evident. Syphilis cases rose from 6 in 1999 to 46 in 2000. In 2002, I treated a gay Dublin man with the rash of secondary syphilis, something I had only previously seen in a colour atlas of disease.

The civil libertarian argument is against the forced screening of refugees for HIV, etc. Nonetheless, I believe that the public health reality is heavily in favour of some disease screening. If people are found to be HIV positive, at least they will receive appropriate treatment in this country. The Department of Justice is in favour of screening, whereas the Department of Health and Children is not. Similarly, the Irish Refugee Council is opposed to compulsory screening as is the Dublin Aids Alliance.

Refugees and racism

In Britain, 29,100 refugees, including wives and children, applied for asylum in the third-quarter of 2002. The average cost in the UK for each asylum seeker given board and lodgings is £6,100 per year. There were 238,000 foreign migrants allowed into Britain in 2001. The net inflow of asylum seekers is running at nearly 104,000 for 2002. The influence of the tabloid press is the probable reason why the study of British Social Attitudes in 2002 found that the public believed that 32 per cent of the population is black or Asian, whereas the true figure is 7 per cent.[4] Interestingly, the numbers that consider themselves not at all racially prejudiced fell from 34 per cent in 1985 to 25 per cent in 2001. The number a little prejudiced has also fallen by about 6 per cent, as has the numbers who are very prejudiced. Older and less qualified people were also more likely to admit racial prejudice. Young people are likely to keep their attitudes as they grow older.

It is clear that the issue of migration is not going to go away. The rich north will attract economic migrants from the poor south. Similarly, Western Europe will attract similar migrants from Eastern Europe, most of whom will have full freedom of movement within a decade. Racism and religious intolerance should be countered in schools. At the very least, history teaching in schools should have modules that recognise the origin of significant emigrant minorities.

HIV testing for NHS staff

In January 2003, the British Department of Health proposed that healthcare workers should be free of HIV and hepatitis B and C before working in clinical areas where there is a risk of blood-borne infection to patients.[5] These may occur with needles or surgical instruments. In the past 14 years, there have been about 24 look-back checks involving thousands of patients as a result of possible contact with a HIV-infected health worker. In only two cases worldwide has there been any suggestion that such an event happened. These involved a dentist in Florida and an orthopaedic surgeon in France.

All entrants to the NHS would be treated similarly, irrespective of origin. Approximately 15,000 people per year would be affected by this measure. In response, the British Medical Association has pointed out that the measures may not be effective. On the other hand, the British Dental Association claimed that there was a strong case for students to

A Cure for the Crisis

be tested before starting training, as most clinical dental activity is prone to exposure. For tests to be meaningful, however, they have to be carried out regularly and must be applied to all relevant staff.

Solutions

1. Screen all visa seekers for infectious diseases.
2. Report results to the subjects directly and to their physicians, where known.
3. In the case of refugees, independent doctors in Ireland should act for the welfare of refugees and ensure that they receive immediate appropriate investigation and treatment, which should comply with current best medical practice.
4. Medical checks must not be used as a means of denying sick people admission to the country or as an excuse for deportation.
5. Healthcare workers throughout the service should be treated equally and be tested for HIV and hepatitis B and C where there is potential risk of contamination.
6. All healthcare workers involved in exposure to blood or body fluids should have hepatitis B vaccination. This should include contract cleaners who are often overlooked.

22

Disturbed children

Mr Justice Peter Kelly has been a very effective advocate for disturbed children from the bench. Ballydowd Special Care Unit in Lucan, Co Dublin was built after an unprecedented High Court order directing the State authorities to take steps to ensure the unit was open and operational by 2000. It was the intention that the unit would provide places for 24 children. However, there were serious problems recruiting staff. The problems were highlighted when a 12-year-old boy caused €20,000 worth of damage to the unit by flooding rooms, ripping up skirting boards, smashing doors, windows, toilets and TV sets. The boy had been in care since the age of five and clearly was deeply disturbed. Mr Justice Kevin O'Higgins, at the request of staff who could not cope with the boy, transferred him to the remand centre Oberstown House saying that the situation at Ballydowd was "well-nigh intolerable".[1] The deputy director of Oberstown, Michael Woodlock, did not believe that Oberstown was an appropriate place for the 12-year-old boy. He would be the youngest in the remand centre and would be mixing with boys who had criminal convictions and a history of repeat offending.

Recruiting staff

In England, people are leaving the very stressful field of child protection. The reasons given were covered in *The Guardian* in statements and vignettes from social workers in the field and they are salutary. Hazel Lamb, a 52-year-old family social worker for 27 years in Sussex, wrote:

> The form filling now required of social services when there are concerns about a child is analogous to offering a family a psychiatric consultation by computerized questionnaire.

> This welter of back-covering paperwork and the inquisitorial approach it entails impedes listening and trust. This is dangerous, because alienating families who could be helped places their children at greater risk.

It is also demoralising for workers whose skills and creativity, like those of teachers, are increasingly bypassed in the interests of providing statistics to demonstrate the apparent achievement of government targets, so that we have become brokers of care packages, while the direct care is provided by others.

A brief example – a family with five children referred to social services.

- For each we have to provide his or her 10 page assessment, a 4 page statement of need, setting out what is to be done, and a 4 page care plan detailing local authority services and undertaking by the parents.
- If a child protection conference is called, a further report on the family with risk assessment has to be done...
- In some cases, each service provider will have an individual service agreement with the family.
- There is also a whole other batch of internal paper work... for a placement for a child...
- Each child going into care will need care documentation with copies to foster parents, parents, children and files.[1]

The issue of recruitment is closely linked to remuneration. In Britain, social worker pay starts at £16,371 and with added qualifications it is currently £21,300. The area of social work in Britain is losing workers rapidly. In Ireland, we usually follow their mistakes after a delay. It is highly likely that the situation will be replicated here. Remember if we had proper child protection in the past, the problems which have come to light regarding clerical and parental child abuse, the Magdalen Launderies, orphanages and industrial schools might not have been so pervasive.

Establishing priority

The State still reneges on its responsibility for disturbed children. Evidence given to the Laffoy Commission shows the silent, secret suffering and brutality which was the lot of children of a particular section of Irish society in the last century. The high cost and potential duration of the inquiries led to Government interference and the resignation of Miss Justice Mary Laffoy. Law changes to allow a French-type inquiry to report would be more effective. Available money should be redirected from a multiplicity of lawyers and targeted at today's children. Steps must be taken to avoid another compensation inquiry in 25 years' time to deal with present-day failings.

23

People with disabilities

About 10 per cent of the Irish population of working age has some form of disability or chronic disease. Despite the economic boom in this country, the lives of people with disability are still closely linked to poverty. How we treat people with a handicap is a litmus test of our civic society. Equality is a clichéd myth but equity certainly is not. Quite simply, a society that does not redistribute its wealth and talents is callous, uncaring and nasty.

An ESRI report in 2002 showed that more than half of households headed by an ill or disabled person were living at or below the 60 per cent poverty line. At least 70 per cent of people with disability are unemployed compared with a national rate of 4.4 per cent. The Central Statistics Office found that 60 per cent of people with a disability or long-standing health problem between the ages of 15 and 64 are unemployed. The chief executive of the Disability Federation of Ireland, Mr John Dolan, claimed that after the 2002 General Election the Government had stated that: "We are committed to building service provision and legislative frameworks which enable people with disabilities to fulfil their potential and make a full contribution to the economic and social life of our country." Mr Dolan wants immediate adequate income support, a comprehensive range of community services and the enactment of rights-based legislation. He pointed out that disabled people had effectively become second-class citizens because they could not operate in everyday society in a way that would be regarded as normal for everyone else. "Their income is significantly below that of other people. If that does not mean they are second-class citizens, what does?"[1]

Legislation and Equality Authority

Disability is specifically included in the Employment Equality Act 1998. Under the Act, employers are obliged to make any necessary changes to enable an employee with a disability to do their job as long as the cost is nominal. The Equality Authority has called for the nominal cost exemption to be removed from public sector employers. In 1977, a target of 3 per cent of workers with disability was set for the public service. Currently the rate is 2 per cent. Disabilities Minister Willie O'Dea TD stated that public service bodies had "a duty to invest the time, effort and resources required to make the target attainable". I am pleased to note that there are a number of people with disabilities that I see most days in Beaumont Hospital working in technical services, portering and administration.

Up to the end of October 2002, 119 cases of disability discrimination had been reported to the Equality Authority compared to 111 cases in the whole of 2001. Fifty-six cases related to discrimination in the workplace and, of these, 29 showed a failure on the part of employers to take account of the needs of their disabled employees in a way that would allow them do their jobs properly. Other problems include not being given information on promotional jobs, being told that their disability makes them unsuitable for promotion, difficulties having contracts renewed, and delays in the offer of employment and dismissal when disability is discovered. In fact, 20 per cent of all discrimination within the workplace relates to disability.

The Equality Authority has also been to the forefront of spearheading change. Issues include access for people with guide dogs to restaurants and pubs, and wheelchair access to hotels, aircraft and shopping centres. The Equal Status Act 2000 requires service providers to "accommodate the needs of people with disabilities through making reasonable changes". The information booklet from the Equality Authority provides advice and information of achieving this objective. According to Christina Whyte of the National Disability Authority, the increase in cases referred to the Equality Authority showed a growing awareness of disabled people's rights, a trend she welcomed.[2]

At the end of 2003, an EU employment directive will become operational and will oblige employers to reasonably accommodate people with disabilities, unless they can prove that this amounts to a disproportionate burden on them. This is a more stringent requirement than the Employment Equality Act 1998.

Other significant developments include the establishment of Ireland's first-ever professor of disability studies. Dr Patricia Noonan Walsh has recently been appointed at UCD, where the chair is funded by the

People with disabilities

National Disability Authority. The application of academic rigour to the life problems of the disabled should result in incremental improvements in all spheres. Clearly, hard evidence and lobbying is the combination that is most likely to succeed. In fact, disabilities and rehabilitation are, like psychiatry, low on the prestige list of medical subspecialties. That is the key reason why such diseases are not properly addressed.

Caring for carers

At present, there are 100,000 carers looking after relatives and friends and only 20,000 currently qualify for the carer's allowance. The weekly threshold for means testing for this allowance is €210 for a single person and €420 for a couple. The respite grant of €735 only benefits about 30,000 carers because it is tied to the carer's grant and the domiciliary care allowance. Since 2000, there has been an increase of 2,000 day care places, 950 residential and 360 respite places, but despite this there are still 1,711 mentally handicapped people on the waiting list for residential care, another 1,014 awaiting respite and 861 waiting for day care services. There are 462 with no service at all and 485 inappropriately detained in psychiatric institutions.

St Michael's House in Dublin has a waiting list of 344 and has no chance of reducing it in the current financial climate. Instead of the €38 million allocated in 2002, only €13.3 million has been allocated for 2003. It is scandalous that there is such an underprovision of places for handicapped people in a wealthy country like Ireland, where untaxed horse reproduction is put before the handicapped.

Solutions

1. Fund the necessary care facilites for the physically and mentally handicapped as a priority.
2. Give all carers a guaranteed minimum of three weeks of annual respite.

24

Depression and suicide

Depression

There remains a stigma attached to depression in Ireland. About 280,000 people suffer from depression and it is twice as common in women as in men. Young males and elderly males living alone are the most likely to commit suicide. A recent MRBI study found that most people think that depression is a weakness rather than a physical illness and 13 per cent of the public would not visit their GP if depressed. Twenty-six per cent of 15–24-year-olds said that they would be unlikely to attend a GP if depressed. More than half believe that depression does not run in families, and 41 per cent believe that there is no permanent cure, despite the fact that 70 per cent respond very well to antidepressants, which are non-addictive. Many also think that antidepressants are addictive. Not surprisingly, 25 per cent wrongly believe that alcohol helps to combat the disease.

In Britain, the number of young people diagnosed with depression has doubled in the last 12 years, according to the Joseph Rowntree Foundation. Socially disadvantaged people aged between 15 and 25 are more prone to clinical depression. In particular, younger people had to face unemployment and labour market collapse in some parts of Britain. Those with college degrees were one-third less likely to be depressed. Furthermore, those who did not complete their education or left early were particularly prone to unemployment and to clinical depression. Suicide is a particular problem for the unemployed.

Suicide

Suicide is a cross-cultural international problem with a rate of 23 per 100,000 in China, where it is the fifth most important cause of death.[1] Among young adults 15 to 34 years of age, it accounts for 19 per cent of all deaths and is the leading cause. The rate in women is 25 per cent

Depression and suicide

higher than in men. Rural rates are three times higher than urban rates. This rate is higher than that in Ireland and underlines why the issue should be treated with the utmost gravity. An OECD survey, published in February 2003, found that Ireland was second only to New Zealand in suicide rates for the under 25-year-olds. The New Zealand rate is 13.6 per 100,000, the Irish rate is 10.3, Finland is 9.9 and the UK rate is 3.3. If these figures are an accurate snapshot of the true position, then we in Ireland have much to worry us. Certainly, we need to explore why our figures are so much worse than those of our neighbours.[2]

National Task Force on Suicide

The Report of the National Task Force on Suicide in 1998 is an excellent document setting out what should be done as well as detailing the extent of the problem in Ireland.[3] Between 1945 and 1995, the rate of suicide in Ireland rose from 2.38 to 10.69 per 100,000. Suicide is the second most common cause of death in young men aged 15–24 years at a rate of 19.5 per 100,000 compared to 2.1 per 100,000 in similar-aged females.

In a study in Cork from 1989 to 1993, only 18 per cent of young 15–24-year-old men who had committed suicide had received psychological treatment in the year before their death, even though 75 per cent had been regarded as mentally ill. It is also known that 15 per cent who suffer from major mood disorders (manic depression) end their lives. The suicide rate in men older than 65 years has risen from 9.4 per 100,000 in 1976 to 17.9 per 100,000 in 1993. In the age group 65–74, there is a far higher suicide rate in men and women than in the 75 years plus age group. In 1995, the overall suicide rate in men was 17.17, whereas it was 4.32 in women.

In Cork, the profile of parasuicide victims was someone living in rented, council accommodation with overcrowding, with minimum education and who is unemployed. A 10-year follow-up of self poisoners seen at A&E departments in Cork hospitals in 1992 found that 60 per cent of the women had a current mental illness, 40 per cent had major personality difficulties, 40 per cent described their childhood as unhappy and almost 50 per cent had significant disadvantages. For the males, alcoholism, personality difficulties and current psychiatric illnesses were factors in over half the cases. Things were generally better than they had been at the time of the attempted suicide in 60 per cent of women and 44 per cent of men.

A Cure for the Crisis

Dealing with suicidal behaviour

There is overwhelming evidence that the reporting and portrayal of sui-cidal behaviour in the press, on television and in films has a negative effect. This is particularly disastrous when a method of suicide is speci-fied and especially when presented in detail. Suicides of celebrities often result in many copycat deaths. Mental illness is a common factor in sui-cides and must be recognised more, especially in the media. The National Suicide Prevention Strategy for England addressed the media question in 2002.[4] Several sets of guidelines have been produced and, unquestion-ably, this issue should be part of the journalism training courses at uni-versities.[5] No clear policy exists at present for "suicide sites" on the internet. The ramifications of media guidelines including interference with freedom of speech was discussed recently in the *British Medical Journal,* as was the existence of the very limited evidence for the effec-tiveness of media intervention.[6]

In Ireland, staff training to deal with suicide is deficient to judge from a December 2002 report from the North Eastern Health Board, where approximately 18 per cent of staff had experienced "client suicide" at some point. Some staff had encountered up to 25 suicides. Forty per cent of staff involved had experienced feelings of anger, guilt and sadness fol-lowed by physical and psychological symptoms associated with trauma. These included insomnia, loss of concentration, and professional self-doubt. Females were more likely than males to be affected. Thirty-six per cent said that no guidelines were available and a further 14 per cent were uncertain as to the existence of such guidelines. Staff felt that they needed special training on how to cope with families of suicide victims. Clearly, this is an issue that should be addressed as a matter of urgency.

25

Drugs of abuse and recreational drug use

According to the Drug Treatment Centre in Pearse Street, Dublin, there are currently 13,000 heroin users in Dublin and 80 per cent of these are hepatitis C positive. A statewide survey by the National Advisory Committee on Drugs (NACD) shows that the number of heroin users in Dublin has fallen since 1996. There are 5.6 heroin users per 1,000 population, 16 per 1,000 in Dublin and 0.9 per 1,000 elsewhere. The numbers of opiate users in the Irish Republic are shown in the Table 25.1.

Table 25.1 Estimated numbers of opiate users in Ireland

Estimated users	1996	2000	2001
Rep. of Ireland	–	14,158	14,452
Dublin	13,461	12,268	12,456
Rest of State	–	2,526	2,225

In a recent Union of Students in Ireland (USI) survey carried out among 250,000 students across the whole island, 51 per cent of students had taken drugs and 66 per cent of these had started in school. Twenty-three per cent of these were in the 13–15-year age group, while 1 per cent were as young as 12-years-old. Curiosity was the motivation in over half the cases. Cannabis was cited as the first illegal drug taken by 98 per cent and is used regularly by 89 per cent of drug users. Ecstasy is taken by 9 per cent and cocaine by 2 per cent.

In 2003, the first drug prevalence survey of households in Ireland conducted by the NACD found 19 per cent claimed to have ever used an illegal drug. Cannabis was the most commonly used illegal drug. Lifetime prevalence rates for cannabis were 18 per cent in the Republic of Ireland and 17 per cent in Northern Ireland, while lifetime prevalence rates for all other drugs were less than 5 per cent. The other most common drugs used were ecstasy and magic mushrooms (each 4 per cent); ampheta-

153

mines, cocaine, LSD and poppers (each 3 per cent); solvents (2 per cent); heroin (0.4 per cent) and crack (0.3 per cent).

Screening for drug use

Two schools in Dublin, St Andrews and Sutton Park, have started to screen their students for drug use if they felt they had cause. Many employers screen for drugs of abuse and indeed the whole area is growing fast at present. This activity has been common in the US for the past decade and many US multinationals have imported the practice to Ireland. The availability of many urine dipstick tests for drugs of abuse has lead to an ease of self-testing; however, the technicalities of specificity, cross reactivity, sensitivity and cut-off levels are often lost on the users.

The Drug Treatment Centre announced that they have plans to introduce specialist training to deal with the subject of screening. In 2001, the Drug Treatment Centre set up a Young Adults in Action programme to provide a medical, therapeutic and life skills service to young adults. This was very necessary when they found that the number of homeless clients they serviced had risen from 129 in 2000 to 166 in 2001. The Centre treated 1,189 drug users in 2001, a 15 per cent increase on 2000, where 97 per cent were heroin addicts.

The potential for the casual criminalisation of the huge number of young soft-drug users, which could be caught by urine drug screening tests in schools, is a cause for concern. It must also be borne in mind that cannabis can be detected by sensitive test for five days after the last exposure. This police activity is not a school function. Indeed, it raises more issues than it addresses. As all the drugs detected are illegal, is the teacher obliged to inform the Gardaí? Who can give consent? Over-16s can give their own consent and may not be consented by parents. Was the consent given under duress? If so, has this got legal implications? Will the student be expelled if he/she refuses to consent? Is that just or is it bullying? Are parents freely willing to have their children involved with the criminal justice system with the consequences for visas, jobs, etc. in the future. Certainly, I would not support such drug screening for the above reasons. However, where parents are suspicious of drug taking, I would be happy to deal with it in strict confidence, but I would not report any findings to a school or employer unless there was freely given written consent.

Drugs of abuse and recreational drug use

There is a steady expansion of the numbers taking heroin and cocaine use is also climbing rapidly. The Drug Treatment Centre laboratory reported a 46 per cent growth in the number of positive cocaine samples and a 20 per cent growth in the opiate numbers. A swab test kit taking samples from the back of the hand and using equipment costing £40,000, which is portable being the size of a briefcase, can be used to detect ecstasy, cannabis, heroin, cocaine, amphetamines and Rohypnol, the so-called date rape drug. The test takes about eight seconds. Police in Cannock and Stafford in England have used the machines to check for drug use in pubs and clubs. This is an extremely questionable use of police powers, but is indicative of the sophistication of modern technology if society wants to apply it to the limits. Such equipment could be useful for police to use if suspicious of drug-impaired driving or for research projects to try to quantify the extent of drug abuse in cities. Figures for the number of users of, for instance, ecstasy seem to me to be guesstimates at best. Public health would be better served by more accurate information.

Economic costs

A study published by the University of York estimates the annual economic costs to the NHS and the criminal justice system due to hard drugs users at between £3.7 billion and £6.8 billion. The social cost of crime to victims and property boost the total cost figure to between £10.9 and £18.8 billion. Recreational class A drug users under 25 in Britain number 400,000, and there are over 1 million older regular drug takers. The problem user is anyone for whom drugs are no longer recreational but have become an essential part of existence. The latter group number about 300,000. Drug treatment and testing orders from courts have a 50 per cent success rate with users. Offenders are given the choice of treatment as an alternative to prison. Clearly, drug use and abuse will not go away. We would be wise to adjust our attitude with regard to public sector job bans and visas.

British Home Office research shows that the average drugs user spends £16,500 each year on drugs. Approximately £13,000 is funded by crime. Heroin is a poverty index drug. The 1998 target of trying to cut drug abuse by 25 per cent by 2003 is now regarded as impossible to achieve. The British government has decided to change its drugs policy for 2003. People who test positive for drugs will be given the choice of treatment or prison. The situation is such that the government now wishes to reduce the amount of drug-related crime and the consumption of class A (hard) drugs. They intend to increase the participation of problem drug users in treatment programmes to 55 per cent by 2004 and 100 per cent by 2008. They intend to reduce poppy cultivation in Afghanistan by 70 per cent within 5 years because 90 per cent of opium used in Britain originates there. How? The government plans to achieve it by "improving security and law enforcement capacity and implementing reconstruction programmes which encourage farmers away from poppy cultivation". From media accounts, Tony Blair gave the Hamid Karzai government £20 million in 2002 to pay Afghan farmers to plant wheat rather than poppies. The farmers pulled up their poppy plants and were then faced with the situation of local warlords grabbing their money. Now the farmers have planted a double poppy crop for the coming year.

Four million people have used illegal drugs in England and Wales in the past year; three million were cannabis smokers. Among 16–24-year-olds, 0.5 million used class A drugs, unchanged since 1994. There has been a rise in the use of cocaine, crack and ecstasy and a reduction in amphetamines, LSD and glue. The guesstimate of the social cost of drug abuse in Britain is between £10 and 18 billion per year. About 250,000 hard drug users are responsible for 99 per cent of this. The target is to treat 200,000 of these by 2008.

Heroin maintenance

Doctors will be encouraged to prescribe heroin for those with a proven clinical need who have failed to respond to methadone. Ironically, methadone causes a greater number of deaths than prescribed heroin. I advocated this harm reduction policy almost 10 years ago for addicts in Dublin. The current British figure of 400 addicts receiving heroin is expected to rise to 1,500 as a result. Currently, there are about 1,000–2,000 very sick addicts among the 25,000 heroin addicts in the Netherlands. The Dutch government is investigating how a nationwide heroin-maintenance programme for heroin addicts, who have failed all attempts to wean them off the drug, could be set up. The heroin programme was tested in six cities and the study found that for about 25 per cent of addicts who smoked and injected drugs, treatment with a combination of heroin and methadone produced improvements in physical and mental health and led to a decrease in criminal behaviour. Participants were at

Drugs of abuse and recreational drug use

least 25-years-old and had a life expectancy of one year or less.[1] Free heroin would cost about €15,000 per year per patient. Switzerland also is to hold a second referendum on the issue of heroin maintenance.

Cocaine

Cocaine addiction is the hardest to treat and the least successfully treated at present. However, vaccines and novel compounds are under development.

Cannabis

There will be a doubling of the number of drug testing and treatment orders made by the British courts for those who test positive for class A drugs when arrested. In Britain, cannabis is now a class C drug and users will only be arrested where there is public disorder or where children are involved. This will, in effect, decriminalise cannabis. This is long over-due but education programmes should be aimed at schools to inform children that there are serious downsides to cannabis use. Opposition to the legalisation of cannabis in Britain has fallen to 46 per cent in 2002 from 75 per cent in 1983. The numbers who want cannabis legalised have risen from 12 per cent in 1983 to 41 per cent now, with a further 15 per cent undecided.

As regards medical uses, 86 per cent now support a change in the law which would allow doctors to prescribe cannabis. Decriminalisation of cannabis is also the position in the Netherlands, Portugal, Spain and Italy where the police do not prosecute for possession of drugs, although the law remains on the statute book. Here in Ireland, I believe that we should cut the hypocrisy concerning cannabis and that it should be graded, licensed, taxed and legalised just like alcohol and tobacco, both social, damaging and addictive drugs. As with tobacco, advertising should be prohibited and the packaging should carry health warnings. In Britain, 90 per cent believe that ecstasy and heroin should remain illegal.

An Eastern Health Board survey in 2000 found that about 30 per cent of secondary school boys aged 15–18 use cannabis on a regular basis, while 12 per cent admitted using an illicit substance other than cannabis in the previous month. Ten per cent of 11–18-year-olds claimed that they used cannabis during the previous month.

Mr Tony Geoghegan at the Merchant's Quay Project has been a consistent advocate of effective addiction treatment policies in Dublin.

There are 5,000 addicts using Merchant's Quay's needle exchange programme, which treated almost 11,000 individuals between 1997 and 2002. Early school leaving and poverty are the key characteristics. According to Mr Geoghegan, "the gateway to heroin use is poverty". At Merchant's Quay, only 40 per cent of the heroin users used cannabis first. In fact, more used alcohol. Then is alcohol the gateway drug, or is it that neither alcohol nor cannabis is a gateway drug? Credit should also be given to the former Junior Minister with Responsibility for Drugs, Eoin Ryan TD, in his efforts to address the drug problem in an honest fashion.

Drug Court

In Dublin, an experimental Drug Court was established in 2001 under Mr Justice Gerard Haughton at the Richmond Courthouse. The primary aim is to reduce crime through rehabilitation, as many drug users are repeat offenders. The issues concerning drug courts were discussed in the Working Group on a Courts Commission[2] and the thrust of the report is being put to the test. The goal for addicts is to stabilise, rehabilitate and then gain employment or further education and training. The Court brings together the Probation Service, Department of Education and Science, the health boards and the Gardaí. Charges can be re-entered if the clients regress and misbehave within 12 months of graduation. The Court has had 88 referrals, 37 of which were deemed unsuitable. Of the remaining 51, 4 are currently being assessed and 14 have been taken out of the programme. Five people have been given drug-free certificates at the end of 2002, and 28 are in various stages of the programme. The five sign on to a postgraduate programme for at least 12 months and keep contact with probation officers and health and education workers. This is much better than the revolving prison door drug-ridden and life-shortening experience of many such people. Judge Haughton's insightful comments are exemplary: "One thing I've learned in the last 18 months is the difficulty coming to terms with and overcoming problems of drug abuse. The participants really did superhuman work."

The real answer to heroin and crime is to address poverty in poor communities. Strategies focused on drugs use only through education, effective treatment programmes in the communities, and through the justice system continue to treat the symptoms, while ignoring and diverting attention away from the causes. The comments of Mrs Justice Susan Denham of the Supreme Court, and chairperson of the Courts Service

Drugs of abuse and recreational drug use

Board, summed up the situation at the graduation of four north inner city drug addicts from the Drug Court. She said:

> Drug abuse is a cancer in our society. It destroys individuals, families and communities. Court lists are filled with drug-related crime. Our prisons are full of inmates who have abused drugs. A cycle of addiction and crime, life and death, has been established around drug abuse.

Interestingly, in January 2003, expansion of the Drug Court was frozen because Government officials did not believe it had been successful. Thirty-three were being assessed or were completing the course. In practice, it may be unrealistic to expect more than a 30 per cent success rate.

Solutions

1. A school programme othe effects of drugs should be instituted without moralising.
2. Link the drug programme with alcohol and tobacco information.
3. Emphasis on personal responsibility for the consequences of one's actions should be made.
4. Legalise, quality control, tax and regulate cannabis usage.
5. Establish a drug quality control caravan in cities for the use of ecstasy users. In my opinion, ecstasy is too dangerous to legalise. It may cause brain damage and depression.
6. Heroin should be made available on prescription.
7. A poor area action plan involving extra schoolteachers, social workers, sports and arts facilitators should be targeted at areas where drug usage is common.
8. Expansion of the Drug Court idea in Dublin to take in other cities and towns should be undertaken.
9. Publicise the dangers of cocaine abuse. Cocaine should never be legalised.
10. Consider decriminalising all personal drug use, which would have to be tightly defined, but keep suppliers illegal with Criminal Assets Bureau-type consequences plus custodial sentences for traffickers. I would prefer to medicalise substance abuse and criminalise the pushers.

A Cure for the Crisis

11. Graduate sentences by toxicity – i.e. crack cocaine, cocaine, heroin, ecstasy, etc.

It is worth noting that the only substance which has positive health effects is the consumption of less than 20 units of alcohol per week. Among men, consumption of alcohol at least three to four days per week is inversely related to the risk of heart attack.[3] None of the other substances has health advantages for the healthy normal. Cannabis may have medical use in multiple sclerosis but this has yet to be proven. Cocaine is used in ear, nose and throat (ENT) disorders for anaesthesia; heroin may have a future role in palliative care. Ecstasy has no therapeutic role whatsoever.

26

Alcohol and tobacco

Alcohol

There is a €700 million annual "subsidy" from the Government to the alcohol industry. The Government Strategic Task Force found that in 1999, the State took in €1.5 billion in alcohol-related revenue, while the payout in alcohol-related social welfare, healthcare costs, absenteeism, crime and road accidents caused by alcohol came to €2.2 billion. Overall, alcohol is a net cost of €700 million to the taxpayer. The least that industry should be is budget neutral. Complaints from the Licensed Vintners Association about their costs are unlikely to include the true cost to the public.

Public opinion and surveys

A poll of 1,000 adults by Lansdowne Market Research in November 2002 found that 40 per cent believed that alcohol taxes should be unchanged, while 30 per cent favoured an increase. Forty-two per cent wanted earlier pub closing, whereas 41 per cent said it should remain the same. Ninety per cent wanted no children in pubs after 7 pm and 66 per cent wanted restrictions on alcohol advertising. Some 83 per cent agreed that random breath tests should be widely enforced all year around. Sixty-seven per cent agreed with a lowering of the legal blood alcohol limit for driving to 50 mg%. A total of 53 per cent believe that the drinks industry should be restricted from sponsoring sports and cultural events.

Another Lansdowne poll of 900 adults by telephone (a doubtful method) found that 68 per cent wanted Irish blood alcohol driving limits reduced from 80 mg%. There is no good reason to reduce the level. If anything, the current levels should be enforced, for the simple reason that speeding is the major cause of deaths on our roads.

One cheery recent fact is the decline in volume of alcohol products sold in Ireland year on year to September 2002. Beer was down 9 per cent to

161

A Cure for the Crisis

14.9 million litres; spirits down 2 per cent; brown spirits down 5 per cent; white spirits down 2 per cent. Cider was down 11 per cent; but wines were up 9 per cent and alcopops up 30 per cent to 334,000 litres.

A survey of 1,000 women by *Company* magazine in Britain found that 10 per cent of women have drunk themselves unconscious. Among 16–34-year-olds, 40 per cent said that they had become so drunk that they had no memory of the night before. That figure rose to 57 per cent among those under 24. One in seven women had had a fight while drinking and 20 per cent had lost keys or valuables during a binge. Half had walked home alone while drunk. Women cannot drink the same volumes as men due to slower metabolism and less tolerance. Those who do, however, put themselves at risk of obvious problems from injury to assault and rape.

Over the period 1989–1999, 10 EU countries showed a reduction in alcohol consumption, whereas consumption in Ireland rose by 41 per cent.

A recent survey by the Department of Health and Children found that 20 per cent of 12–14-year-old boys had experimented with alcohol. At 15–16-years-old, 50 per cent of girls and 66 per cent of boys are regular drinkers. About one-third of 15–16-year-olds indulge in binge drinking. This is defined as having five or more drinks in a row, three or more times per month. Among Irish secondary school pupils, 89 per cent drink alcohol, by far the highest rate of youth alcohol consumption in Europe.

Ill effects of alcohol

Disorder, violence and rowdiness in the streets are obvious accompaniments of heavy drinking. Happy hours and cheap booze offers fuel disorder and crime on city streets. Indeed, the prohibition on "happy hours" in the Intoxicating Liquor Act 2003 is not before time. In 2001, the number of teenagers arrested for being drunk and disorderly increased by 45 per cent. Alcohol-related offences were up by 85 per cent in the same year and the number of prosecutions for alcohol more than doubled. Ten per cent of adults drink to excess and one-third of admissions in A&E departments are alcohol related. In the Mater Hospital in Dublin, 30 per cent of male and 8 per cent of female inpatients had alcohol problems in 2001.

Being drunk, nauseated, dizzy, incapacitated, ataxic and sick is not really "cool". Paul Gilligan of the Irish Society for the Prevention of Cruelty to Children (ISPCC) has stated that "there is a misconception

Alcohol and tobacco

that teenagers who drink heavily or take drugs are those who have many friends and enjoy a good social network. In fact, kids who misuse are generally socially isolated with poor self-esteem and often encounter family problems." To help counter these misconceptions, the ISPCC is running a Nationwide Drug and Alcohol Prevention Programme with the support of the AIB Better Ireland Programme. Similarly, the Department of Health has started a campaign to try to reposition alcohol in Irish life through a National Alcohol Awareness Campaign.

However, the alcohol lobby is very powerful in Ireland. There are 60,000 full-time jobs in the drinks industry and €3.3 billion was spent on drink in 2001. In 2001, VAT returns on drink were €790 million. The average pint costs €3.30, of which 24 per cent goes to the brewers, 45 per cent to the pub and 31 per cent to the Exchequer. The tax take on alcohol will be €1.6 billion in 2003. It is clearly in their interests to sell booze. Their success is highlighted by the huge prices that pubs command at auction. Furthermore, the extent of drinking and smoking is shown by the fact that the tax take on these two activities could have funded 43 per cent of our health services.

Alcohol advertising and sponsorship

Sponsorship of sports by alcohol companies is pervasive and should be phased out, because it gives an enormous positive influence for alcohol. Headline examples include the Guinness All-Ireland Hurling Championship, the Heineken European Cup, the Harp Lager FAI Cup, the Amstal Beer sponsorship of the Champions League in soccer, the Worthington Cup in soccer, etc. Similarly, in the Eircom National League, Budweiser sponsors UCD and Smithwick's sponsors Derry City, etc. Junior soccer teams are also sponsored by Guinness, among others. Carlsberg sponsors Liverpool FC and there are many other soccer examples. Fosters sponsors the Aussie Compromise Rules team. Alcohol has nothing to do with being a better player (it makes you worse!), nor is it necessary to enjoy the game. The problem is that fashion and increased wealth have made excess alcohol drinking nearly a normal event. The pervasive influence of alcohol is regrettable. Personally, I am not anti-booze and indeed have highlighted the benefits of drink in moderation.

A positive development is the Department of Health's concern to introduce legislation, if necessary, to control alcohol advertising. Recently, the Advertising Standards Authority of Ireland banned an alcohol advert for

A Cure for the Crisis

showing that drink encouraged feats of daring. The Guinness volcano advert featured a man walking over lava to save a cask of Guinness from damaging a building. Likewise, the Authority banned the following adverts: a Carlsberg one for portraying an attractive, alcohol-linked holiday as this would appeal to underage male drinkers in particular; a Heineken one which showed three young men prompting a hesitant pal to approach the bar and accept a glass of Heineken while a beautiful woman looked on; another Carlsberg one for using Robbie Keane, the international footballer, because he is under 25, and also Jason McAteer another Irish soccer international because he would particularly appeal to youths under 18 years of age; a Guinness billboard which had "Goodness" printed on it, as it is considered misleading to portray alcohol as goodness.

The Department of Health's Task Force on Alcohol reported that alcohol advertising "has a strong attraction for teenagers, as it portrays lifestyles and images which are part of their social setting".

There are many reasons why today's youth drink more than ever. Many drink to get totally "blotto". Some drink to appear cool to their friends, others from peer pressure, others because they are unsure and shy others because they are deeply troubled and unhappy, others because it is an available escape from boredom, others because they think it is a rite of passage to adulthood.

In Budget 2003, taxes on spirits rose by 20 cents and alcopops rose by 35 cents. The Government described this as a measure to combat drinking by young people. Rubbish! What the Fianna Fáil government fail to realise is that kids drinking their heads off in parks carry around bags full of 500 ml cans of lager and cider. Why ignore the reality?

Solutions

1. It is probably a good idea to ban alcohol advertising, including the sponsorship of hurling, football and rugby. Anything that deglamorises alcohol is now a good thing.

2. Treatment of alcohol and other drug addictions works and saves society money. About 40 per cent of alcoholics treated in hospital remain abstinent at two years compared to 20 per cent who attend Alcoholics Anonymous and other groups.

3. Increase alcohol taxes to make the industry at least budget neutral.

4. Reduce pub trading hours during weekdays in the winter.

Alcohol and tobacco

5. Prohibit alcohol sales at petrol stations.

6. Support school and youth participation sports by paying grants to teachers and coaches from hypothecated alcohol taxes.

Smoking

Mortality and morbidity levels

There are 7,400 smoke-related deaths in Ireland every year. That is 10 times the number killed on our roads. In Europe, there are 215 million smokers and 1,500 people die every day from smoke-related disease. Tobacco kills about 4.2 million people annually and WHO reckons that it will kill over 10 million per year by the late 2020s, if robust steps are not taken to curb the smoking epidemic immediately. About 25 per cent of smokers die prematurely due to the habit and those that die lose an average of 10–15 years of life.

About 25 per cent of deaths from heart disease are caused by smoking. Smoking also causes peripheral arterial disease and gastrointestinal ulcers. Smoking is the major cause of 90 per cent of lung cancer deaths and 75 per cent of the deaths from bronchitis/emphysema. Smokers also cough more frequently, get more chest infections and breathlessness. Non-smokers exposed to passive smoking have at least a 35 per cent increased risk of lung cancer and an increased risk of cardiorespiratory symptoms. Smoking increases the risk of death from colon cancer by 34 per cent in men and 43 per cent by women. Bladder cancers are also a problem.

Young children living with smokers have more respiratory symptoms than those in a smoke-free environment. Only 15 per cent of cigarette smoke is inhaled by the smoker, the rest is offered free to those around. Of the 4,000-plus chemicals in cigarette smoke, at least 60 are known to cause cancer. The risk of lung cancer from passive smoking is small but is 50 to 100 times greater than the risk of lung cancer from exposure to asbestos (see Ash Ireland website: *www.ash.ie*). Attempts by the tobacco industry to generate a study to refute the 1981 Japanese study – which concluded that wives of heavy smokers had twice the risk of developing lung cancer as wives of non-smokers – while disguising their involvement, has recently been exposed.[1] Research has shown that there is a significant association between lung cancer and smoke exposure from a spouse. The excess risk is 20 per cent for women and 30 per cent for men. It also shows that there is a 16–19 per cent excess risk of lung cancer

A Cure for the Crisis

from smoke exposure at work. However, at present there is insufficient evidence that children exposed to parental smoke have an altered risk of developing any cancer.[2] Nonetheless, the tobacco industry will fight hard and dirty to maintain its vast toxic addiction empire.

By 2003, about 24 per cent of the Irish population over 15 years smoke and between half and one-third of these will die as a consequence. This is down from the early 1970s when 44 per cent of Irish adults smoked. Seventy per cent of 15–18-year-olds have smoked at least one cigarette and more than 28 per cent are regular smokers. Defining a smoker as someone who smokes at least once per week, then 20 per cent of secondary school students smoke.

The British General Household Survey in 2001 found that 27 per cent of adults are smokers and 24 per cent are ex-smokers. Research by Nicorette found that the number of heavy smokers has risen from 51 per cent to 62 per cent since 1993. Fifty-three per cent of smokers are women. In 1997, 73 per cent tried to stop smoking but the figure fell to 61 per cent in 2002. The number of smokers who said that they would quit for their family's health has risen from 8 per cent to 13 per cent. Nicotine replacement and anti-smoking therapy is available on the GMS, but this is unknown to 79 per cent of smokers. Certainly, GPs are fully aware that these therapies are publicly funded.

The number of women in Ireland dying from lung cancer is rapidly catching up with the numbers dying from breast cancer. One in four cancer deaths in women was from lung cancer. The five-year survival after diagnosis is less than 10 per cent. Most women get lung cancer 20 years after starting to smoke. Because so many young women are starting smoking, we are facing a lung cancer epidemic in the 35–45-year age group. The National Cancer Registry figures for the years 1994 to 1998 show that 634 women died from breast cancer while 521 women died from lung cancer. Women become more dependent on nicotine than men making quitting more difficult. Women smoke to aid weight loss, and 25 per cent of women smoke throughout pregnancy.

Fifty-two per cent of smokers state that neither price increases nor smoking bans would induce them to quit smoking. However, significant price increases result in fewer teens smoking and people will smoke less and more will stop. A doubling of the price of cigarettes is backed by 46 per cent of the Irish population.

The taxes raised on tobacco in 2003 are projected to be €1.65 billion. Cigarette sales continue to rise, despite 3,000 new cancer cases in Ireland

Alcohol and tobacco

each year. In the first nine months of 2002, cigarette sales rose by 3.9 per cent to a massive 5 billion cigarettes consumed during this period. The figures show an extra 190 million cigarettes consumed in 2002 compared to the first nine months of 2001. Some of this increase may be exaggerated due to a squeeze on smuggled cigarettes, obviously not quantified.

Weight gain

Over 100 years ago, the association between body weight and smoking was known. In a study reported in 1991[3] of 1,157 men and 1,496 women in the US aged 25 to 74 years, who were followed for 10 years, the average weight gain in those who stopped smoking was 2.8 kg in men and 3.8 kg in women. Weight gain was greater than 13 kg in 9.8 per cent of men and 13.4 per cent of women. Males reached the average weight of age and sex matched non-smokers. The number of cigarettes smoked was directly proportional to the weight gained on quitting. The authors concluded that weight gain is not likely to negate the health effects of smoking cessation, but its cosmetic effects may interfere with attempts to quit. Nicotine lowers the body weight set point so that weight gain is physiological (i.e. normal).[4] Each cigarette utilises 8 kcal by stimulation of the sympathetic nervous system.[5] Gain in weight is also evidence of a continued abstinence from smoking.[6] Weight is a major concern of young females and has to be addressed as part of the totality of a quit smoking programme. There is some evidence that using fluoxetine (Prozac) appears to have a role in forestalling post-cessation weight gain and may help in some circumstances.[7]

Quitting

Norma Cronin, anti-tobacco consultant with the Irish Cancer Society, has pointed out that there is support in the form of quit lines, smoking cessation counsellors, nicotine replacement therapy and drugs such as buproprion (Zyban). In my experience, the patient-led demand for Zyban quickly followed its media advertising. There is interest in quitting smoking when patients are pushed in that direction. It is important to enquire from ex-smokers if they are still in that category because life's vicissitudes often induce ex-smokers to relent. About 70 per cent of smokers see a GP every year, where 35 per cent admitted they have tried to quit. Only about 15 per cent were offered assistance by a doctor and only 3 per cent had a tobacco addiction follow-up visit. Yet a 3–10 minute counselling session by a doctor results in about 16 per cent quitting.[8]

Nicotine vaccine

Animal experiments have shown that nicotine vaccination works. A nicotine vaccine substantially reduces the rewarding effects of nicotine but also prevents nicotine relieving the distress of nicotine withdrawal. It sequesters nicotine in the bloodstream, preventing it entering the brain. It may have fewer side-effects than drugs such as buproprion, which work directly on the brain. In addition, it may be most effective for relapse prevention in those trying to kick the habit.

Advertising and smoking bans

Smoking is responsible for about 20 per cent of deaths in Britain. From April 2003, cigarette advertising on hoardings and in the media was banned in Britain. "Light" and "mild" cigarette brands are also banned as their names are purposely misleading and aimed at the youth market. Ministers in the UK aim to cut the number of young people smoking from 13 per cent in 1996 to 9 per cent by 2010. Eleven per cent of girls and 8 per cent of boys are regular smokers.

Commenting on the difficulties in implementing smoking reduction measures, the former Health Minister Alan Milburn has said "if there's one thing I know and have learnt over the course of the last five or six years, it is that the tobacco industry will be absolutely relentless in delaying and preventing any measures which are necessary to protect the public". The EU Court of Justice in December 2002 upheld the ban on the use of the words "light" and "mild" on cigarette packs. There are also limits on levels of tar, nicotine and carbon monoxide in tobacco smoke. The ruling followed an appeal by Imperial Tobacco Group and British American Tobacco against the EU directive on the manufacture, sale and presentation of tobacco products. This is a most welcome blow to the tobacco lobby.

Here in Ireland, in response to the Report on the Health Effects of Environmental Tobacco Smoke from the Health and Safety Authority in January 2002, and the recommendations of two separate reports from the Oireachtas Committee on Health, smoking will be banned in all workplaces, including restaurants, pubs, nightclubs, trains, taxis, and all public service vehicles from February 2004.

Alcohol and tobacco

Evidence of the detrimental effects of smoke on public service workers is wide-ranging. Irish bar workers have up to 20 times more metabolised nicotine in their bodies than non-smokers. Environmental tobacco smoke killed 150 bar workers in Ireland in 2002. Passive smoking in pubs cannot be dealt with by ventilation unless a breeze is created. Even with air displacement ventilation, which is the most effective space cleanser, exposure levels 1,500 to 2,500 times the acceptable level for hazardous air pollution remain. Seventy per cent of pub customers and bar workers do not smoke.

In Australia, a pub worker received AUS$500,000 compensation for tobacco-related illness from the pub owner. In Spain, the regional government in Andalucia filed a lawsuit against six tobacco companies that control more than 90 per cent of the Spanish market. They are seeking €1.77 million to pay for the Andalucian health service costs of treating 135 patients with smoking-related diseases in 2001. If compensation is not offered, the claims will ratchet up to €306 million, about 9 per cent of the Andalucian health service's annual budget.

More bad news for the tobacco industry from Malaysia is the ban on advertising. In place for nine years, the ban is being tightened in 2003 to include sports events because more than half the adult males and 35 per cent of adult women smoke. Cigarette companies spend US$26 million on indirect advertising campaigns there.

In Budget 2003 in Ireland, the price of cigarettes rose by 10 per cent making a pack of 20 John Player cigarettes retail at €5.71. True to form, the tobacco industry described the increase as an unfair burden on smokers. In my view, the whole tobacco industry is an unfair burden on society. Minister Micheál Martin has cast a blow for the rights of people to work in and frequent public hostelries without being poisoned. When the prohibition on pub smoking was announced, Frank Fell of the Licensed Vintners Association claimed that because 45 per cent of drinkers smoke, the ban would hit the trade hard and tourism would also be affected. He also warned of serious political fall-out. These are nothing more than vacuous, predictable threats!

Solutions

1. All countries (including the US) should sign the 2003 Framework Convention on Tobacco Control (FCTC), sponsored by the World Health Organization. The text covers tobacco taxation, smoking pre-

A Cure for the Crisis

vention and treatment, illicit trade, advertising, sponsorship and promotion and product regulation.

2. The Irish 2004 smoking ban in public places, including pubs, clubs, workplaces and public transport must be enforced.

3. Taxes on cigarettes must be ratcheted up to reduce sales.

4. Tobacco should be removed from the consumer price index calculations.

5. The EU must be stopped from subsidising tobacco farmers to the tune of €1 billion annually.

6. EU anti-smoking campaigns must be stepped up. Currently only €18 million is spent on this health priority. The gap between sponsoring a death-wish habit and discouraging it is stark. It is shame on the European bureaucracy and the politicians, especially in France and Spain.

7. Smoking advertisements and sponsorships must be banned in Europe. By July 2005, Member States will have to comply with a general ban on tobacco advertising in print media, radio and on the internet. This law will also ban tobacco sponsorship of Formula One motor racing.

8. Anti-smoking treatments should be made available at minimum cost.

9. Anonymised graphic images of smokers dying from lung cancer, emphysema and coronaries, and of gross specimens of lung tumours, etc. should be printed on cigarette packages, etc.

10. The next never-smoking barman who gets lung cancer should sue the employer and other responsible organisations.

11. The Health and Safety Authority should close pubs and clubs that do not enforce the smoking ban as smoking is a health risk to staff.

12. Personal responsibility for one's actions and their consequences regarding smoking, alcohol and drugs should be underlined. They may be fashionable but are not sexy, healthy or a good thing.

13. Doctors should identify smokers at every visit, urge them to quit, determine their willingness to try, aid with a plan, counselling, medications and educational materials, and schedule a follow-up contact.

27

Mental Health Act Ireland

Doctors have always had grave concerns about psychiatric services and, at last in 2001, a new Mental Health Act was passed. The Act was summarised by my colleague Dr Brian O'Shea in the *Irish Medical Journal*.[1], in which he noted the legal changes in respect of admission orders, time limits, duration and renewal of admission orders, consent to treatment and finally bodily restraint and seclusion.

Admission orders can be made where:

- The person is likely to cause immediate and serious harm to self or others.
- Judgement is so impaired that without admission significant deterioration is likely or appropriate treatment would not be possible.
- Admission would materially help the patient or alleviate the disorder.

Time limits:

- The applicant must have seen the subject not more than 48 hours before applying.
- The doctor making the recommendation must examine the patient within 24 hours of receiving the application.
- The recommendation is valid for seven days.
- The decision to detain at an approved centre must be made within 24 hours.

Duration and renewal of admission orders:

- Initially to last for 21 days.
- Can be renewed for up to three months.
- Then can be renewed for up to six months.
- Then can be renewed for periods of up to 12 months at a time.

A Cure for the Crisis

- A Mental Health Tribunal's decision on admission must be made within 21 days.

Consent to treatment:
- Free and informed consent should be the norm.
- Treatment can be given without consent if the patient is incapable of giving consent.
- Psychosurgery requires written consent from the patient and authorisation from a tribunal.
- Electroconvulsive therapy (ECT) requires written consent from the patient and by two consultant psychiatrists, one being the treating consultant.
- After three consecutive months of giving drug therapy, written consent from the patient for further such treatment is required or it can be authorised by two consultant psychiatrists, one being the treating consultant (three-monthly renewal thereafter).

Bodily restraint and seclusion:
- Subject to rules to be made by the Mental Health Commission.

Criticism of new legislation

In response, a critical viewpoint was written by Dr BD Kelly.[2] It addresses two key issues – involuntary detention and mechanisms for assuring standards. The Act does not detail the procedure for voluntary admissions to hospitals nor does it define a minimum standard of care entitlement. Persons admitted involuntarily will be reviewed by a Mental Health Tribunal consisting of a consultant psychiatrist, a solicitor or barrister and another person, within 21 days. The criteria for the selection of the third person are not defined. These tribunals will be appointed by a Mental Health Commission whose remit is the maintenance of high standards and good practice in the delivery of mental health services. The Commission is to protect the interests of the detained person. It will consist of 13 people – one barrister or solicitor, three doctors including two psychiatrists, two nurses, one social worker, one psychologist, one member of the general public, three representatives of voluntary bodies and one representative of the CEOs of the health boards.

172

The Mental Health Commission will be responsible for the administration of the legal aid scheme involving the tribunals, the registration of approved centres (an accreditation function) and the appointment of an inspector of mental health services. The inspector must visit mental health services on a yearly basis and can take evidence under oath. A doctor can make a "recommendation" for involuntary admission of a patient.

Patients have been given explicit rights to information regarding their detention and review and to automatic legal representation at a tribunal. Personality disorder, social deviance and substance abuse are not grounds for involuntary admission per se. Gardaí can enter a premises by force if necessary, where there are serious concerns about a patient and can be requested to escort a detainable person to an approved centre.

Consent is also addressed and involuntary inpatients sign a consent form for psychiatric medication, which has continued for longer than three consecutive months. There is an automatic review of involuntary status. However, there is need for clear guidelines about confidentiality.

The policy has been to move patients into new units or out into the community. There are 18 new-style units in place and there are developments due in Beaumont Hospital, St Vincent's University Hospital, James Connolly Memorial Hospital, Blanchardstown, Portiuncula Hospital, Ballinasloe, and Nenagh, Portlaoise and Sligo Hospitals.

There are serious resource and logistic shortcomings with the new legislation. In 1999, there were 2,729 involuntary admissions to Irish psychiatric hospitals or inpatient units.[3] According to Dr Kelly, "If 60 per cent of these are still inpatients after 21 days, there will be 1,637 Mental Health Tribunal hearings for these patients in any one year. If involuntary status is maintained for three months, a further hearing is necessary."[4] This may result in about 2,000 tribunals per year. This has resource implications for psychiatrists in clinical practice but is an excellent development. However, who will cover the psychiatrists when the tribunals are in session?

Protection of patient rights

The Mental Health Tribunals should provide a forum to protect the rights of the patient and provide a platform for patients to express their views, however unwell and psychotic they may be. New Zealand has a similar system with a judge present to make final decisions based on the

A Cure for the Crisis

contributions of the patient, the family, psychiatrist, nurses, social workers and other stakeholders. The Tribunal can discharge the patient, allow the admission order to run its course, or extend the order by periods of 14 days. The patient or solicitor can appeal the Tribunal's findings to the Circuit Court within 14 days of the decision. A medical or nursing member of staff can hold a voluntary patient for up to 24 hours, if deemed necessary. The patient must then be either discharged or have a second consultant opinion.

Making use of pyschiatric patients in clinical trials is also covered under current Irish legislation: "Notwithstanding section 9(7) of the Control of Clinical Trials Act, 1987, a person suffering from a mental disorder who has been admitted to an approved centre under this Act shall not be a participant in a clinical trial."

The stipulations on consent for psychosurgery are a good innovation as they protect all involved. I would also suggest that prisoners with psychiatric conditions are not overlooked. There are so many mentally ill prisoners that a special effort should be made to improve mental health services in prisons.

28

Exercise and obesity

In the past 10 years, there has been an alarming rise in obesity worldwide. Ireland is by no means an exception to this trend. The North/South Ireland Food Consumption Survey conducted by the Irish Universities Nutrition Alliance investigated habitual food and beverage consumption, health, lifestyle and demographic information, attitudes to food and health, restrained eating patterns, physical activity and anthropometric measurements in a representative sample of 1,379 adults aged 18 to 64 during 1997–1999. The sample was representative of the population as a whole with regard to age, sex, location, social class, marital status, and socioeconomic group.[1]

- The prevalence of obesity was 20 per cent in men and 15.9 per cent in women.
- A further 47 per cent of Irish men and 33 per cent of women are overweight.
- Since 1990, obesity has more than doubled in Irish men and increased from 13 per cent to 16 per cent in Irish women.
- The highest prevalence of obesity (30 per cent) was in women aged 51 to 64 years.

Lack of exercise

Physical inactivity is now the most common risk factor in cardiovascular disease, being responsible for one-third of cardiovascular deaths every year. It is more of a problem than smoking or obesity and is responsible for about 45 per cent of strokes and 33 per cent of colon cancer deaths. Inactive adults are also at increased risk of hypertension, coronary artery disease, diabetes, osteoporosis, various cancers, anxiety and depression. A decrease in activity of only 10 kcal per day can add a pound in weight per year. This can cumulate to be significant.

A Cure for the Crisis

The mechanism underlying the benefit of exercise is unknown but it may result from increased insulin sensitivity in muscles and other tissue. Exercise has positive cardiovascular effects outside of weight loss. It increases the size and decreases the amount of the "bad" LDL (low-density lipoprotein) cholesterol and increases both the size and amount of the "good" HDL (high-density lipoprotein) cholesterol. The intensity of exercise is not as important as the amount. Those jogging for 20 miles per week were better than those doing 12 miles per week.[2]

Physical activity levels are low among Irish adults. Almost one-quarter of people in Ireland take no exercise at all. Men spent 1.7 hours per week in vigorous recreational pursuits compared with 1.0 hour per week for women. Both men and women spent 19 hours per week watching TV. Men were twice as physically active at work than women. About 25 per cent of adults spent at least 25 hours per week watching TV. Walking was the most popular exercise, where 41 per cent of men and 60 per cent of women walk at least once a week. Gardening and floor exercises are the next most popular. One-quarter of our national "couch potatoes" do not even want to try to get fit.

Obesity

Obesity is also associated with an excess risk of colorectal cancer in males, breast and ovarian cancers. Weight loss is associated with a worsening of gall stone disease. Fatty liver from obesity is not a benign entity. Obstetric complications include the development of diabetes, impaired glucose tolerance, pregnancy-induced hypertension, pre-eclampsia, thrombophlebitis, postpartum haemorrhage and wound infections. Macrosomia (birth weight >4,000 g) in the baby is also common as are labour problems.

Body mass index (BMI: weight in kg ÷ height in metre^2) of around 21–22 is associated with the lowest mortality. The risk of death doubles at a BMI of 29.0 to 31.9. The BMI at 18-years-old predicted overall and cardiovascular mortality in middle age.[3]

Benefits of 10 kg weight loss in a 100 kg subject are:[4]

- Mortality   20–25% reduction in premature death
- Blood pressure   10 mmHg reduction in systolic pressure
                   20 mmHg in diastolic pressure

Exercise and obesity

- Angina   Reduced symptoms by 91%
             33% increase in exercise tolerance
- Lipids   10% reduction in total cholesterol
             15% reduction in LDL
             8% increase in HDL
             30% reduction in triglycerides
- Diabetes   Reduction in risk of type 2 by 50%
             30–50% reduction in elevated blood glucose
             15% reduction in glycosylated haemoglobin

In Britain, the government's belief is that up to one-third of cancer and heart disease could be prevented by a better diet. At present, treating ill health from obesity costs the NHS £2 billion each year.

Worldwide, there is a worrying rise in obesity. Rates of overweight and obesity have increased 2.3-fold to 3.3-fold over 25 years in the US, 2- to 2.8-fold over 10 years in England, and 3.9-fold over 18 years in Egypt. In China, the number of overweight men has tripled in eight years and doubled in women with hypertension rates similar to the US. In Egypt, 50 per cent of women are overweight and the rate of diabetes is similar to the US. In Mexico, overweight and obesity are 35.2 per cent and 24.4 per cent among women, respectively, where the diabetes rate is the same as the US. In Tanzania, overweight and diabetes rates are rising. Clearly, obesity is a global health crisis.[5]

Lifestyle changes

Lifestyle changes can prevent the development of diabetes in high-risk people. Doctors can do this for patients by following the prescription of the Finnish Diabetes Prevention Group, which successfully used individual counselling aimed at reducing weight, total intake of fat, and intake of saturated fat and increased intake of fibre and physical activity. Average weight loss was about 3.5 kg in the intervention group compared to 0.8 kg in the controls. In people with impaired glucose tolerance, after 3.2 years' average follow-up, 11 per cent of the intervention group had developed diabetes compared to 23 per cent of the comparison control group.[6] This is a 58 per cent reduction in the incidence of diabetes. Thus, we should make every effort to address obesity in patients.

A Cure for the Crisis

Childhood obesity

Childhood obesity could be prevented and treated by the following measures:

1.	Mothering	Encourage breastfeeding.
2.	Home	Set aside time for healthy meals and physical activity, limit TV viewing.
3.	School	Fund mandatory physical education. Impose strict standards for school lunches. Remove soft drinks and sweets, bars, etc. from vending machines. Provide healthy snacks as an alternative.
4.	Urban design	Preserve open spaces. Build footpaths, cycle lanes, playgrounds and pedestrian zones.
5.	Healthcare and media	Improve insurance cover for effective obesity treatment. Encourage GPs to target obesity.
6.	Marketing	Add a tax on fast food and soft drinks. Subsidise fruit and vegetables. Require nutrition labels on fast food packaging. Ban fast food marketing directed at children. Increase funding for public health campaigns for obesity prevention.
7.	Politics	Regulate political contributions from the fast food industry.

These suggestions are to prevent the spiral of childhood obesity. A type 2 diabetes epidemic with heart attacks in the paediatric age group is possible, if we ignore the inexorable trend of obesity worldwide and at home.

Breastfeeding protects against the development of obesity in children and adults. It is also associated with lower blood pressure, improved cognitive development and other benefits.[7] Television campaigns should encourage its use. In this respect, soap opera discussion of the subject could be effective.

29

Cardiovascular Strategy: Building Healthier Hearts

Ireland has one of the highest rates of cardiovascular mortality in Europe, with almost one in two deaths attributable to heart disease. About 25 per cent of deaths from heart disease are caused by smoking. Smoking cessation reduces the risk of recurrence of heart attack by 50 per cent in two years and is the most avoidable factor. For this reason, it is disgraceful that cigarettes form part of the consumer price index. In effect, it prevents governments vigorously taxing the cancer sticks due to the Maastricht Stability Pact corset.

Fuel smoke is also a major factor in the global burden of disease. Tánaiste Mary Harney's order in 1990 banning the marketing, sale and distribution of bituminous smoky coal in Dublin has earned her a place amongst those who have struck an effective blow to improve the health of the population. Dr Luke Clancy's collaborators have shown that the coal ban has resulted in about 116 fewer respiratory deaths and 243 fewer cardiovascular deaths per year in Dublin since 1990.[1] Clearly, this ban must be extended to all urban areas in the country.

Secondary prevention

The report of the Cardiovascular Strategy Group "Building Healthier Hearts" recommends (R6.21) "secondary prevention of most patients with cardiovascular disease should be provided in the general practice setting". The Department of Health and Children along with the Irish College of General Practitioners (ICGP) and the Irish Heart Foundation have started the initial implementation phase of the National Programme in General Practice for the Secondary Prevention of Cardiovascular Disease, called the "Heartwatch Programme". The patient groups targeted are those with a proven history of myocardial infarction, coronary artery bypass surgery or coronary angioplasty and, I presume, stents. The overall aim is to reduce morbidity and mortality due to cardiovascular disease.

A Cure for the Crisis

In excess of 60 per cent of the population visit their GP in any one year and 95 per cent do so within the course of five years. Patients will be recruited from GPs' practices using disease registers from computerised lists where they exist, from a review of practice records or opportunistically or through drug data at local pharmacies or hospital discharge records. The specific objectives are:

- To examine the baseline levels of risk factors and therapeutic interventions relevant to secondary prevention and their trends over time.
- To examine the processes involved in implementing the programme, including the referral process and patient retention.
- To record the incidence of cardiovascular events in patients participating in the programme.

The methods used will be four visits to the GP per year with a protocol to be followed. The Strategy reckons on 30-minute consultations and will involve a GP and a practice nurse. Data will then be returned to an independent national data centre. The GPs are selected from 20 per cent of the national total of 2,200 current full-time equivalent GPs.

Parameters
- The patient to live as full and active a life as possible.
- To record blood pressure, smoking, cholesterol and produce a risk score.
- To review diet, exercise and obesity.
- To record the adequacy of diabetic control where relevant.
- To review current medication, compliance and the need to prescribe.
- To intervene as appropriate or arrange referral for intervention by other specialist services based in the practice, the hospital or the community.

The IMO negotiated a deal in which the GPs are paid €1,250 on entry to the programme. Then there is a €50 payment for each of the four quarterly visits for GMS patients and an additional €50 bonus where greater than 80 per cent of all data items are compiled and returned accurately. There is a national quota and, when reached, doctors will be told that no further patients will be recruited. Each practice has to recruit at least 15 patients to the programme. There is a formal contract with the health

Cardiovascular Strategy: Building Healthier Hearts

board involved, one of whose stipulations is, "where the CEO of the Board has reason to believe that the care of any eligible person is being put at risk or that the General Practitioner is in material breach of any term of this Agreement, the CEO may carry out such investigation as is warranted by his suspicion".

Cardiovascular end points to be notified include fatal or non-fatal myocardial infarction, stroke, heart failure, non-cardiovascular mortality including sudden or unexpected cardiovascular-related hospital admission, revascularisation, cardiovascular-related referral to outpatients, new or recurrent angina and other cardiovascular events.

The aims of this programme are to implement and evaluate the first phase of a structured programme of secondary prevention of cardiovascular disease. It will adhere to internationally recognised cardiovascular prevention guidelines – *Prevention of Coronary Disease in Clinical Practice 1998* from the Second Joint Task Force of European and Other Societies on Coronary Prevention. The guidelines will be used to:

- Determine the risk factors to be used in follow-up.

- Determine the interventions to be pursued to achieve control.

- Determine the clinical events to be monitored for the purpose of evaluating progress.

The targets for risk factors and intervention are shown in Table 29.1.

Table 29.1 Cardiovascular risk factors and intervention

No.	Risk factors	Intervention
1	Smoking	Cessation
2	Systolic blood pressure	140 mmHg
3	Diastolic blood pressure	90 mmHg
4	Total cholesterol	<5.0 mmol/L
5	LDL cholesterol	<3.0 mmol/L
6	HbA1c	<6.5%
7	Exercise	>210 min/week (3.5 hrs+)
8	Body mass index	<25 kg per m^2
9	Waist circumference	<94 cm in male, <80 cm in female
10	On aspirin	Unless contraindicated
11	On betablocker	If indicated
12	On ACE inhibitor	If indicated
13	On lipid lowering	If indicated
14	On antihypertensive	If indicated

A Cure for the Crisis

Consent must be formal to enter the programme. This should include a careful explanation and written information. The practice must also agree to a call and recall system for all patients within their practice who are recruited to the programme. The GP will agree to abide by the clinical protocol agreed for this programme. The apparent need to train GPs for the study comes as a surprise, given that the exercise appears to be standard clinical practice.

There are no details on how weight reduction is to be achieved – if medication is involved, e.g. is sibutramine contraindicated? Will fish oils be part of the diet and what are those details? A recent paper on exercise training on sedentary overweight men found a mean compliance of 86 per cent with a "high amount" exercise regime of 200 minutes per week. The actual amount of time spent exercising was 174±35 (mean±sd) per week. Exercise affected the HDL and the sizes of the LDL, VLDL (very low density lipoproteins) and HDL in a positive direction, but has no effect on the total cholesterol or LDL values without reducing weight.[2] Increased insulin sensitivity is likely to be a central mediator of the beneficial effects of exercise.

Protocol shortcomings

There are a number of problems with this protocol. First, the biochemical parameters measured are following a 1998 protocol – ancient history in the face of the relentless progress of evidence for therapeutic intervention in cardiovascular disease. Serum B_{12} or folate status, whether red cell folate or serum folate, are not included. Neither is HDL – an important omission. Is the measure of triglycerides inferred as the values are often used to calculate LDL? The recommended blood pressures for diabetics, which are lower than the figures used in the table, are not specified. Current blood pressure targets in diabetics recommended by the American Diabetes Association are <130 mmHg systolic and <80 mmHg diastolic.[3] The target values that are quoted for lipids in diabetics are shown in Table 29.2.

Table 29.2 Target lipid values in diabetics

Lipid	Target value (mmol/L)
LDL cholesterol	<2.60
HDL (men)	>1.15
HDL (women)	>1.40
Plasma triglycerides	<1.70

Cardiovascular Strategy: Building Healthier Hearts

However, in Britain, the Medical Research Council/British Heart Foundation (MRC/BHF) study commented on using target values of LDL cholesterol where under-treatment may occur:

> .... current guidelines may inadvertently lead to substantial under-treatment of high-risk patients who present with LDL cholesterol concentrations below, or close to, particular targets (such as the 3.0 Second European Joint Task Force or 2.6 ATP 111 guideline)... In this trial, a 1 mmol/L reduction in LDL cholesterol from about 4 mmol/L to 3 mmol/L reduced the risk of major vascular events by about one quarter, but so too did reducing it from about 3 mmol/L to 2 mmol/L.[4]

Best practice is just that. Thus, as the project was started from scratch in September 2002, the protocol should have been amended. Who will publish this work? What group will the effects be measured against? Should not all patients with proven coronary artery disease not have their lipids lowered, be put on homocystine lowerers,[5] and after a myocardial infarction be placed on a statin, aspirin or warfarin, an ACE inhibitor, betablocker and possibly niacin if their HDL is low?[6]

Schynder *et al.* found that by using folic acid 1 mg, B_{12} 400 mg and pyridoxine 10 mg daily, the degree of renarrowing after angioplasty was reduced from 48.2 to 39.9 per cent, and the rate of restenosis was reduced from 37.6 to 19.6 per cent, while the need for revascularisation of the target lesion was down from 22.3 to 10.8 per cent. Some impressive improvement for such a simple non-toxic remedy! In the simvastatin and niacin paper, the average stenosis progressed 3.9 per cent with placebos, 1.8 per cent with antioxidants and 0.7 per cent with niacin plus antioxidants and simvastatin, but regressed with niacin plus simvastatin on their own. The frequency of clinical end points was 24 per cent with placebos, 21 per cent with antioxidants on their own, 14 per cent in the group with simvastatin plus niacin plus antioxidants and 3 per cent with simvastatin plus niacin on their own. Most consumers would have one of the latter and perhaps B_{12} and folate and pyridoxine.

The laboratory aspect has also not been addressed. Where and how are the cholesterol and LDLs going to be measured? If "point-of-care-testing" is being used, what are the analytical standards required for use of the machines? By which method is the HbA1c going to be measured? LDL is often derived from the Friedewald equation, but can be measured directly. Targets for LDL cholesterol vary from <3.0 in Europe to <2.6

183

A Cure for the Crisis

from the National Cholesterol Education Programme in the US. In the MRC/BHF-HPS study, a 1 mmol drop in the LDL led to a 25 per cent reduction in the relative risk of coronary heart disease and strokes overall. Clear benefits were also seen in those with LDL below 2.5 mmol/L. Reducing the LDL from 2.5 to 1.7 mmol/L was safe using simvastatin, where it produced a risk reduction about as great as that seen among those presenting with higher LDL concentrations.

There are even problems with the aspirin part of the study. Short-term use of aspirin and long-term use of oral anticoagulants are effective in patients who have had a myocardial infarction. Compared with placebo, antiplatelet treatment with aspirin reduces vascular events by 25 per cent after myocardial infarction, and long-term treatment with coumarins (warfarin) reduces vascular events by 35 per cent. The ASPECT-2 study has shown that:

> In patients recently admitted with acute coronary events, treatment with high intensity oral anticoagulants (INR 3.0–4.0) or aspirin with medium intensity oral anticoagulants (INR 2.0–2.5) was more effective than aspirin (80 mg) on its own in reduction of subsequent cardiovascular events and death. The end point was reached in 9 per cent on aspirin, 5 per cent on anticoagulants and 5 per cent on the combination. Major bleeding was 1 per cent on aspirin and anticoagulants and 2 per cent on the combination. Minor bleeding was 5 per cent with aspirin, 8 per cent with anticoagulants and 15 per cent with the combination.[7]

The additional benefits of clopidogrel are ignored. This drug reduces the relative risk of ischaemic stroke, myocardial infarction or death from vascular causes by 8.7 per cent as compared to aspirin alone. In acute coronary syndromes, clopidogrel plus aspirin reduced the risk of death from vascular causes by 20 per cent over aspirin alone.[8]

In support of the Cardiovascular Strategy study protocol are the data conveniently summarised in a *Lancet* commentary (see Table 29.3).[9]

184

Cardiovascular Strategy: Building Healthier Hearts

Table 29.3 Potential cumulative impact of four simple secondary-prevention treatments

Treatment	Relative risk reduction (%)	2-year event rate (%)
None		8.0
Aspirin	25	6.0
Betablockers	25	4.5
Lipid lower by 1.5 mmol/L	30	3.0
ACE inhibitor	25	2.3

Smoking cessation lowers the risk of recurrent myocardial infarction by about 50 per cent. To calculate cumulative risk reduction, multiplicative scale is used. Two interventions each reducing the event rate by 30 per cent would be expected to have about 50 per cent relative risk reduction $[1-(0.70 \times 0.70)]$. No interactions in treatment effects are seen in trials suggesting that proportionate risk reduction of specific drugs in the presence or absence of other effective interventions would be expected to be similar. Therefore, a smoker with vascular disease who quits and uses the four drugs would expect around an 80 per cent reduction in relative risk.

It is my belief that all GPs should try to ensure that all cardiac patients have their lipids done, are prescribed statins, betablockers, aspirin or warfarin and ACE inhibitors as part of their professionalism. Smoking cessation with the use of all aids, including Zyban, is a priority. They should also have the niacin, B_{12}/folate cocktail as above. This is an obvious first audit in practices. I do not believe that GPs should accept fees for entering patients into a programme that should be standard care anyway.

Unquestionably, the pace of evidence-based change in cardiology is phenomenal. For example, it is now clear that the discontinuation of statins after the onset of coronary symptoms leads to an increased risk of death from coronary events (adjusted hazard ratio 2.93 per cent).

Summary

- Update the protocol.
- The ICGP should organise its own audit of all practices for secondary prevention and other screening activities such as thyroidism.
- Be professional – do not accept extra payment for what one should be doing anyway.

A Cure for the Crisis

- Seek out all "at risk" patients in one's practice by doing fasting blood glucose in all candidates, as 50 per cent of type 2 diabetics are undiagnosed in the community and obesity is increasing quickly in the Irish population.

- Statin therapy is expensive but, as can be seen from the findings of Schnyder *et al.*, the benefits are undoubted. Much of the cose discussion is based on cost. The side-effect profiles of simvastatin and pravastatin are minimal. Liver-enzyme rises in the MRC/BHF study were 0.09 per cent with simvastatin and 0.04 per cent with placebo. Muscle aches occurred in 32.9 per cent of simvastatin-allocated and 33.2 per cent of the placebo-allocated patients. However, there were rare cases of severe myopathy with simvastatin.

Secondary prevention of heart disease survey

Some Irish figures for secondary prevention were recently published from the TCD Medical School Group and Dr Emer Shelley in the Department of Health and Children.[10] They found that since 1994, more patients now smoke, take no exercise and are overweight. The prevalence of type 2 diabetes has increased by 70 per cent. Certainly, we can improve medical therapy but we must focus more on lifestyle intervention. The figures in Tables 29.4 and 29.5 are baselines for considering the progress and outcome of the new Cardiovascular Strategy. The 2000 European and Irish figures are taken from the EUROASPIRE II Study of 2000.[11]

Table 29.4 Comparison of the prevalence of risk factors and physical activity in Irish patients in 1994 and 2000 and in 15 European countries in 2000

Risk factor	Ireland 1994 (%)	Ireland 2000 (%)	Europe 2000 (%)
Smoking men	19	26	22
women	19	30	18
BP >140/90 mmHg	48	48	50
Overweight BMI >25 kg/m^2	60	75	79
Obese BMI >30	–	27	
Diabetes	7	12	28
Cholesterol >5.0 mmol/L	68	54	58
Regular strenuous activity	2	5	18
Irregular/infrequent non-strenuous activity	89	80	72
No exercise	9	15	10
Rehab programme	16	54	43

Sources: TCD Medical School Group/Department of Health and Children. EUROASPIRE II Study Group, 2000

Table 29.5 Comparison between drug therapy used in secondary prevention in Ireland in 1994 and 2000 and in 15 European countries in 2000

Drug therapy	Ireland 1994 (%)	Ireland 2000 (%)	Europe 2000 (%)
Statins	18	62	61
Betablockers	15	47	63
Aspirin	85	92	86
ACE inhibitors	27	27	38

Sources: TCD Medical School Group/Department of Health and Children. EUROASPIRE II Study Group, 2000

Emergency care

Emergency medical technicians are still unable to administer emergency cardiac care drugs more than two years after a Government strategy recommended that they be allowed to do so. Dr Vincent Maher, medical director of the Irish Heart Foundation, has criticised the Government's inaction: "This is despite the fact that at least half of patients dying of fatal coronary heart disease are dead within two hours of the onset of symptoms, a fact recognised by the Cardiovascular Strategy."

Two observational studies from Britain, the United Kingdom Heart Attack Study (UKHAS)[12] and the Southern Heart Attack Response Project (SHARP)[13] can be used to illustrate how reckless this inaction is. Overall in the 3,972 patients who received medical care, resuscitation was successful in 257 (6.5 per cent) and fibrinolysis prevented death in 63 (1.6 per cent). In both studies, about 80 per cent of lives saved were attributable to resuscitation from cardiac arrest and about 20 per cent to fibrinolytic treatment. Of the patients whose lives were saved by resuscitation, 36 and 39 per cent respectively had had their first arrest outside hospital and so *owed their lives primarily to the ambulance service.* These results show the superiority of resuscitation from cardiac arrest over fibrinolytic treatment in terms of lives saved, at least for the first 1–4 weeks after the onset of a heart attack. Fibrinolytic treatment has been estimated to save twice as many lives, if given in the first hour after the onset of symptoms.

The time-dependent figures for fibrinolytic therapy in heart attack are 65 lives saved per 1,000 patients treated within the first hour of onset of chest pain, 37 per 1,000 for those treated in 1–2 hours after the onset of pain, 29 per 1,000 for those treated in 2–3 hours, 26 per 1,000 in 3–6 hours, 18 per 1,000 in 6–12 hours and 9 per 1,000 in 12–24 hours after

A Cure for the Crisis

onset. An average figure is 30 lives saved per 1,000 patients, which means that delays in treatment are commonplace.[14] In the UKHAS and SHARP trials only 2 per cent of patients received thrombolysis. A European Society of Cardiology working party concluded that only about 55 per cent of patients with myocardial infarction were eligible for thrombolysis.

In 1992, the Grampian Study (GREAT) was the first trial to show a significant reduction in mortality with prehospital treatment in the UK.[15] At one year, the absolute difference between home-treated and hospital-treated groups was 11 per cent. The time saved by GP home injection was over two hours because of the rural setting. Eleven years later, rural GPs in Donegal were the first in the Republic to put this evidence into practice.

Primary angioplasty

Meta-analysis has shown that for every 1,000 patients treated with primary angioplasty (a catheter with an inflatable balloon fed into the blocked blood vessel in the heart) rather than thrombolytic therapy, an additional 20 lives are saved, 43 reinfarctions are prevented, 10 less strokes occur, and 13 intracranial haemorrhages are avoided.

Even with the huge organisational efforts required for a policy of primary angioplasty, the strategy of prehospital fibrinolysis with accelerated alteplase (with transfer to an interventional facility for possible rescue angioplasty) has been shown in a French study to be equally as good as primary angioplasty in the treatment of early (within six hours) myocardial infarction. The death rate was 3.8 per cent for prehospital fibrinolysis and 4.8 per cent with primary angioplasty.[16] Thus, the case for early clotbusters by paramedics is unanswerable. In the French study, there was a doctor in each rescue mobile emergency care ambulances with ECGs and defibrillators.

In Ireland, I could not see that measure being possible, but using paramedics on a protocol is likely to save lives, as would the use of early aspirin. In all likelihood, there will be delays in treatment using primary angioplasty in routine hospitals, and we are causing unnecessary deaths at present by the delays in implementing the policies as agreed. Delays to primary angioplasty in the US are about 2 hours and 1 to 1.5 hours in Europe. Some hospitals in Ireland are now using primary angioplasty when staff are available. Angioplasty has been shown to reduce the composite rates of death, reinfarction or stroke compared to tissue plasmino-

Cardiovascular Strategy: Building Healthier Hearts

gen activator, even if it took three hours to reach the intervention centre. Primary angioplasty is a superior method of reperfusion for evolving acute myocardial infarction. This was reinforced by meta-analysis of 23 randomised trials which concluded that primary angioplasty is more effective than thrombolytic therapy for the treatment of ST-segment elevation acute myocardial infarction.[17]

Dr Gregg Stone put the current cardiology case strongly when he wrote in *The Lancet:*

> Thus, until the large trials of facilitated PTCA are completed (none of which have even begun enrolling), the best therapy for most patients with evolving acute myocardial infarction should no longer be debated: administer antiplatelet therapy (aspirin, thienopyridine and possibly abciximab), withhold thrombolytic therapy and transfer the patient for primary percutaneous coronary angioplasty regardless of whether the nearest catheterization suite is three floors or three hours away. To do less should no longer be considered standard care. Strong words, yes, but it is time for a wake-up call.[18]

Subsequently, a randomised trial of 1,572 patients comparing angioplasty to accelerated treatment with alteplase clotbuster concluded that transfer of patients with a heart attack for angioplasty is superior, provided the transfer takes two hours or less.[19]

The use of sirolimus-eluting (drug secreting) stents in therapeutic angioplasty reduces the overall rate of major cardiac events from 26.6 per cent with standard (cheaper) stents to 5.8 per cent with the sirolimus stents.[20] Stopping the use of the latter stents was on the well-publicised list of Beaumont Hospital potential cuts in the spring of 2003. That, as well as the threat to dialysis services, explains the public medical uproar at the time. Thus, we have some way to go in Ireland to have a world-class health service.

Cardiac arrest and public access defibrillation

The majority of cardiac arrests occurs at home but up to one-quarter occurs in public places and are often witnessed by trained personnel who attempt resuscitation. The survival rate is almost 100 per cent, if ventricular fibrillation is treated immediately. After a delay of 4 to 5 minutes, the survival rate decreases to 15 to 40 per cent and after 10 minutes or longer, 95 per cent die. As most cardiac arrests are unpredictable, it is wise to have defibrillators available and to encourage bystanders to use

A Cure for the Crisis

them. There are automatic external defibrillators which are designed for use by minimally trained users. They cost about $2,500 each. All restrictions on their usage should be removed in the interests of saving lives and they should be available in shops, public buildings, small businesses and along thoroughfares, analogous to lifebelts hanging on side walls or placed on the banks of rivers and lakes.

The experience at O'Hare Airport in Chicago had added evidence that bystanders with no previous training can use these defibrillators safely and effectively. This calls into question the requirement for formal training. Defibrillators were installed throughout passenger terminals at O'Hare, Midway and Meigs Field Airports in Chicago, which together serve more than 100 million passengers per year. The use of defibrillators was promoted by public service videos in waiting areas, pamphlets and media reports. Over a two-year period, 21 people had cardiac arrest, 18 with ventricular fibrillation. With two exceptions, defibrillator operators were Good Samaritans, acting voluntarily. In four of the patients with ventricular fibrillation, defibrillators were not used within five minutes and the patients died. Three others remained in fibrillation and eventually died, despite the use of a defibrillator within five minutes of the collapse. Eleven with ventricular fibrillation were successfully resuscitated and eight of these regained consciousness before hospital admission. No shock was delivered in four cases of suspected cardiac arrest and the device correctly indicated that the problem was not due to ventricular fibrillation. The rescuers of six of the 11 successfully resuscitated patients had no training or experience in the use of automated defibrillators, although three had medical degrees. Ten of the 18 patients with ventricular fibrillation were alive and neurologically intact at one-year follow-up.[21]

Another study showed that sixth-year school students, after reading nothing more than the instructions included with the device, were able to deliver a shock in a clinical mock-up after 90 seconds which is only 30 seconds longer than it took emergency medical personnel to administer a shock.[22] Interestingly in Ireland, eight of the customer care staff at Blanchardstown Town Centre were trained in public access defibrillation at the local hospital. This was the first such venture in Ireland. At present, Dublin Airport and Blanchardstown have portable AED (automated external defibrillator). In September 2003, the West of Ireland Cardiology Foundation, *Croí*, planned to install public access defribillators at seven locations. The first two will be located at Galway Airport and Galway Shopping Centre.

190

Cardiovascular Strategy: Building Healthier Hearts

Inhospital treatment

Cardiology audits were published from Our Lady's Hospital, Navan[23] and St James's Hospital, Dublin[24] on the management of heart attacks. At St James's Hospital, the fatality rate was 16 per cent, confirming the higher mortality in clinical practice than in thrombolytic trials. Revascularisations went up from 34.9 per cent in 1992 to 72 per cent (5 per cent primary angioplasty, 67 per cent thrombolysis) in 1996–99. Aspirin or warfarin were given in 99 per cent and betablockers in 67 per cent in line with international trials, and ACE inhibitors in 34 per cent and statins in 28 per cent, which could be improved upon. The cost has risen by 51 per cent with angiography or angioplasty gone from 32 to 50 per cent, but the hospital bed stay has fallen from 11.9 days in 1994 to 7.8 days in 1999. Efficiency and technology developments have increased costs. The costs in 1999 were IR£3,976, taking operative costs into account for those needing coronary bypass surgery.

In Our Lady's Hospital, Navan, the period studied was 2000 and the inhospital mortality was 12 per cent. At discharge, aspirin was prescribed for 81 per cent, betablockers in 41 per cent, statins in 35 per cent and ACE inhibitors in 44 per cent. Women were less likely to be given betablockers. Thrombolytics were administered to 93 per cent of eligible cases, up from 70 per cent in 1998. In discussion, the authors state:

> This study highlights the failure in implementing in everyday practice the evidence from clinical trials that identify the most effective drug treatment. There is evidence of the potential to achieve even better long term outcome with a secondary prevention policy that utilizes proven effective drug treatments.

It is almost certain that these hospitals will improve their performances in the immediate future. Indeed, GPs are well placed to correct omissions in post-infarction drug therapy.

Solutions

1. Defibrillators with simple instructions should be placed prominently in public thoroughfares like Grafton Street and O'Connell Street in Dublin, shopping centres, airports, railway stations, and in all other urban areas in the State.
2. Cardiopulmonary resuscitation courses should be widely available for the public.

A Cure for the Crisis

3. Television and press campaigns to demonstrate the use and benefits of this innovation and to ensure the public acceptance of lay-person use must be a priority.

4. Legal and administrative barriers need to be abolished. Liability protection for all users will have to be safeguarded.

5. In some rural areas, ambulance crews should be trained to follow an emergency drug injection protocol for heart attack to save more lives. They should be indemnified by the State and rewarded for their skills.

6. GPs on emergency calls and out-of-hours co-ops should consider giving emergency thrombolysis where appropriate, unless there is a local hospital policy of primary angioplasty.

7. 24/7 primary angioplasty should be the standard of care for those with heart attacks in all our large general hospitals and for those within a two-hour transfer time.

8. The roles of aspirin, clopidogrel, warfarin, betablockers, statins, ACE inhibitors and analgesia must not be ignored.

9. Patients should be given a discharge protocol, preferably agreed by the Irish Cardiac Society/Irish Heart Foundation, explaining the use and evidence for rehabilitation, and drug therapies after heart attacks.

10. GP surgeries should have a supply of these protocols to give to patients and to ensure that their patients are being optimally treated and educated.

11. The impact of the protocols should be audited and the results published.

30

Screening for disease

Screening is defined as tests done among apparently well people to identify those at an increased risk of a disease or disorder. Those identified are usually offered a test or procedure or a treatment or a preventive medication. Looking for additional illnesses in those with medical problems is called case finding. However, screening per se is limited to the apparently well. Undoubtedly, screening can improve health. Beneficial examples are cervical cytology, blood pressure in adults, screening for hepatitis B, syphilis and HIV in pregnant women, urine culture at 12 to 16 gestation, galactosaemia, thyroid-stimulating hormone (TSH), phenylalanine and other amino acids in newborns.

There are also downsides. Screening can have false positives as well as false negatives with unfortunate consequences in both directions. Women labelled with gestational diabetes reported deterioration in their health and that of their infants over the five years after diagnosis. Clofibrate treatment of hypercholesterolaemia led to a 17 per cent increase in mortality in middle-aged men given the drug, resulting in more than 5,000 deaths in the US alone. Prostate biopsies are recommended for a high prostate specific antigen (PSA), but sometimes no cancer can be found. Screening can be unpleasant often involving sigmoidoscopies and colonoscopies. In assessing the results of screening, there are also the questions of lead-time bias (in breast cancer) and length bias.[1]

If one gets a clinical specialist society together, the question of recommending screening for their diseases is sure to come up. Using a computer model to assess cost-effectiveness, the American Thyroid Association has recommended TSH screening using a sensitive laboratory method every five years in patients older than 35 years.[2] However, the American College of Physicians recommends thyroid screening in women older than 50 years, but not in older or younger men.[3]

A Cure for the Crisis

Cancer treatment

There are now 16 oncologists in Ireland compared with three only seven years ago. Twenty-five per cent of all inpatient and day cases in the ERHA are taken by cancer patients and the cost of drugs has risen from €10 million in 2000 to €15 million in 2002. Almost half of the cancer treatments nationwide in 1999 were carried out in the Eastern region, with almost 50,000 discharges recorded in that year. The ERHA Public Health Department estimate that the death rate from cancer in that area decreased by 8 per cent in men and 9.7 per cent in women between 1992 and 1999. Death rates from breast cancer decreased by more than 20 per cent, while hospitalisation for breast cancer treatment increased by 45 per cent.

St James's Hospital, Dublin has 34 oncology beds and claim that they need 80. At their day unit, 1,100 patients were treated per month in 2003 compared with 400 per month only four years ago.

Waterford Regional Hospital is the regional centre for oncology in the South East, serving a population of 40,000. Yet it has no oncology ward, only 12 designated oncology beds, no palliative care beds, no pharmacy facilities for constituting chemotherapy and no radiotherapy.

Approximately 22,000 cancer cases occur in the country every year, of which 11,000 should have radiotherapy but only 6,000 can be treated. Dublin and Cork are the only places with treatment facilities at present, so obviously people in other regions have the added burden of extensive travel placed upon them. Clearly, regional cancer treatment centres are needed. The issue was addressed in the Report of the Expert Working Group on Radiation Oncology Services published in October 2003. Treatment centres were recommended for Cork, Galway and two for Dublin.

Prostate cancer

Due to prostate specific antigen (PSA) screening, the lifetime risk of a diagnosis of prostate cancer is about 16 per cent, whereas the risk of death from prostate cancer is about 3.4 per cent. This is because prostate cancers have a slow doubling time of about three years or more and the diagnosis is often made in older men who die from another disease. In England and Wales, 1 in 13 men is affected and death rates have trebled over the last 30 years. Even though prostate cancer is common, only 5 per cent is hereditary. In England, less than 10 per cent are diagnosed by screening. Most present with symptoms and the median age of presentation is 72 years. The natural history of prostate cancer is variable and

Screening for disease

unpredictable. However, early prostate cancer is often diagnosed by rectal examination. Digital rectal examination (gloved finger in rectum) is insufficient for screening as its positive predictive value is only 11 to 26 per cent.[4]

As a general statement, PSA is raised in prostate cancer, prostatitis (inflammation of the prostate) and in around 30 per cent of people with benign prostatic hypertrophy. PSA testing has false negatives and false positives. In the US, the incidence of prostate cancer in white men has doubled from about 55 per 100,000 in the period 1983–87 to 110 per 100,000 in 1993–95. About 75 per cent of the cancers would not have been diagnosed without screening. It is unclear whether such screening has improved survival, because US death rates have fallen both in high and low PSA screening rate areas.

The downsides of PSA testing are the side-effects of aggressive treatment (incontinence and impotence). In addition, if PSA is positive and cancer is diagnosed, there is anxiety associated with a false positive result and the burden of dealing with cancers that otherwise might never have become evident. A PSA has a sensitivity of 46 per cent for identification of prostatic cancer occurring within 10 years, where the specificity is 91 per cent.

The probability of a raised PSA was 5 per cent among men in their 50s, rising to 25 per cent among men in their 70s. The probability of prostate cancer remained about 30 per cent, given that the age-related increase in the prevalence of prostate cancer was inversely proportional to the decline in the specificity of the test. PSA detected 45 per cent more cases of cancer than digital rectal examination alone, whereas digital rectal examination detected 18 per cent more cases of cancer than PSA test alone. Each test detects cancers missed by the other.

Traditionally, a PSA of 4 ng/ml has been used as an upper limit of normal. However, biopsies on men with PSA values of 2.5 to 4.0 and normal digital rectal examination found prostate cancer in 12 to 23 per cent. Men with suspicious findings on rectal examination and a PSA of 4.0 or less have a probability of cancer of at least 10 per cent and biopsy is usually recommended. As a result of the PSA test being suboptimal, about 74 per cent of men undergoing a prostate biopsy because their PSAs are from 4.0 to 10.0 do not have cancer. To improve the specificity, three PSA measurements over one year can be done and this will give a better indication.

Free PSA can also be measured because prostatic cancer is associated with a lower percentage free PSA than benign prostatic hyperplasia. The

A Cure for the Crisis

probability of prostate cancer at biopsy among men with a PSA value of 4.0 to 10.0 with normal digital rectal examination ranged from 56 per cent with a free/total PSA ratio of up to 10 to 8 per cent of men with a ratio more than 25 per cent. Nonetheless, 8 per cent of men with a ratio over 25 per cent still have prostatic cancer, so is there a real role for the measurement of free PSA/total PSA ratio? If one intends to biopsy those with risks of 8 per cent or greater, then the answer is no. When prostate cancer recurs after radical prostatectomy, the rise in PSA precedes symptoms by a median time of eight years except for those symptoms caused by the knowledge of the increased PSA.[5]

There is mathematical evidence for screening at 40–45–years old every two years and stopping at 65 for those with persistently low values and at 75 for the rest. Convention is to offer the test to those between 50 and 75 years. However, there is no published randomised trial answering the question of whether screening for the early detection of prostate cancer has a clear benefit or harm. Currently, there are two trials underway. The US trial is due to report in 2009, while the European trial is expected to be completed between 2004 and 2009.[6]

Until then, national screening programmes should be put on hold. That should be borne in mind when one hears proponents of PSA screening pushing their views on TV and radio. The American Cancer Society supports PSA testing, however, in asymptomatic men 50 years or older and in younger men with established risk factors.

Table 30.1 Estimated probability of prostate cancer in men with normal digital rectal examination according to the PSA level

PSA level (ng/ml)	Probability of prostate cancer (%)
0–2.4	Uncertain
2.5–4.0	12–23
4.1–10.0	25
>10.0	>50

For clinically localised prostate cancer, a 1994 report found that watchful waiting had the same survival result as those who had radical surgery, and also to that of an aged matched population without prostate cancer.[7] As you can see, prostate cancer is a medical minefield.

Radical prostatectomy for localised prostate cancer will in many cases remove the risk of death from the disease, but how can this procedure be justified in otherwise healthy men? After surgery, 2–5 per cent of men

Screening for disease

will have severe incontinence and 10 to 90 per cent will become impotent with an average of about 70 per cent.[8]

Breast cancer

Breast cancer accounts for about 4 per cent of all deaths annually. However, even a 21 per cent reduction in breast cancer mortality as claimed in some trials will not have much of an effect on all-cause mortality. The risk of breast cancer increases with age and the one in eight lifetime risk is the lifetime risk for a newborn who lives for 90 years. At least half the women given a diagnosis of breast cancer survive, regardless of the use or non-use of screening. From politicians like Dr Gerry Cowley to professors like Niall O'Higgins, the public have the impression that screening mammography will save lives. This fact is axiomatic and indisputable. But is it true? Where is the evidence?

In 2000, Gøtzsche and Olsen reviewed the mammography trials using the Cochrane Library Data Base and published their report in *The Lancet*.[9] Cochrane was selected as it is an organisation that commissions detailed analyses on numeric data. Having identified eight trials, the authors claimed that six studies had baseline imbalances and four had inconsistencies in the number randomised. Only two were adequately randomised.

New York study

The New York study involved pairs of women matched and the pairs randomised. The patients were allocated thus: every nth woman was placed in the study group and the paired (n+1) woman was placed in the control group. This should ensure equal numbers in both groups, however, the numbers of women in the study group were "about 31,000", i.e. 30,000, 30,131, 31,092, 30,239 and in the control group the figures published were 30,756, 30,765 and 30,565.

There were post-randomisation exclusions – if breast cancer was diagnosed before the trial entry. Thus, status was ascertained more fully for the screened group. The final cohort was 30,131 v 30,565. Therefore, there was *bias in favour* of the screened group. There were highly significant imbalances for previous breast lump ($p<0.0001$) and menopause ($p<0.0001$) and less so for education ($p<0.05$). Consequently, there was inadequate randomisation.

A Cure for the Crisis

Edinburgh study

Patients from 87 GP practices were cluster randomised and the allocation was later changed for three. The screening and control groups dif-
fered significantly. At baseline, only 26 per cent of the control group but
56 per cent of the screened group were in the higher social class group.
Randomisation was inadequate even for clusters.

Canadian trial

All 39,405 women were randomised individually and were recruited from
January 1980 to March 1985. Names were entered successively on allocation lines and the intervention noted in each line. Randomisation could
have been subverted, but possible subversion was reviewed and they concluded that there could not have been enough cases to affect the results.
There was no data on age distribution. However, both groups were similar at baseline for lumps, family history of breast cancer, number of live
births, menopause, education, birthplace and marital status.

Malmö trial

Each birth cohort was randomised by computer program and those on
the first half of the lists were invited for screening. No baseline data were
available. Malmö II is a follow-up but cannot be used because follow-up
data from the original trail is mixed with new data and some were not
randomised. As a result, Malmö II is not suitable for meta-analysis.

Stockholm study

In this study randomisation was by birth date. Women born on 11–20th
of any month were put into the control group. Inexplicably, the control
group was increased from 19,943 to 20,651. Exclusions should lead to a
decrease. The age difference in the study group was 0.18 years younger
than the controls ($p=0.006$ Mann–Whitney test). The conclusion is that
there was inadequate randomisation.

Göteborg study

Randomisation was partly by date of birth (18 per cent) and partly individual. The study group was significantly younger 0.09 years ($p=0.02$). It
is reasonable to conclude that the randomisation may have been inadequate.

Screening for disease

Kopparberg and Östergötland study

The population was divided into 19 blocks and then subdivided into two or three groups by unspecified criteria. These groups were then randomised by an unstated method, possibly cluster randomisation. In Kopparberg, the study group was 0.45 years older than the controls ($p<0.0001$), i.e. this is a highly significant bias in favour of more tumours in the study group. Similarly, the Östergötland study group was significantly 0.27 years older ($p<0.0001$). The numbers randomised to the study groups were 39,034 or 38,491 in Östergötland and the total numbers in the two trials were 134,867 or 133,065. What was the problem in counting?

Swedish meta-analysis

The mean age of the screened group was 55.05 compared to the controls, 54.54 years. The standard deviation of the ages in the Swedish group is 10 years. These are very wide and disparate age spreads. The age difference is highly significant ($z=12.7$, $p=3\times10-37$). There was a highly skewed distribution incompatible with a truly chance distribution to either group. The data showed that screening lowered the mortality by 29 per cent in women aged 50 to 69 years.

The conclusion was that only the Malmö and Canadian trials were unbiased. Both had adequate randomisation and consistent numbers of patients (see Tables 30.2 and 30.3).

Table 30.2 Malmö and Canada studies: adequate randomisation

Study	Screened	Controls	Deaths in screened group	Deaths in control group	Relative risk (95% CI)
	66,013	66,105	183	177	1.04 (0.84–1.27)
Malmö	21,088	21,195	63	66	0.96 (0.68–1.35)
Canada	44,925	44,910	120	111	1.08 (0.84–1.40)

Table 30.3 Randomisation NOT adequate

Study	Screened	Controls	Deaths in screened group	Deaths in control group	Relative risk (95% CI)
Göteborg	11,724	14,217	18	40	0.55 (0.31–0.95)
Stockholm	40,318	19,943	66	45	0.73 (0.50–1.06)
Kopparberg	38,589	18,582	126	104	0.58 (0.45–0.76)
Östergötland	38,491	37,403	135	173	0.76 (0.61–0.95)
New York	30,131	30,565	153	196	0.79 (0.64–0.98)
Edinburgh	22,926	21,342	156	167	0.87 (0.70–1.08)
Total	182,179	142,053	654	725	0.75 (0.60–0.83)

A Cure for the Crisis

In these trials, Gøtzsche and Olsen claimed that the mammography screening was futile. Not surprisingly, it gives rise to scepticism about such screening programmes here in Ireland.

In 2000, the Canadian National Breast Study 2 was published in the *Journal of the National Cancer Institute* by Miller for the study group.[10] These were 13-year results of a randomised trial in women aged 50–59 years, which did not show any benefit for screening. All were taught breast self-examination. One group had mammography plus a detailed 10-minute breast examination. The other group had a detailed 10-minute breast examination only. At the first annual screen, the differences were that 21 per cent of cancers were greater than 20 mm when found by mammography alone; 46 per cent of cancers found by physical examination in the mammography plus physical examination group were greater than 20 mm; 56 per cent of cancers found by physical examination alone were greater than 20 mm. Finding smaller cancers did not make any difference to the 13-year outcome. The authors reached the following conclusion: "In women aged 50–59 years, the addition of annual mammography screening to physical examination has no impact on breast cancer mortality."

Conclusions

However, just when you have reached your own conclusions, Dr Lennarth Nyström and colleagues published an updated overview of the Swedish mammography trials to 1996 and concluded that breast cancer benefits started to emerge at four years and continued to increase for 10 years. In the *Lancet* he claimed that the "recent criticism against the Swedish randomised controlled trials is misleading and scientifically unfounded".[11] Dr Peter Gøtzsche came back with a vigorous mathematical riposte four months later.[12] He concluded by stating that "a meta-analysis from independent researchers is therefore crucial, based on the raw data from all the screening trials, using total mortality as the primary outcome". This strikes me as slightly illogical. Why write that, if you really believe that the randomisations were truly and meaningfully incorrect? A 2003 clinical practice review of mammography in the *New England Journal of Medicine* by Fletcher and Elmore concluded that the Gøtzsche/Olsen criticisms had been answered: "In-depth independent reviews of the criticisms concluded that they do not negate the effective-

Screening for disease

ness of mammography, especially for women older than 50 years of age."[13] I remain sceptical.

The downside is that about 11 per cent of screening mammograms are read as abnormal. Breast cancer is found in about 3 per cent of abnormal mammograms (0.3 per cent of all mammograms). On average, a woman has a 10.7 per cent chance of a false positive result. After 10 mammograms, about 49 per cent will have had a false positive result, which will have led to a needle biopsy or an open biopsy in 19 per cent of cases, according to Fletcher and Elmore. There is also the possibility of false positive diagnosis of breast cancer; however on balance, diagnosis of even ductal carcinoma *in situ,* which has an excellent outlook, is an advantage because some progress to invasive cancer.

BreastCheck Ireland

BreastCheck screening mammography is unlikely to be available nationwide until September 2004 at the earliest, when the planned units in the west at University College Hospital Galway (UCHG) and in the south at the South Infirmary Hospital, Cork open. Total annual operating costs for the programme will be €21,285,328 at a cost of €73 each for the screening and diagnosis of 291,232 women in the national target population. The Health Boards Executive took over the management and governance of BreastCheck in March 2003.

Geography plays a role in breast cancer treatment, which is a national disgrace. While 40 per cent of patients nationally have radiotherapy, only 24 per cent have radiotherapy for breast cancer in the Western Health Board area. By November 2002, Michael Kelly, secretary general of the Department of Health and Children, claimed that 65,011 women had been screened, which constituted 74 per cent of the relevant group.

My conclusion is that every woman should have a detailed regular physical breast examination and any suspicions should be seen by a specialist breast surgeon. And I certainly would not march on Dáil Éireann for BreastCheck. In the midst of this, however, there is some good news in the form of a reduction of nearly 30 per cent in breast cancer mortality since 1990. How much is due to screening and early diagnosis and how much to better treatment is unknown. Meanwhile, the medical literature keeps publishing further data – the latest from the Östergötland and Kopparberg counties in Sweden in April 2003 claims that "mammography screening is contributing to substantial reductions in breast cancer

A Cure for the Crisis

mortality in these two Swedish counties". The details in the paper are convoluted and what one can conclude for certain is that breast cancer survival in those aged 40 to 69 years at diagnosis has improved dramatically from the period 1958–69 to 1978–97.[14]

Fortunately, the American Society for Clinical Oncology and the US National Cancer Institute are currently looking again at screening mammography. Meanwhile, we must support the oncologists in demanding better treatment of cancer patients. Also, breast cancer must be kept in perspective. Heart disease in women is more lethal by some distance. Table 30.4 outlines the chances of the development of and cases of death from breast cancer within the next 10 years in a sample of 1,000 women.

Table 30.4 Probabililty of developing breast cancer within 10 years

Age (yrs)	Cases of invasive breast cancer (No.)	Death from breast cancer (No.)	Death from any cause (No.)
40	15	2	21
50	28	5	55
60	37	7	126
70	43	9	309
80	35	11	570

Colorectal cancers

The National Cancer Registry shows that 1,900 people are diagnosed with colorectal cancer in Ireland per year and over 900 people per year die from the disease. One in 20 men and 1 in 32 women will develop bowel cancer in their lifetime. Obesity doubles the risk in pre-menopausal women.

Most tumours evolve from normal gut mucosa (the inside lining) to adenomatous polyp to invasive cancer, where survival is directly related to the extent of the disease at operation. That is why screening works in this case. Colonoscopy is the best screening method but may still miss 6 per cent of adenomas 10 mm or larger. Anybody with a first-degree relative or two other relatives with colon cancer should have a colonoscopy. The risk of colon cancer is 2 per cent with no risk factors and 1 in 17 with a first-degree relative involved. Colonoscopy should be done at 10 years earlier than the index case in a first-degree relative or at the age of 45, whichever is earlier. A recheck should be done after 10 years. If a patient has hereditary non-polyposis colon cancer or adenomatous polyposis, they should be checked every two years.

Screening for disease

The American Gastroenterology Society suggests that everyone should be screened at the age of 50. Ninety-four per cent of all cases of colorectal cancer occur in people over the age of 50 years. Symptom-free people who have no risk factors should have an annual faecal occult blood test. Many gut cancers and polyps bleed intermittently. So blood is unevenly distributed through the faeces. Occult blood tests fail to detect 20 to 50 per cent of cancers and up to 80 per cent of polyps.

The American Cancer Society recommends a sigmoidoscopy every five years, a barium enema every 5 to 10 years and a colonoscopy every 10 years. Those with a close relative with either an adenomatous polyp or a colorectal cancer should have annual faecal occult blood testing at 40 and more frequent colonoscopy.

This is clearly a resource problem, which is the reason why nurse endoscopists have been and are being effectively trained in some centres. Virtual colonoscopy using CT scanners with and without bowel preparation can be used in patients at high risk to detect polyps that are 6 mm or more in diameter.[15] I have no doubt that this and other developments in MRI technology will change the face of gut screening in the future.[16] Current practice for surveillance of colonic polyps at the Royal Infirmary of Edinburgh is available online at *www.mph.ed.ac.uk/endo/downloads/colpolguide.htm*

Flexible sigmoidoscopy is safer and less costly than colonoscopy and is often considered as a first-line screening test. However, it misses the right half of the colon where 30–40 per cent of tumours are found. There is an argument for the use of barium enema, but it only detects polyps and cancers over 1 cm in size. The risk of radiation is insignificant in older patients. Annual faecal occult blood tests supplemented by barium enema every three to five years has been suggested as the most cost-effective of a variety of screening strategies, but using colonoscopy and sigmoidoscopy can be therapeutic as well as diagnostic.[17] A single flexible sigmoidoscopy between the ages of 55 and 60 has been suggested as an effective screening strategy.[18] For those interested in the details of this excellent paper, screening for asymptomatic colorectal cancer is available at *www.bmj.com*, where Dr Diarmuid O'Donoghue from St Vincent's University Hospital is one of the authors.

A Cure for the Crisis

Cervical cancers

The lifetime risk of developing cervical cancer is 1 in 25 for Irish women and approximately 70 women per year die from the disease. It is detectable, preventable and treatable. Smear tests can detect around 90 per cent of cases. It is thought that about 60 per cent of cervical cancer deaths could be prevented by mass screening of women over 25 years. The Mid Western Health Board launched a pilot screening scheme in October 2000 to screen all women aged between 25 and 60 years at least every 5 years and paid a fee of €40.19 per smear. The Department of Health and Children agreed to extend the scheme to all GMS patients as soon as practicable. Given the class basis of the burden of this disease, the official attitude is tardy and feckless.

By 1994, cervical smears covered 85 per cent of the target population in Britain. This was a terrific achievement. Financial incentives were offered to GPs in 1990 and this increased the uptake of smears. In Britain, the intention is to screen the target group every three years. The death rate fell about 7 per cent per year through the 1990s, but there is controversy as to whether this can validly be attributed to the cervical screening programme. In a paper published is 1997, the number of new cases of invasive cervical cancer had fallen by 50 per cent in 10 years and most new cases were diagnosed at an early stage where there is an 85 to 95 per cent cure rate.[19]

Five human papilloma virus (HPV) types 16, 18, 31, 33 and 45 are responsible for most cervical cancers and there are 15 and possibly 18 high-risk types. HPV types 16 and 18 are the nastiest ones. Being a smoker, being HIV positive, having multiple sexual partners, or if the male partner has had multiple partners, having abnormal smears and having cancer of the vagina and uterus are all risk factors. In the US, most young women become infected with HPV within a few years of becoming sexually active. About 10 per cent of the HPV-infected women remain infected for five years. It is this small group that is at a greater than 50 per cent risk of developing high-grade pre-cancerous changes in the cervix or cervical cancer. Because 90 per cent of HPV infections are cleared, a test for HPV would cause needless anxiety in most women who would be reported as HPV positive.[20] The American Cancer Society recommended that HPV testing be carried out no more frequently than every three years in women 30 years or older.

Screening for disease

There is a downside to smear testing. The delay in reporting cervical smears has caused anxiety. Beaumont Hospital has a turnaround time of about four weeks at present. An "abnormal smear" result, even if followed by a negative result on recall, may cause long-term distress and anxiety, difficulties in obtaining life insurance, worries about the effect of treatment on subsequent reproductive ability and psychosexual trauma. Discussion on the details of benefits for younger women is contained clearly in a paper in the *British Medical Journal* from the UK National Cancer Registry.[21] The smear test has low sensitivity and specificity and many are technically unsatisfactory. Testing for HPV DNA is now recommended for most women with atypical squamous cells of undetermined significance.

In the future, vaccination is the likely answer. To date, HPV 16 vaccine has been shown to be effective and multivalent vaccines are being tested. HPV 16 is present in 50 per cent of cervical cancers and at least 25 per cent of abnormal smear cells. Vaccines could reduce the risk of cervical cancers by 85 per cent and reduce deaths by 95 per cent.[22] It would also reduce the incidence of genital warts and anogenital cancers. Because cancer-forming HPVs cause cancers in the vulva, penis, larynx, nasopharynx, nailbed and conjunctiva, a case can be made for vaccinating everyone.

31

Irish medical morale and job satisfaction

It is fair to say that medical morale across all categories of doctors is at an all-time low. In an Irish Medical Organisation (IMO) survey *Turning Vision into Reality* in 2000, 42 per cent of the country's doctors regretted their career choice as did a quarter of both GPs and consultants. Thirty-six per cent of female doctors and 24 per cent of males said that they would reject the career choice of medicine, if they were back at school.

Workload was a major concern of all doctors. Sixty-nine per cent were concerned at the increase in workload, while 60 per cent claimed that more productivity was being sought when they were already at full capacity. Nearly half the doctors expressed difficulties in participating in continuing medical education (CME) due to pressure of work. In addition, they cited the absence of planning at a national level as a major problem. Some 77 per cent overall were concerned by litigation and 83 per cent of GPs rated litigation a priority concern.

Twenty-two per cent of junior doctors and 18 per cent of consultants were concerned about bullying in the workplace. Consultants had experienced bullying behaviour from hospital management as well as from administrators and politicians. In my own experience, I have witnessed bullying of junior doctors by consultants and of consultants by other consultants. However, overt bullying by doctors is much less obvious than it was 20 years ago.

Ten per cent of doctors were concerned about racism in the profession. Working in Beaumont and Blanchardstown hospitals with so many foreign students and staff, I have seen racism among patients but not from the staff. Patients' over-optimistic expectations were a major problem for 52 per cent of doctors, while 30 per cent believed that they had suffered a loss of personal esteem and patient respect.

Underfunding and inadequate resources for the job undermined medical morale and also the morale of nursing, paramedical and other staff. On this point, IMO chief executive George McNeice's words are apt:

Irish medical morale and job satisfaction

"Each profession is swimming against the tide, and they can't continue to do so. There is a definite need for change, which is heightened by demographic shifts, patients' expectations, and working time legislation."

Earnings and training costs

Imbucon Ireland carried out a recent professional earnings survey of doctors, engineers, solicitors and barristers. The professional salaries are shown in Table 31.1.

Table 31.1 Professional earnings

Salary	Doctor (€)	Engineer (€)	Solicitor (€)	Barrister (€)
Starting	25,370–31,000	23,254–27,482	35,520–42,180	–
After 10 years	67,650–87,370	58,490–67,650	105,705	91,608

In addition, senior business managers average €60,947, with directors of a major function earning €90,711. Arts graduates in teaching earn €50,000 after 25 years with an allowance of €7,780 for principals. The cost of educating graduates is in excess of €9,000 per student in Medicine and Engineering, about €8,000 per Science student and €6,000 per student in Arts, Law and Business. Therefore, dissatisfaction in medicine is not down to income.

The Higher Education Authority (HEA) published education costs for the year 1999–2000. The costs in medicine do not include clinical training costs. However, they do show that the taxpayer has a legitimate interest in service return for the investment made. The same goes for dentists who recently took industrial action.

Table 31.2 Education costs 1999–2000

Faculty	Cost (IR£)	Cost (€)
Dentistry	17,283	21,945
Veterinary medicine	14,288	18,142
Engineering	6,437	8,173
Medicine	6,121	7,772
Science	5,697	7,234
Arts/Law	4,197	5,327
Business	4,041	5,131

Source: Higher Education Authority

32

Consultants: gongs and chairs

There are various motivating factors at work which drive people to work harder and compete. These vary over time and context. Now only the high fliers can enter medicine screened by the Leaving Certificate meritocracy. No buzzing chimney-hopper pilots need apply! The era of the chronic medical student drinking in Hartigans and O'Dwyers on Leeson Street is long gone.

Power, prestige and money are the modern aphrodisiacs but what ever changes? Standing in the social pecking order has an important place in society and drives many people's life choices. Medicine came to be seen as a high-prestige, high-pay job in relative terms. Now, high-flying barristers, corporate lawyers, city financial dealers and IT experts are the real movers and shakers. The autonomy of medicine has been under attack and professionalism has been undermined to some extent by strike action of junior doctors in Ireland, GPs in France and elsewhere.

Civic or academic honours

In the UK, members of the medical establishment almost invariably end up with gongs of some description – MBE, CBE, peerages, etc. Civic recognition as a substitute for money gives a prestige boost to the individual ego. It also ensures a steady stream of sycophants who are only too willing to do the bidding of civil service mandarins and politicians. In certain parts of Europe, title-itis is epidemic. You need to be Herr Professor, Herr Doktor and Direktor of something before you are considered worthy of being taken seriously.

Many years ago professors occupied the rarified academic stratum. In medicine, professors headed the major subject departments: Medicine, Surgery and Pathology were the senior chairs. There were others in Anatomy, Physiology, Biochemistry, Pharmacology, Paediatrics, Obster-

Consultants: gongs and chairs

ics and Gynaecology, Psychiatry, ENT, Microbiology (bacteriology), Public Health and Forensic Medicine.

Now there is no limit and I think that the "Professor" moniker has been devalued. UCD and TCD have a committee to evaluate the curriculum vitae of prospective candidates who can put themselves forward for elevation to a chair. You do not even need to have an endowment as "The Smelling Salts Professor of Resuscitation" now. Besides, plain doctor seems to be the new prestige title. If you're a long time in your job in Dublin without a chair, then you must be in the wrong club. Alternatively, the club might just consider you an "also ran", a mediocrity. Try the Knights or the Masons or certain golf clubs instead. You can go to the US, get your Prof title over there and import it. Then you have no need for any embarrassing scrutiny of CVs, etc. A professor in UCD, now retired, said in 1972 "call me doctor – a professor is a piano player in a whorehouse". I wonder how he knew!

Sometimes, things are not quite what they appear. Some surgeons place a high value on being members of the Council at the Royal College of Surgeons in Ireland. However, professors at the College cannot become Council members or stand for election as president. So certain ambitious surgeons have an interest in retaining their surgical misters. Undoubtedly, some of these would be otherwise enthroned on their own gold-plated chair.

The other Irish "Knighthoods" are the conferring of honorary doctorates and the "Freedom of the City" on distinguished citizens and foreigners. Gay Byrne, Michael Smurfit, Mick Galwey and many others have all been honoured academically, while Nelson Mandela, Bill Clinton and Mikhail Gorbachev can graze their sheep on St Stephen's Green. For their huge contribution to medicine, Maurice Neligan and Risteard Mulcahy are my medical candidates.

Consultant job interviews

Power, pride, jealousy and prejudice are powerful forces in moulding the attitudes and behaviour of some members of interview boards. An objective analysis of consultant appointments in some voluntary hospitals, using a mathematical model of attributes ideally required of candidates for the post together with an impact computation of the value of their publications, would make interesting reading.

A Cure for the Crisis

At an ENT academic interview, a professor on the panel suggested that any candidate who had submitted work for a higher degree should be treated as though they already had the distinction, so negating any advantage those conferred with MD/PhD/MCh might have had. Certainly, I can think of indefensible decisions in pathology, medicine and surgery where I am certain that injustice was done. Indeed, a recent appointment provoked a hospital board member to remark to me personally that the decision was scandalous. Fortunately within a matter of months, the doctor involved, at the receiving end, was appointed to an identical post in another hospital.

With the requirement for 3,500 new consultants in the near future, competition for posts is certain to lessen and controversy also. True best practice should be used in recruitment as per the intention in the Health Strategy.

Solutions

1. All consultant appointments should be structured through the Local Appointments Commission (LAC) with strong input from the appointing hospital, which must be represented by a same-specialty representative, a consultant from a related specialty and two other doctors from other areas in the hospital, one external assessor and the CEO or head of personnel with two appointments from the LAC.

2. Academic appointments that are partly public should also have a LAC input. We should stop pretending that pre-ordained bias and "reddy-ups" do not happen.

3. The methodology should be formulaic and the job description and local requirements should be the criteria used to select the particular candidate. Public appointments must be above Carlton Club black balls!

33

Scientists in medicine

Good scientists of virtually all disciplines have played pivotal roles in the development of medical investigations and treatments. At present, there are two non-medical scientific streams in hospital laboratory medicine: medical scientists (formerly technologists) and biochemists. The educational requirements for entry to training at present are similar – both require university Bachelor of Science (BSc) degrees.

The Expert Group Report on Medical Laboratory Scientists, 2001 recognised that biochemists and medical laboratory scientists performed the same jobs up to very senior levels and should have a uniform pay structure. Both require an honours primary degree as a basic entry requirement. There is a coherence in the Report but the secret benchmarking exercise in the public sector extraordinarily failed to take the observations of the Expert Group into account and recommended a 10–14 per cent increase for biochemists, whereas the medical laboratory scientists were given a ridiculous 4 per cent!

Apparently, the biochemists were linked with the group including occupational therapists and audiologists, whereas the medical laboratory scientists were a marker grade in a different group. The moral of the story is – never trust a secret deal. Somebody is always "screwed"! I am passing no judgment on the pay awards but just on the anomaly of two jobs essentially interchangeable being weighted differently. Demarcation is being eroded elsewhere in the health services, except apparently in the minds of our benchmarkers.

Solutions

1. I believe that there should be an Institute of Pathology within the Royal College of Pathologists with membership open to all scientists whether biochemists or medical scientists. The Royal College of Pathologists would then preserve the integrity of both groups.

A Cure for the Crisis

2. The Association of Clinical Biochemists in Ireland (ACBI) and the Academy of Biomedical Sciences should ultimately amalgamate. There is a difficulty because in the UK the ACB also functions as a trade union, although many of its members are also members of ASTMS. In Ireland, most biochemists are members of the trade union IMPACT, whereas the medical scientists have an association attached to SIPTU.

3. There should be a separate paramedical scientists pay spine independent of medical staff to include medical scientists, biochemists, medical physicists, dieticians, geneticists, molecular biologists and non-medical immunologists and microbiologists.

4. High fliers should receive merit awards on the basis of explicit criteria of excellence in performance and in peer-reviewed publications.

34

Continuing medical education/ continuing professional development

Professional misconduct in Bristol has raised serious questions as to how the medical profession monitors its activities. Rather than dealing with the issue in an even-handed fashion, it seems to me that the British over-react to medical scandal. Nowadays, the British medical establishment wishes to appease administrators and politicians first and deal with the problems second. They seem cowed and bullied into absurdity. Yet there is much at stake. Medicine is a long undergraduate course. It is five years plus one in pre-registration. There is also a premedical year for the sciences, unless the student is exempt. Some medical schools now have shorter, more compressed courses and others take graduate entry students.

For a consultant post, another seven years' training is required at a minimum. Most consultants are in their mid-30s when appointed. In Ireland to date, there has usually been fierce competition for most consultant posts. So having reached a certain standard of independent practice in their mid-30s, doctors must now retrain to the equivalent of a new degree every five years.

However, not having some continuing medical education (CME) or continuing professional development (CPD) programme is unthinkable. A lay assessor who was involved in 11 assessments for the General Medical Council in London, involving a range of medical specialties, wrote that doctors who were found to have seriously deficient performance in one or more areas shared the following characteristics:

- An erroneous perception that they were up-to-date and performing well.
- Little recognition of the importance of regular education.
- Lack of understanding of medical audits and their place in improving standards of care for patients.

A Cure for the Crisis

- A significantly inaccurate view that they had no need to undertake regular education because their current knowledge and skill base was good, or in some cases excellent.[1]

Public accountability and outcome audits are the best way forward. The General Medical Council has been running pilot studies on appraisal and revalidation in recent times. In their October 2002 newsletter, they identified four areas where they were short of data. These were working with colleagues, relationships with patients, health and probity. This is heading in the direction of being over-intrusive.

The control freakery in Britain is obvious in the rigid requirements for pre-approval of educational activities before credits can be gained:

> Only approved educational activities gain credit for the scheme. Physicians are required to undertake a variety of kinds of educational activities. These points are reflected in the regulations for meeting the minimum credit requirements. The CPD website has a database of forthcoming approved educational activities. Physicians are required to plan their development, both over a yearly and five-yearly cycle. This will cover both their clinical and non-clinical roles and will indicate the specific learning objectives that will form the CPD for the coming year. Approved educational activities designed to meet these objectives can then be selected.[2]

For example, for consultants, in case they are not "on message" from the establishment, the Royal College of Physicians' educational credits include the stipulation that there should be 25 non-clinical educational credits of the 250 required over a five-year period. You might call that rounding – I call it brainwashing.

Irish Medical Council and CME

The Irish Medical Council set out the framework for CME in 2002. The Medical Council has also followed the British in declaring "it is essential that the educational activity be approved in advance, that participation is verified, and that some form of audit of the effectiveness of the intervention be undertaken". The implication is that doctors are not to be trusted and have to be treated like children with sign-ins, paper trails and pre-approval to remove any spontaneity. As professionals, we must be mad.

The Medical Council stipulates that, in any one year, a maximum of 60 points is allowed with a minimum of 40 points required. At the end of the

Continuing medical education/continuing professional development

five-year period, the points will be distributed as follows – 60 per cent CME points, 20 per cent for peer review of competence, and 20 per cent for performance review. There is no peer review at present nor is there any formal inspection of audit.

CME activity is recorded by the hour. One unit is the equivalent of one unit of "real education time". This excludes travel time, meal breaks, refreshments, etc. A whole day counts as five hours, seven hours if an evening session is included. A half-day study counts as three hours.

Requirements

- A five-year CME/CPD cycle, during which doctors must accumulate 250 points, with an average of 50 points per year, to maintain their names on the specialist register.
- Clinical audit and/or peer review at least twice during the five-year CME/CPD cycle to be phased in from 2005.
- Performance appraisal for "at risk" doctors.

There are four categories for points. These are listed as five-year minima below:

1. Internal – not less than 50 points.
2. External – not less than 100.
3. Personal learning – at most 50.
4. Research, postgraduate examining, training and supervision – at most 100.

For doctors with accreditation in more than one specialty, it is recommended that at least 30 per cent of credits should be relevant to each specialty area of practice. For part-time doctors, full participation in CME is required. The same applies for doctors on leave, whether sabbatical or extended sick leave.

There is also the question of variability in the type of course. It is not acceptable to earn all the points in the same type of course. Peer review of competence will also take place. This has not been finalised but will probably occur on the basis of small groups of peers undertaking practice visits, review of protocols and case review. Valid protocols and procedures for such peer review must be developed.

A Cure for the Crisis

Consultant CME points

For consultants, the following points' quotas are in operation from 2000 to 2004. The external points requirement of 20 per year is interesting. Some systematic audit of practice activity with effective peer comparison would be included. The audit must be meaningful and associated with a strategy to affect change, if appropriate. Is this on top of the points or does this activity count as points? As the system has been introduced for most doctors in January 2003, the CME points section was the only part ready to go, therefore, 40 of those points for everyone is the minimum.

There may be 20 personal learning points per year (a joke valuation – some doctors do that in a bad month). Perhaps a little research, maybe for some of us! The odd five points for a peer-reviewed publication! I am being sarcastic. Listening to some of the external material that counts for points is dreadfully boring. I am and would be much better off studying the *New England Journal of Medicine, The Lancet, Clinical Chemistry* or *Annals of Clinical Biochemistry.* Where does the other 40 per cent for peer review and audit come in? The Medical Council intends to phase these in from 2005, if there is covering legislation.

The Royal College of Physicians of Ireland (RCPI) stipulates that "external CME usually requires study leave or protected time and is not part of the participant's routine or everyday work. It is likely to include, for example, attendance at regional/national/international conferences and workshops, external courses and seminars, etc". This has financial implications. Who pays? At present, consultants with the common contract are entitled to €1,270 per year with a rollover. This is likely to be inadequate for many who will have to fund some of their activities themselves. The RCPI notes quite sensibly that meetings which are not formally accredited may be accepted as valid CME activity. Such cases should be recorded in the annual return; if in any doubt they can be discussed with the education office. In a later circular, this is defined thus:

> In order to have CME credits awarded, the delegate should send evidence of attendance, and details of the programme to the Education Committeee, Royal College of Physicians of Ireland. If approved, confirmation of the number of CPD credits awarded will be sent to the delegate.

There is an obvious anomaly here. Under Category E, Research, only five points are allowed for the preparation and publication of any one peer-

Continuing medical education/continuing professional development

reviewed article. Most of us who try to do research work consider this paltry allocation a joke.

Activities which do not qualify for CME include "lecturing which has not involved substantial new learning". To lecture properly, it is necessary to stay up-to-date. The purpose of the CME/CPD activity is to stay current. Also "articles in peer-reviewed journals, chapters in books, reports and official documents where new learning and substantial writing has not been undertaken by the author" are disallowed. This is illiberal and mistaken. If you write an editorial for the *Irish Medical Journal* or a commentary for *The Lancet,* is that not requiring new learning? Learning itself is always new, even it is relearning what you have forgotten! With this accreditation system, I can envisage organisational problems in the Irish health services for consultants in hospitals with low numbers of doctors. How are they going to get the required time to stay up-to-date?

GP CME points

For GPs, I consider the 50 CME points per year as an over-requirement. Ten hours are allowed for personal studying. GP meetings are not usually held during the periods from the end of May to mid-September, the three weeks over Christmas and the two weeks at Easter, which leaves about 32 weeks for the accumulation of CME meetings points. This is more than one hour every week even in the middle of an epidemic. It is not feasible and will have to be negotiated to sensible levels. Single-handed GPs in rural areas will be particularly affected and life will be made impossible for them. In fact, this issue will have to be resolved before the new Medical Council legislation is enacted. Revision of the legislation on registration of doctors, nurses and other health professionals has a target date of 2003 in the Health Strategy.

CME and CPD are necessary but the details of how these should be implemented need greater thought and flexibility. At the very least, the system has to be minimalist and user friendly. It should also be based on professionalism and trust. Up to 2002, participation in CME/CPD had been voluntary and approximately 12 per cent of those eligible had complied with CME/CPD requirements at the RCPI.

A Cure for the Crisis

The big stick

It is interesting to note that the following stipulation is also made: "external meetings – certificates of attendance/registration receipts/scientific programmes are **required**" [their emphasis]. "If a doctor who is audited cannot produce confirmatory documentation of his/her CME record, a certificate of compliance with CME will not be issued by the College until satisfactory evidence of CME is forthcoming." The consequence will be loss of specialist registration.

Solutions

1. Reduce the minimum requirements to 200 CME points in five years. External minimum should be 80 and internal minimum should be left at 50. This would encourage the reluctant to attend hospital medical conferences and audit meetings. It would also allow steps to be taken to remedy obvious clinical problems.

2. If 250 points in five years is immutable, then the suggestion of the Irish Hospital Consultants' Association that the distribution should be CME/CPD (40 per cent), peer review (20 per cent), performance review (20 per cent) and the remaining (20 per cent) flexible. This is a more adult requirement.

3. Reduce GP points to 30 CME per year with a peer review audit of issues set out in cycles by the ICGP. It is most unwise to set an unattainable goal.

4. Practice audits should be limited to one per year.

5. Video conferencing should become an acceptable norm and qualify for a significant number of the points required. This would be useful for some overseas meetings. It would also provide an easy link for rural and single-handed GPs.

6. Distance learning should be formally recognised as part of the scheme.

7. MCQs like the *CPD Bulletin* approved by the Royal College of Pathologists could be used as a template for CPD points. Three credits can be gained per issue.

8. Peer reviews for GPs should concentrate on the treatment of the major life-shortening diseases in the first instance.

35

Salaries and economic incentives

In 1988, the then editor of the *New England Journal of Medicine,* Dr Arnold Relman, wrote a commentary on the consequences of the change in medical earnings from fee-per-item to a salary. At that time, about 35 per cent of male and 60 per cent of female doctors under the age of 35 years in the US were salaried, whereas for doctors older than 50 years, about 18 per cent of men and 30 per cent of women were salaried. Relman claims:

> In principle, primary and specialized care can be more effectively integrated in salaried group practices. Education, peer review, record keeping and the reporting of clinical outcomes can also be facilitated. Freed of the administrative burden of piecework reimbursement, salaried doctors ought to be less influenced by perverse economic incentives and therefore better able to concentrate on their patients' medical needs.

> But whether these potential advantages of salaried practice are realized depends heavily on the character and objectives of the organization hiring the physicians.... When fee-for-service is used, management may pressure medical staff to run up the bill. Conversely, when payment is per capita, management may try to constrain the use of even beneficial services. In addition, organizations lacking in managerial competence are likely to make the day-to-day tasks of caring for patients harder rather than easier, whatever the payment system.[1]

Dr Relman offers the following as idealised practice guidelines:

1. Doctors, whether salaried or not, must first of all be advocates for their patients. The economic interests of the employer should not be allowed interfere with this basic responsibility. Neither should the economic interest of the physician.

2. Salaried physicians should where possible work for a self-regulated, physician-managed professional group and not be direct employees

A Cure for the Crisis

of a business organisation. This helps the precedence of proper care and professional values over the business imperatives.

3. Doctors should work only for non-profit institutions and avoid direct employment by investor-owned businesses and hospitals.

4. No doctor should enter into any arrangement offering rewards for withholding services or for increasing the use of services.

As medicine becomes more overtly business-like and industrial, Dr Relman made the following further suggestions for the guidance of conscientious physicians:[2]

1. Doctors should limit their practice incomes to fees or salaries earned from patient services personally provided or supervised.

2. Doctors in private practice should avoid any arrangement which rewards them for choosing a particular facility or service for their patients or restricts the choices they can make.

3. Doctors should avoid direct employment with a for-profit medical organisation and should be self-employed or part of a self-managed or self-regulated medical group. Doctors must give their primary allegiance to the patient and not the corporation.

4. Doctors must not enter into any deal which rewards them for withholding services from patients.

Doctors must be vigilant that their patients' interests are put first and must do their utmost to preserve their patients' trust. The Irish Medical Council's *Guide to Ethical Conduct and Behaviour* states in section 11.3 on indicative drugs budgeting that "doctors should be careful about how they exercise indicative drugs budgeting. They should continue to re-educate themselves on the principles of best practice and rational prescribing by referring to published guidelines and by availing of various continuing medical education activities". I do not believe that this item should be included in an ethical guide. The activity in its essence rewards a doctor for being below a calculated figure for drug cost per patient and the reward can be considerable in financial terms. I believe that the scheme is contrary to point 4 in Relman's guide above. Ethical guides should be above politics. When statins were proven so efficacious, their use skyrocketed, as did the expense. The Government then made these drugs budget neutral and continued the scheme. If the initial pur-

Salaries and economic incentives

pose was to induce doctors with mega drugs bills to rein in their prescribing habits, there must have been better ways to operate.

Under section 11.1 on prescribing, the *Guide* states: "...the manner in which doctors are remunerated, or the financial interest they may have in the pharmaceutical or allied industry, must not be taken into consideration when recommending therapy for their patients."

Pharmaceutical companies have been stellar performers on the stockmarkets for years. Clearly, doctors are the major targets of their advertising campaigns. I do not believe it should be ethical for practising doctors to hold shares in the industry as it might create a conflict of interest between the financial interest of the doctor, no matter how miniscule the benefit, and the best drug for the patient. As a practising physician, one would be better informed regarding the potential impact of new drugs and thus able to make informed stockmarket choices in that area.

For-profit medicine in the US

Malfeasance may be a problem when the profit motive surpasses professionalism. The US Department of Justice is investigating whether some of the cardiac surgery performed at the Redding Medical Center in San Francisco was unnecessary. In an affidavit filed in November 2002, FBI agent Michael Skeen alleged that 25 to 50 per cent of the clinic patients underwent unnecessary procedures including angioplasties, coronary bypasses, cardiac catheterisations and heart valve replacements. Tenet, the second largest private hospital group in the US, owns the facility. It has 116 properties in 17 states. Its chief operating officer and chief financial officers resigned and $17 billion was wiped off its stock value in early November 2002. The two doctors being investigated are Chae Moon, director of cardiology, and Fidel Realyvasquez, chairman of the hospital's cardiac surgery programme. The claim is that healthy patients were operated upon to claim fees from Medicare and from private health insurers.

"God heals and the doctor takes the fees"

Most illness is self-limiting and Benjamin Franklin's comment that "God heals and the doctor takes the fees" is apposite. Pages of broadsheet newspapers are taken up every week by articles and advertorial about medical services, treatments and disease. Many people have unrealistic expectations of medicine. Most think and expect that doctors can cure anything and cure it quickly. However, what should the doctor do and what should the patient realistically expect? Donald Irvine set out a list in the *Lancet,* with which I concur.[3] The doctor is expected to:

- Be clinically competent and up-to-date.
- Listen to the patient.
- Respect the patient's views.
- Treat the patient with kindness and consideration.
- Explain things clearly.
- Give advice without being patronising.
- Be honest and keep secrets safe.
- Have integrity and the confidence to admit to fallibility.
- Act in the patient's best interests and involve the patient in his/her own treatment.

CMA and professionalism

The Canadian Medical Association (CMA) issued a policy statement on professionalism in July 2002.[4] It announced that doctors could protect their professional status by "reflecting the values of the medical profession in their practice and by contributing to the efforts of organized medicine to maintain and enhance the ethic of service, clinical autonomy, and self regulation". Evidently, some physicians have not upheld the values of the profession. A few put their interests or the interests of third parties above the interests of their patients. The CMA in particular is concerned with reports of physicians sexually abusing patients, receiving gifts from pharmaceutical companies or participating in industrial actions, all of which have undermined society's trust in physicians to put the interests of patients above their own.

Many Canadians believe that doctors abuse their clinical authority "by making unilateral treatment decisions", and that educators encourage medical students to practise procedures on patients without the patient's consent. There is also the belief that self-regulation serves to shield doctors rather than to protect the public from incompetent and unethical practitioners.

Salaries and economic incentives

External threats to professionalism include:

- Financial cutbacks.
- Increasing commercialism.
- Enticements from pharmaceutical firms, such as aggressive promotion of drugs, provision of free samples, entertainment, consultancies, paid travel to conferences, payment for post-marketing "research" and other benefits.
- Market mentality within medicine in which the patient is viewed as a client or consumer.
- Governments or insurance companies or other corporate interests determining who should receive treatment because of the spiralling costs.
- Industrialisation threatens clinical autonomy where medical care is being dissected into component parts and distinct acts. Managers are assigning each act to a particular health profession, usually the lowest skilled and lowest paid who are able to perform the act. The consequence of which is that doctors lose control over their work and become a cog in the assembly line care of patients with multiple needs.

In response to the threats, the CMA urges a public campaign on the values of professionalism, improved medical education on its precepts, and more vigorous self-regulation. The medical profession must "continue to demonstrate its commitments to the tasks required by self-regulation, including setting and enforcing high standards of behaviour for both individual physicians and medical associations".

I endorse these views and the effects of financial cutbacks, commercialism, widespread drug company sponsorships of ordinary hospital meetings, the market in medicine and stripping of care into component parts with nurses, outreach clinics, hospice care, hospital clinics doing the work of primary care, which are all evident in Ireland.

As the CMA document states, many doctors deny that their relationships with drug or equipment companies compromise the independence of their judgment as to what is best for their patients or department, but research suggests otherwise. Hospitals and governments should fund inservice education to a greater degree. Physicians groups should draw up a policy procedure for hospital meetings.

A Cure for the Crisis

Solutions

1. For GPs, the Irish College of General Practitioners should have an expert committee set up to hear complaints from the GMS Payment Board about an individual practice, if their drug bills, excluding cancer chemotherapy and statins, appeared chronically excessive by comparison with peer practices.

2. Such a system would prevent progressive GPs from being penalised for being clinically effective while providing a mechanism to audit apparent anomalous practices. The grant-type aid from the central indicative drug scheme should be given to practices under new ethical criteria.

3. No doctor practising clinical medicine should hold shares in pharmaceutical companies.

4. Doctors who own an interest in equipment-supply or reagent-supply companies should declare their interest to their hospital management so that the integrity of the tender system is protected.

5. Hospital medical boards should draw up a code of practice for consultants' relationships with pharmaceutical and equipment-supply companies.

6. Doctors' fees should be displayed in their waiting rooms in the interests of clarity and open competition.

36

Medical errors

After the Blood Bank scandal, the Drogheda obstetric cases, the Rotunda Sexual Assault Unit cases and the furore over the premature birth and death of the Livingstone baby after referral from Monaghan General Hospital to Cavan General Hospital among others, medical errors are an important issue.

The Institute of Medicine in the US claimed that 44,000 to 98,000 deaths per year are caused by medical errors. US medical errors occur in 2.9 to 3.7 per cent of admissions leading to death in 6.8 to 13.6 per cent of cases. There is much controversy concerning the accuracy and implications of these findings.[1] However, there is another argument that medical errors do not cause as much damage as failure to control blood pressure properly in hypertensives or to screen for colorectal cancer in much more than half the population. Often clinical quality, cost efficiency and patient safety are regarded as in competition.

In practice, there are three main areas of medical errors, underuse, overuse and misuse. Underuse is when flu vaccines are not given to the elderly or when statins are not given to coronary patients; overuse is classically when antibiotics are given for viral respiratory infections; and misuse is when penicillin is given to a known penicillin-allergic patient.

How do we, as doctors, deal with errors?

A recent US study demonstrated the difference between doctors and the public in relation to doctors dealing with errors. Eighty-six per cent of doctors believed that reports of errors in hospitals should remain confidential, whereas 62 per cent of lay people believed that any report should be released publicly. According to the authors: "Physicians believe that confidentiality will promote openness among colleagues; lay people favour 'transparency' and the pressure of public accountability."[2] If you are in the openness and transparency camp on this issue, then you must remember the likely consequences. Doctors will be ultra-defensive and will question the validity of any data which cast doubt on their work. Lots of reasons will be offered why something was or was not done. These may be valid but not the whole story. In the US about 50 per cent of the lay public want suspension of the doctors as an effective way to reduce errors, whereas only 3 per cent of physicians felt that this was the best way to go. Also, 71 per cent of the public believed that reporting hospital errors voluntarily to a state agency would be effective, whereas only 21 per cent of doctors thought so. If medical errors of all three types can be addressed without the threat of public humiliation, the assessment is more likely to be open and honest.

There are sufficient studies published to recognise the extent of the medical error problem. A study of the incidence and types of adverse effects in Utah and Colorado in 1992, involving 15,000 patients, found that adverse effects occurred in 2.9 per cent of hospitalisations in each state. Between 27 and 33 per cent of these were judged by an independent doctor to be due to negligence. Death occurred in 6.6 per cent of all adverse events and 8.8 per cent of negligent adverse effects. Operative adverse events comprised 44.9 per cent of all adverse events, and of these 16.9 per cent were negligent and 16.6 per cent caused permanent disability. Adverse drug reactions (ADR) were the leading cause of non-operative adverse events, i.e. 19.3 per cent of all adverse events of which 35.1 per cent were negligent and 9.7 per cent caused permanent disability. Most adverse events were attributed to surgeons (46.1 per cent with 22.3 per cent negligent) and physicians (32.2 per cent with 44.9 per cent negligent). The authors' conclusion was that improving the systems of surgical care and drug delivery could substantially reduce the burden of medically caused injury.[3] A second report on the Utah/Colorado data found that adverse events were more common in elderly patients. Preventable drug side-effects, falls and procedure-related morbidity should be the focus.[4]

In Britain, more people are suing for medical negligence. Complaints to the UK General Medical Council have increased from 1,500 in 1997 to 4,500 in 2000. There are 285,000 annual medical adverse events that result in death or serious injury, of which 1.5 per cent result in a claim. The total including less serious medical adverse events exceeds 900,000, of which about 0.5 per cent sue. The UK Department of Health accepts that immediate medical treatment of the resultant injuries occupies six

Medical errors

million bed days per year at a cost of £2 billion. This is five times the annual cost of compensating the victims. The 66 per cent lower adverse rate in the US suggests to solicitor Simon John that litigation has actually made for a safer hospital environment.[5] The NHS is committed to reducing by 40 per cent the number of serious prescription errors by 2005.[6] Pharmacists at a London teaching hospital identified 88 potentially serious prescribing errors and interviewed the prescribers who made 44 of these. Inattention to detail and not following rules were the main causes, with contributing factors being the work environment, workload, whether it was their own patient or not, communication within the medical team, physical and mental well-being of the doctor and lack of knowledge. To reduce such errors, hospitals should train junior doctors in the principles of drug dosing, before they start prescribing, and enforce good practice in documentation.[7]

Good practice

Good practice should include a drug chart which stays with the patient, clear writing only, minimal transcription, and all medication orders should be checked by a pharmacist. Prescription errors could be reduced further by documenting the reason for the drug prescription in the patient's notes, detailing allergies on the chart and adhering to the hospital's prescribing policy. Community pharmacists in Ireland should be welcomed by doctors when they query a prescription detail. They are performing an important function in protecting the patient. The over-70s medical card scheme has exposed the bad handwriting of many consultants to GPs because of the requirement to rewrite the consultant prescription on a GMS form. Clearly, pharmacists are often frustrated by the illegible handwriting of doctors. Prescription computerisation in general practice will eliminate some of these difficulties. If patients attended one GP practice only, it might also help to prevent drug-induced mishap.

Undeniably, the medical profession usually avoids conflict. Doctors are busy and are orientated towards individual professional autonomy rather than towards organisational effectiveness. I do not believe, however, that doctors have earned enough trust to deal with all quality of care issues privately. Furthermore, no organisation dealing with the public should be immune from routine open scrutiny. Suppression of awkward truths and findings is mistaken.

A Cure for the Crisis

Complaints

The Irish Medical Council deals with about 200 to 300 complaints against doctors annually. In 2002, there were 241 complaints, 14 (6 per cent) of which led to a full inquiry; 148 complaints were against GPs, 75 against consultants and 13 against junior hospital doctors. Twelve related to alcohol, drug abuse or irresponsible prescribing, 52 concerned professional standards, 10 about failure to attend at surgery or a house call, 35 about communication or rudeness, 14 about failure to supply medical records, 4 about inappropriate advertising and 2 were for mental or physical disability. Some complaints are withdrawn, some are deemed not the business of the Medical Council and in the vast majority, a decision is made that the doctor has no case to answer.[8] Many are vexatious. I was privy to the correspondence in two cases and the complaints were so outrageous that I firmly believe the patients should have been countersued. However, the Medical Council has never dealt with a case where the doctor subsequently sued for nuisance, harassment and libel.

Dr Michael Johnson wrote to the *GMC News* on 15 December 2002 about a malicious complaint. He wanted the GMC to write to the doctor involved and tell the doctor that having investigated such a compliant that the GMC had found it to be groundless or malicious, and that the doctor's reputation was intact. These cases are not rare.

Variations of no-fault compensation for medical injuries have been suggested in an attempt to find an alternative to litigation. One suggestion eschews individual blame and makes the institution rather than the individual primarily responsible for an injury. It is suggested that avoidable or preventable injuries rather than negligent ones should be the focus.[9] Adverse incidents may have devastating effects on the patient and on family members, but they also have serious and underappreciated effects on the staff members involved, who should be offered appropriate support by colleagues. A report in the *New England Journal of Medicine* in 2003 highlights the impact of adverse incidents on staff:

> After making a mistake, caregivers may experience shame, guilt, and depression; litigation and complaints impose an additional burden.... doctors or nurses may become very anxious about practising clinical medicine, seek out a specialty with less direct patient contact, or abandon medicine entirely.[10]

In August 2002, new legislation in Germany makes it easier for patients who suffer ADRs to get compensation from pharmaceutical companies.

Medical errors

Patients no longer have to prove that the drug caused an unexpected side-effect. From now on, the drug manufacturer must prove that the adverse effect was not caused by the product in order to avoid paying compensation. To prove liability, patients must identify medical evidence proving that the drug can cause an ADR. The law gives patients the right to make enquiries about adverse effects before starting legal action. The manufacturer and licensing agency must respond with complete disclosure. The new law compensates patients for the cost of extra healthcare as a result of their illness. It also establishes the right to additional damages for pain and suffering even when negligence is not established. The pharmaceutical industry has protested that they should be allowed a mutual right of enquiry to get information on the claimant about previous medical history or other drugs that he/she may be taking. This seems reasonable as everyone must have the right to defend him or herself properly. The government's objective is to strengthen the position of patients and to improve enforcement of patient rights.[11]

The European Working Time Directive and the limits on work hours in the US will require better co-ordination of care, as this is a recognised risk factor in medical error. Formal structures should be developed for handovers of patients. In many cases, handovers of patients lead to the recognition of an unrealised problem by the fresh incoming doctor, which is to the patient's benefit.[12] It must be remembered that fatigue can cause depression and anger and result in detachment and a lack of compassion for patients.[13] A recent health policy report from Harvard listed seven characteristics of a successful reporting system; non-punitive, confidential, independent, expert analysis, timely, systems-orientated and responsive.[14] My tailored suggestions are the following:

Solutions

1. Hospitals should work on standard protocols for as many common conditions as practicable. These should be reviewed formally every year.
2. Formal written and verbal communication is essential as is medical team leadership.
3. Medical communication with other professional staff – nursing, social workers, dieticians, therapists, pharmacists, etc. – should be formalised.
4. Medical audit will reduce errors.

A Cure for the Crisis

5. Hospitals should have clear guidelines for discussing errors with patients and there should be an institutional policy on open disclosure.

6. Errors will be reduced by concentrating difficult procedures into high-volume hospitals where staffing levels should be optimal.

7. Errors will also be reduced by increasing the number of consultants and reducing the working time of junior doctors. All doctors make mistakes but tired doctors make more. Reduced time with patients due to heavy workloads leads to increased error as does inadequate laboratory and administrative support.

8. Any shift work should move in the day, evening to night direction which is more physiological.

9. The role of pharmacists in the defence against prescription errors should be encouraged and developed.

10. Computer-generated prescriptions will also reduce error.

11. Addressing any error as it occurs in the process of clinical care, whether it is in the portering, nursing, imaging, theatre laboratory, ICU or ward areas, will minimise recurrence.

12. Training, continuous education and development of present staff must be prioritised.

13. New staff should have an introductory apprenticeship to familiarise themselves with a new institution. The length should be determined by the complexity of the job.

14. Hospitals should link with primary care protocols to ensure continuity of care.

15. Hospital morbidity and mortality conferences should be reinstated and a review of all inpatient deaths should formally be undertaken. I believe that three members of the public should be invited to attend to preserve transparency. These people should have a two-year term of office.

16. Internal complaints against doctors should be investigated in the first instance by a committee consisting of three doctors from a panel of five nominated by the medical board of the institution (the defendant making the choice) and two lay people from a list of volunteers in the local community (again with the defendant able to object to individuals) and a member of the hospital personnel department. This committee should have the power to dismiss the complaint if vexa-

Medical errors

tious. It may decide that the complaint is relatively trivial and advise the doctor how best to avoid a reprise. If there is a minor case to answer, the committee may admonish the doctor. If the issue is more serious, then the whole case must be referred to the hospital management for formal deliberation.

17. For small hospitals, a number of nearby hospitals may be linked to achieve the same committee structure.

18. Doctors found to be making vexatious complaints against colleagues should be warned and admonished. They should be asked to withdraw unsustainable allegations and apologise.

19. Some patients deemed to have made a vexatious complaint against a doctor to the Medical Council should be sued *pour encourager les autres.*

20. Risk assessors should be available to doctors to determine what to do when the doctors consider that patients' welfare is being put at risk by the actions or often the inaction of hospital management.

21. If the risk assessors or the doctors cannot get a satisfactory response to the problem from management, this fact should be made public through medical administration in the hospital.

22. Tort changes and an amendment to the Freedom of Information Act (FoI) are needed to aid error reporting. Only documentation relating to an issue which has been judged serious should be available under the FoI.

23. A system of no-fault compensation to compensate patients where there is proof of practitioner fault should be devised.

24. Errors are often obvious in many clinical cases because the reduction of uncertainty is the core pursuit in medical diagnosis. The differential diagnosis is a list of likely causes of the patient's complaints ranked in order of likelihood. Sometimes the right diagnosis may only become apparent over time, often years. Is this process full of error? This issue can easily be reduced to absurdity. Medicine and biology teaches us humility. We often think we know but we are just scratching the surface. The question WHY? still rules OK in medicine.

37

Organ retention inquiry

The Report of the Alder Hay Children's Hospital, Liverpool followed the discovery of hundreds of retained organs of children after autopsies in 1988–95. There was a similar practice in Bristol and an investigation found that around 40,000 organs were stored in hospitals in Britain. The focus then switched to Ireland. The heart and lungs of a child were taken in 1985 at postmortem in Our Lady's Hospital for Sick Children, Crumlin and retained. In 1999, the child's mother discovered this fact and said that it had been done without the family's consent. A support group called Parents for Justice was set up in December 1999 by four mothers who discovered that a hospital had also retained organs without their knowledge or consent. Their efforts forced an investigation into how hospitals retained the organs of people after autopsy without the specific permission of relatives. The support group was reported to represent more than 1,906 parents and now has around 2,500 members. The manner in which organs were disposed also caused upset to some parents. Hospitals returned some organs to families, where requested. Burials at local cemeteries in Angels' plots were also arranged by hospitals.

The question of medical negligence in these cases is not supportable. Prof JCE Underwood of the Royal College of Pathologists (RCPath) in London explained that organ retention was conducted, not through arrogance, insensitivity or malice, but to advance the study of disease and to help bereaved families have a better understanding of the reasons for their loss.

Dunne Inquiry

In Ireland, the Dunne Inquiry was set up in April 2000 as a private inquiry chaired by barrister Ms Anne Dunne to look into postmortem practice back to 1970. This is not a very wise course of action because the procedure for postmortem examination back then was laid down in an

Organ retention inquiry

anatomical fashion. Permission from relatives was broad-ranging as the overwhelming majority of caring doctors would be reluctant to foist a discussion of the details of the autopsy procedure on grieving relatives, particularly at the time of their bereavement. No permission with formal consent is required for coroners' cases. Pathologists in practice in 1970 would have been at least 30-years-old when appointed and would now very likely be retired, nearing retirement or dead. Histopathology records may be able to reveal what the diagnosis was at the time, as formal reports are likely to be extant.

The Department of Health was concerned that the pace of progress over the first 18 months since the Inquiry began in March 2001 was so slow that the whole operation could continue for many years. The cost during that period was €4.4 million, with the chairman barrister Anne Dunne paid over €1 million. Ms Dunne and senior counsel are being paid €1,904.61 per day and junior counsel are paid €1,206.25 daily. Thus far, €1.189 million has been paid to Parents for Justice and their lawyers. In that period, 78 parents were heard and there are still 324 remaining. A similar inquiry in Northern Ireland was completed in 14 months. Parents for Justice withdrew their co-operation in November 2002 demanding that the Inquiry be placed on a statutory basis. It may cost €20 million to complete at the present pace. In Ms Dunne's Interim Report, dated 2 October 2002, 62 signed memoranda from hospitals had been received and 6 of 11 hospitals named in the terms of reference had responded. Meanwhile, the rate of hospital autopsy has fallen significantly to the ultimate detriment of patient care and medical education. The Minister is likely to ask Ms Dunne to concentrate the investigation on the hospitals and centres around the country with paediatric and maternity facilities only. This inquiry should be simple and brief.

Questions raised

Meanwhile 15 families, who claim that their deceased children's organs were removed without parental permission, have asked the Gardaí to intervene. They wish criminal prosecutions to be instigated by the Gardaí. I presume this is against pathologists or is it against hospitals?

The following questions need to be answered. Is there or was there a standard operating procedure for autopsies? The answer is yes and no. The Royal College of Pathologists in London published a detailed procedural document in 2002, openly available on their website. The Irish pathologists would normally followed these procedures.

A Cure for the Crisis

The question of what happened in the 1980s to pituitary glands collected to extract human growth hormone for therapeutic use in growth hormone deficient dwarfs and other patients needing replacement also needs clarification. Was payment made? To who and by whom? Were relatives informed? This extraction procedure occurred before the advent of recombinant human growth hormone. Was there inappropriate hoarding of organs, or body parts or tissues? If so, were these labelled? What consent was sought and given? Were all deaths of children registered? Was the coroner informed of every death from anaesthesia or within 24 hours of surgery or admission?

In 2002, the *Irish Examiner* published a comment by Ms Fionnuala O'Reilly of Parents for Justice, who said that hospitals were under investigation for failing to notify the coroner of children's deaths. They alleged that 11 hospitals were guilty of breaches of the relevant legislation. The parents have claimed that less than half of the accused hospitals have supplied the necessary information. Under the Coroner's Act 1962, hospitals are obliged to notify the coroner of any death from anaesthesia or within 24 hours of surgery. Ms O'Reilly claims there are hundreds of cases where that did not happen.[1] Furthermore, Parents for Justice intends to petition the Attorney General to order inquests, which they say should have been conducted on children up to 15 years ago.

Dr Michael Madden, Dean of the Faculty of Pathology at the Royal College of Physicians in Ireland, was also critical of the slow progress of the Inquiry and wondered why the blame should lie with any individual pathologist or hospital:

> The inquiry is private and Ms Dunne has not told us of anyone not co-operating. But I don't understand why the hospitals and people involved cannot co-operate. There is no information that is not in the public domain. We, as pathologists, do not keep information that is separate from hospital notes and the hospitals are ultimately under the control of the Minister so I'm sure he can make that information available.
>
> Once you get into an inquiry, you get bogged down in legal teams, which may be part of the reason, but I certainly don't see any reason why any individual pathologist would be in a position to withhold information.

Interestingly, Ms Anne Dunne brought her concerns that a number of hospitals had failed to co-operate with the Inquiry to the Minister in a progress report that has remained unpublished, but which was seen by

Organ retention inquiry

The Irish Times. Will the Minister take action? Fergal Bowers, editor of *irishhealth.com,* discovered that Our Lady's Hospital for Sick Children, Crumlin had sought State indemnity from all claims by parents before it participates in the Dunne Inquiry. Crumlin want an indemnity against all civil claims, including claims in defamation that might arise out of submissions or evidence given to the Inquiry, and an undertaking that any evidence given to an inquiry will not be admissible in any future legal proceedings of any kind.

In response, Minister Martin gave assurances that statements made to the Inquiry in good faith would attract qualified privilege and that the risk of being sued would be rather remote. No witness would be obliged to give statements or material which they are *bona fide* advised would tend to incriminate them. The Minister refused to give the indemnity sought, writing that he has been advised that he has no legal authority to grant an undertaking on the admissibility of evidence at any future legal proceedings.

The *Irish Examiner* reports Fionnuala O'Reilly as saying that she is not sure whether the problem is with doctors, hospitals or lawyers but she is certain that "something has become log-jammed".[2] How can there be demands for criminal prosecutions when there is such uncertainty? It does not make sense to me. Unless either Parents for Justice or Minister Martin blinks, the Inquiry seems be heading into an impasse.

In November 2002, Parents for Justice asked that the Dunne Inquiry be stood down and replaced by a statutory inquiry with the same terms of reference. In December, Minister Martin quite rightly refused. By March 2003, Parents for Justice had received €514,000 from the Department of Health for start-up costs and administration expenses in addition to €665,000 for legal expenses. They had instituted 50 High Court actions for compensation and were planning an avalanche of litigation. Damages of at least €40,000 each were being sought from the State.

In February 2003, British parents settled their cases for £5,000 and an apology in similar circumstances. If the Irish cases proceed and compensation less than the High Court threshold of €40,000 is awarded, the litigants will be exposed to the costs of the cases.

Impact on research

The Alder Hay organ scandal in England has had a very negative effect on research into children's cancer. A national tumour bank for children's

A Cure for the Crisis

cancer had been set up prior to the organ report. Donations fell from more than 200 every six months to fewer than 100 in the last six months of 2001 and are still down. The UK Department of Health has failed to come up with clear and simple guidelines about consent for the use of stored tissue, both slides and small pieces of human tissue. Pathologists had become reluctant to release stored tissue as they did not know if consent had been given. Ten of 35 approved high-quality cancer projects could not proceed because of the non-release of stored tissue. Dr Richard Sullivan, head of clinical programmes at Cancer Research UK, said "two years ago, paediatric pathologists were allowed to do their jobs but now they spend their time reading 200-page departmental edicts [Department of Health]".[3]

Consent as core issue

Consent and how informed this should be are the key issues. Society changes and expectations of information and explanations evolve. In my limited personal experience, I respect the shock and grief of relatives when a loved member of a family dies. Even where there has been family conflict, death often has the effect of instantly wiping clean much unpleasantness. Giving details of autopsy procedures in this context is difficult for doctors and for the relatives, but *now* has to be done. I have always encouraged people to agree to a postmortem in the interests of their own families. It is worth remembering that unrealised significant new information is found in about 6 per cent of autopsies. The Bristol Inquiry accused doctors of professional arrogance and being misguided. You cannot hurt the dead, however, only the living. Cultural values and ideas of body integrity evolve and medical practice must parallel such changes.

Interestingly, the Royal Victoria Hospital in Belfast defended the retention of children's organs as "standard practice". Parents were upset and accused the hospital of "playing God". There were 361 children's organs retained at the Royal Victoria and other organs were retained in other hospitals in Northern Ireland. Some were retained with consent and many without. Now explicit consent is mandatory.

I believe that paternalism has a role in medicine even though this characteristic is much criticised. Some people are deeply repelled by details of autopsies. Others are resentful at aspects of treatment by hospitals and doctors. The level of litigation in this country is an incentive

236

Organ retention inquiry

to cover-up and secrecy. Having no clinical postmortems will ensure that the 6 per cent surprising findings remain undiscovered. The quality of medicine suffers but the public and the doctors are none the wiser. Coroner's autopsies, to determine the cause of death where this is unknown, do not require consent and are now the main reason for the performance of postmortem examinations.

Our Lady's Hospital for Sick Children, Crumlin has approved new consent forms seeking approval for the use of residual human material for education and research by medical staff. One copy will be given to the parent or guardian, another will be kept by the hospital and a third will go to the pathologist.

Justification for Inquiry

In Britain, an organ retention report has been produced. Most Irish anatomic pathologists received training in Britain. Lessons for Ireland could have been absorbed at minimal cost. The question of whether there should have ever been an inquiry in Ireland is debatable. I believe that the concerns of many parents could have been addressed without an inquiry. The RCPath/Faculty of Pathology postmortem standard operating procedures could have been adopted in Ireland. Besides, new consent procedures are in operation. What is the purpose of continuing this Inquiry? Who is going to gain or lose? In the UK, the 1961 Human Tissue Act will be reformed, making it a criminal offence to ignore informed consent.

38

Aberrant clinical behaviour

...a conspiracy not a profession.... Every doctor will allow a col-
league to decimate a whole countryside sooner than violate the
bond of professional etiquette by giving him away.

George Bernard Shaw

In Ireland in the past decade, two medical scandals in particular have come to light that have undermined public confidence in the medical profession. Both involve aberrant clinical behaviour, where the health and well-being of patients was seriously compromised, with fatal consequences in some cases. The obstetric scandal in Our Lady of Lourdes Hospital, Drogheda, where unwarranted Caesarian hysterectomies were performed, and the Irish Blood Transfusion Service scandal, where large numbers of patients (mothers and haemophiliacs) were infected with hepatitis C and HIV as a result of infected blood products, serve as warning to the medical profession that its monitoring and regulatory practices were inadequate.

Unwarranted hysterectomies

Dr Michael Neary, an obstetrician/gynaecologist who worked at Our Lady of Lourdes Hospital, Drogheda, Co Louth, was found guilty at the High Court in November 2002 of unnecessarily removing the uterus of Mrs Alison Gough by Caesarian hysterectomy during the birth of her first child in 1992, when aged 27 years. She was awarded €150,000 for general damages to date, €100,000 for the future and €25,223 special damages plus costs of an eight-day hearing.

In his judgment, Mr Justice Richard Johnson found that on the balance of probabilities, Mrs Gough's bleeding could have been stopped and the surgery would not have been necessary. For a Caesarian hysterectomy to be performed on a young woman without having complicating condi-

Aberrant clinical behaviour

tions, such as cancer or placenta praevia, occurred in the region of 1 in 100,000 cases.

Dr Mary Wingfield of the National Maternity Hospital, Holles Street and Prof John Bonnar of TCD gave evidence that had Dr Neary persisted longer with conservative methods, on the balance of probabilities, the hysterectomy would not have been necessary. During the years 1990 to 1998, no first-time birth woman had a Caesarian hysterectomy in Holles Street. In his deliberation, Mr Justice Johnson said that he had had the opportunity to observe Dr Neary in the witness box and, noting the manner in which he gave evidence, the words he had used, his body language and tone, he found that he was very unconvincing in his explanations. There was "no indication whatsoever of any emergency" in the woman's medical notes. Judge Johnson found it "inconceivable" that what should have been a less than 1 in 100,000 case would not have merited a clinical note from either Dr Neary, the anaesthetist or from the nursing staff. He appreciated the depths of despair of Mrs Gough and found that the experience had been "catastrophic" for her. A psychiatrist Dr McCarthy had treated Mrs Gough for despair and distress.

Mrs Gough's attitude, as detailed in an excellent report on the case in *The Irish Times,* is exemplary.[1] She thanked the judge, her legal team and her husband and son, whom she said was "the one good thing to come out of this".

In July 2003, the Supreme Court ruled against Dr Neary and the hospital's claim that Mrs Gough's action was statute barred. However, the Supreme Court reduced the award of €100,000 for pain and suffering by 50 per cent. Mr Justice Brian McCracken ruled that Mrs Gough's psychiatrist expected her to make a full recovery from her depression and consequently the payment of €100,000 for general damages into the future was not sustainable.

Originally in 1998, Dr Neary's rate of Caesarian hysterectomy was brought to the attention of the North Eastern Health Board (NEHB) by two student midwives through their solicitor Gary Byrne. The NEHB, after a preliminary review, asked Dr Neary to stop working. He refused but agreed to take annual leave. Dr Neary's solicitor later produced a review of nine cases by three obstetricians from the IHCA, which concluded that his work was "without fault and acceptable". However, an external review of nine cases by Dr Michael Maresh from St Mary's Hospital, Manchester alarmed the NEHB authorities and Dr Neary was placed on administrative leave. In January 1999, the Institute of Obstetri-

A Cure for the Crisis

cians and Gynaecologists carried out a review at the request of the NEHB into 39 cases dating from 1992 to 1998. They found that the Caesarian hysterectomies were acceptable in 41 per cent, doubtful in 12.8 per cent and unacceptable in 46 per cent. Their report recommended that Dr Neary undergo "a supervised post-graduate programme for a continuous period of six months" in another hospital. They also advised that for one year Dr Neary be obliged to consult a colleague before he could perform a Caesarian hysterectomy. This would be almost impossible to implement in practice.

Prof John Bonnar said that there was only one recorded case of Caesarian hysterectomy in 100,000 pregnancies in the Dublin area. Dr Neary's rate of Caesarian hysterectomy was 20 times higher than that found in the Dublin maternity hospitals. Caesarian hysterectomy in the years 1993–98 was performed 1 per 600 in the Coombe Women's Hospital, 1 per 405 in Holles Street, 1 per 42 in Drogheda and 1 per 20 by Dr Neary. Hysterectomy as a proportion of total births in that period was 1 per 4,373 in the Coombe, 1 per 3,847 in Holles Street and 1 per 179 in Drogheda. Dr Neary was suspended from the medical register in February 1999 following a High Court hearing and erasure was confirmed in July 2003.

The NEHB has confirmed that 65 legal actions are being taken by women who made allegations against Dr Neary. Some of them had their ovaries as well as their uterus removed. In October 2000 the Medical Council's inquiry into allegations that Dr Neary had performed unnecessary Caesarian hysterectomies began. This was more than 18 months after Dr Neary had been suspended from the medical register. By December 2002, the Medical Council had heard 37 complaints about the professional conduct of Dr Neary. They judged that 21 complaints warranted the holding of an inquiry under the Medical Practitioners Act. They began substantive hearings into 15 of the complaints in October 2000. During the course of the inquiry, the committee decided that Dr Neary had no case to answer in whole or in part in relation to the complaints made by five patients. A further six complaints will be heard at the completion of this inquiry.[2]

According to Sheila O'Connor of the pressure group Patient Focus, no records are available for 20 per cent of the women who are concerned at their treatment. However, notes missing for outpatient visits are common problems with any paper system. There is a possibility that a public inquiry to investigate the removal of uteri from up to 90 women will be set up.

240

Aberrant clinical behaviour

Dublin GP Dr Tony O'Sullivan, who is associated with Patient Focus, called for a system that facilitates patient advocacy: "We need a system that allows whistle blowing. To some extent there are some signs of an improvement as this is the first case I'm aware of where Irish expert witnesses stood up in court against a fellow consultant, and you give them credit for that."

Future practices

In a brief commentary in *The Irish Times*, medical correspondent Dr Muiris Houston asked whether such events could happen in the present day. He wrote:

> It is unlikely for several reasons. Teamwork within hospitals has replaced a system of "doctor knows best". Doctors in all specialties now undergo continuous medical education, part of which includes the analysis and discussion of cases randomly picked from their practices.[3]

I agree that a recurrence of inappropriate Caesarian hysterectomy is most unlikely. It is quite possible for other procedures, however, to be used inappropriately with very late or no detection. Medical practice is still relatively autonomous. However, in hospitals like Beaumont, I would hope that specialty conferences and the grapevine would apply the brakes to anything too aberrant. Another important factor is the phasing out of single consultant practice and inspections by the Irish Committee for Higher Medical Training and its surgical, radiological, pathological and psychiatric equivalents.

Nonetheless, mistakes and wrong practices can never be totally eliminated because we are all human. Often what is correct practice varies over time and depends on the availability of equipment and expertise.

Solutions

- The best means of keeping some check on practices is that each consultant has to present his/her work at clinical conferences in hospitals.
- Consultants must also turn up to explain the investigations and treatment of the cases and not leave the task to juniors.
- Continuous medical education requires attendance at such meetings and registration will depend on these in the future.

- Tort reform is also necessary to allow more open discussions of practice problems where the procedure employed is the problem and not the resources.

An interesting book has yet to be written on the internal medical wars in the first decade of Beaumont Hospital's existence. Staff members from consultants to nurses to administrators to junior doctors were adversely affected and it took more than five years and the appointment of an overwhelmingly new uninvolved staff for the hospital to settle down and recover. Casualties included neurosurgeons Mr Padraig O'Neill, Mr Sean O'Laoire, anaesthetist Dr Kate Flynn, gastroenterologist Prof John Fielding and non-consultant neurosurgeon Cristos Georgopoulis.

Blood Bank scandal

Details of the extent of the Blood Bank scandals were first exposed by the Tribunal of Inquiry into the Blood Transfusion Service Board set up in 1996, chaired by Mr Justice Thomas Finlay. A second inquiry set up in May 2000, chaired by Judge Alison Lindsay, specifically looked at haemophiliacs infected with hepatitis C and HIV from infected blood products.

Dr John Murphy, editor of the *Irish Medical Journal,* summarised the story of the haemophilia tragedy after the publication of the Lindsay Tribunal Report in September 2002.[4,5] The families' justifiable bitterness and hurt is not discussed here. Nothing anyone can say at this point would make much difference. The Lindsay Tribunal sat in public for 196 days, and heard 146 witnesses giving oral evidence. There were 64 personal testimonies given by haemophiliacs or members of their families.

Infections

HIV	Haemophilia A	– 97 patients positive
	Haemophilia B	– 7 patients positive
Hepatitis C		– 217 positive, of whom 69 were also infected with HIV
		– 148 infected with hepatitis C only

- 1967 – first treatment for haemophilia – cryoprecipitate, a partially thawed form of factor VIII.
- 1968 – Haemophilia National Co-ordinating Committee (HNCC) set up comprising Blood Transfusion Service Board (BTSB) personnel,

Aberrant clinical behaviour

Irish Haemophilia Society (IHS) members and medical directors of the treatment centres.

- 1974 – imported commercial factor VIII became available. It was suitable for home use, which would reduce time lost from work and school and cause less inconvenience. The IHS and the doctors wanted to use it, but the BTSB was reluctant.
- BTSB wanted self-sufficiency with an Irish donor group and was unhappy with the potential consequences.
- HNCC introduced the imported product. They knew of the risk of non-A non-B hepatitis and viewed the risk as acceptable at the time.
- During the mid-1970s, the BTSB tried to reestablish some degree of self-sufficiency through the provision of freeze-dried cryoprecipitate. There was a three-year delay over lack of funding and the BTSB position on self-sufficiency was weakening over this time.
- Custom fractionation of plasma from Irish donors was tried using a commercial company in the manufacture of factor VIII. The yields were insufficient. Judge Lindsay felt that custom fractionation should have been pursued with greater urgency, particularly in collaboration with the Scottish Blood Transfusion Service.
- 1983 January – seven haemophiliacs in the US had developed AIDS and blood products were suspected as the cause of the infection. It is likely that HIV infection occurred from 1980 onwards in the US.
- The Tribunal considers that 66 per cent of the Irish cases became infected by mid-1983 and the remaining third between mid-1983 and the end of 1984.
- 1984 May – the AIDS virus was identified. At the time there was discussion of the value of heat treatment as a method of inactivating the virus as factors VIII and IX were thought to be highly labile. There were concerns about inhibitors and the risk of thrombosis.
- 1984 October – evidence that HIV could be inactivated by heat first published.
- 1984 November – first Irish haemophiliac was diagnosed with AIDS.
- 1984 December – consultant haematologist Prof Ian Temperley sent a letter to the BTSB stating that the doctors would only use heat-treated commercial products and that locally produced products should be heat-treated.
- 1985 January – unheated commercial factor VIII replaced.

A Cure for the Crisis

- 1985 February – unheated commercial factor IX replaced.
- 1985 February – BTSB supplying both heat-treated commercial factor IX and its own non heat-treated factor IX. Some BTSB people thought that local heat treatment of factor IX would cause thrombosis.
- 1985 October – heat-treated BTSB factor IX became available.

The Tribunal felt that the BTSB should have introduced heat-treated factor VIII sooner, but noted the production difficulties and that the non heat-treated factor IX should have been withdrawn earlier. Seven HIV infections in haemophilia B patients could have been prevented. The Tribunal's major criticism of Prof Temperley was that he took sabbatical leave between May and November 1985.

The Tribunal was critical of the way haemophiliac patients were tested for HIV and then informed of the results. There were delays in transmitting results and there was a lack of counselling after the patients had been informed. In addition, the Tribunal noted the lack of social workers and counsellors: "One possible conclusion from this Tribunal is that pioneering doctors who set up a new medical service for patients without comprehensive finances and supportive services are vulnerable if any unforeseen long-term complication occurs."

HIV infection in the blood supply is a worldwide problem and politicians have been held responsible and convicted in France. Prof Temperley's experiences are often used as a reference for spurring action to safeguard patients and prevent mishap. Putting the patient and not the system first is the first duty of the doctor. We must always communicate with the patient to inform them of any new risks that arise when these are discovered.

The BTSB, recently restructured as the Irish Blood Transfusion Service (IBTS), has now ensured the development of a safe blood supply with a high standard of product. There has been much trauma within the organisation, which still has some time to serve before matters are resolved.

Reaction to Tribunal Report

The Irish Haemophilia Society expressed profound anger and disappointment at the contents of the Lindsay Report. IHS chairman, Mr Brian O'Mahony, felt that all the evidence was not heard at the Tribunal. An opinion piece in the *Bar Review* said that the report contained criticisms of the Blood Transfusion Service Board and of certain doctors but stopped short of placing the blame on any one individual or entity. The judge recommended that the report should not be referred to the Director of Public Prosecutions. According to the *Bar Review,* the judge's conclusions had been described as "weak" and "limited", mainly because no one had specifically been made accountable. "Sometimes there are no straightforward answers and no convenient cast of villains. Sometimes, it is not possible to squeeze the events of years into a pithy executive summary."[6]

The article claimed that Judge Lindsay was handed a thankless and complex brief and in the absence of a conclusion, i.e. fingering a specific fall guy, her report was always unlikely to find favour with the victims and their families. The *Bar Review* also noted that the judge was constrained from publicly defending her report against criticisms. It concluded that it was unfair to condemn a report because it did not amount to a "heads will roll blockbuster". Mr O'Mahony totally disagreed with the *Bar Review* article, particularly as the IHS had always maintained that not all the evidence had actually been heard. He found the opinion piece patronising and disagreed with the assertion that "the public must be constantly reminded that the aim of the tribunal is not to establish guilt or innocence".[7]

International product suppliers

The State is committed to an inquiry into the role of international drug companies in the Blood Bank scandal, despite the comment of Mr Michael McDowell, Minister for Justice and Law Reform, that a new inquiry would be a "monumental" waste of State resources. The Lindsay Tribunal found that as a matter of probability, a young Irish haemophilia sufferer, who has since died of an AIDS-related disease, was infected by an Armour clotting agent. In Canada, the Royal Canadian Mounted Police after a five-year investigation brought multiple criminal charges against Armour Pharmaceuticals, one of the companies involved in the Irish debacle.

Criminal proceedings

In 2003, Dr Terry Walsh, a former medical consultant at the BTSB, and Ms Cecily Cunningham, a principal grade biochemist, were charged under Section 23 of the Offences Against the Person Act that they had

A Cure for the Crisis

"unlawfully and maliciously caused a noxious agent... infected anti-D to be used on seven mothers, which caused them 'grievous bodily harm'". These charges arose as a result of the Finlay Tribunal.

The bill

Almost €450 million compensation has been paid out to 1,590 people as a result of the Blood Bank scandal. The legal bill was more than €55 million to mid-2003 with the average case costing €36,000 in fees. The average award has been €202,000, excluding legal costs. Almost 80 people have died as a result of infection.

39

Whistle blowing in the Irish health service

Dangerous games

Shoot the messenger is a frequent reflex. Kathryn Bolkovac, a UN police officer, was unfairly fired for blowing the whistle on colleagues involved in the Bosnian sex trade. She was employed in a £30,000 per year job with DynCorp, which supplied officers to the UN Bosnia mission. She won her unfair dismissal case at a tribunal in Southampton, England against the US company and was awarded £110,000. Panel chairman, Charles Twiss, declared that her dismissal was a "very serious blight on her ability to apply successfully for posts in international organisations".

To administrators and politicians, I commend the French physician JJ Guillotin, who died in 1814, to their attention. He recommended the heavy knife machine to behead citizens during the revolution in 1789. In Irish politics, Ruairí Quinn famously went to Albert Reynolds looking for a head and I'm sure that many administrators would dearly love the heads of some of medicine's awkward brigade!

However, there is an upside too. *Time* magazine made three female whistleblowers – Cynthia Cooper of Worldcom for exposing fraudulent accountancy practices, Coleen Rowley of the FBI for questioning the FBI's inaction on information on the terrorist Zacarias Moussaoui looking for 747 flying lessons before the 9/11 World Trade Center attack, and Sherron Watkins of Enron, who exposed the hiding of debt mountains of billions of dollars in that company – joint Persons of the Year in their special double issue of 30 December 2002/6 January 2003. All is not lost yet!

Irish whistleblowers

A trawl through the many health and hospital crises and scandals that have beset the Irish State in recent times brings many health professionals to the fore for their efforts at patient advocacy.

A Cure for the Crisis

Dr Joan Power

Dr Joan Power is the consultant haematologist in Cork who helped reveal the contamination of the anti-D blood products with hepatitis C virus in 1994. As a consequence, the Tribunal of Inquiry into the BTSB was set up. She has had a public conflict with the Department of Health and suffered suspension from her post for a period in 2002, but was reinstated after one week. She may be investigated for a delay in informing 28 people in the mid-90s who tested positive for hepatitis C virus. She accepted that she should have made personal contact with patients rather than just speaking to lawyers for the support groups, and expressed regret at the Finlay Tribunal over this issue. On another matter, she was most influential in securing the Cork Blood Bank from closure. I respect her courage and grit.

Mr Patrick Plunkett

Mr Patrick Plunkett is an A&E consultant at St James's Hospital, Dublin. In 2001, Mr Plunkett resigned from the Board of Management of St James's to free himself from the restraints of board confidentiality. He spoke out about the crisis in A&E where elderly patients were kept on trolleys overnight because no beds were available. Waits of 24 hours were common and patients had died waiting. Mr Plunkett called it "lunacy". Yet again in January 2003, Mr Plunkett reiterated: "The whole issue of it being a winter crisis is a load of rubbish. It's essentially the same all the time." He called on the entire Cabinet to be collectively responsible for the state of our hospitals and if change didn't come soon, people could expect a "third-rate health service".

Dr Garrett FitzGerald of Waterford

Dr Garrett FitzGerald is a regular columnist with *Medicine Weekly,* a trade paper. He succinctly and devastatingly outlined the problems for doctors of trying to do their jobs in the face of inadequate beds and resources. In particular, he has railed against restrictive practices in medicine. His article on the illogicality of allowing the death of the internal medicine consultant in this country was timely and appropriate. He noted that the American-style internist has a role as a hospitalist, allowing the superspecialist to continue to be super. In his assessment, he is absolutely correct.

Dr Maurice Gueret

TCD graduate, columnist in *Medicine Weekly* and editor of the *Irish Medical Directory*, Dr Gueret has questioned the expenses and activities of junketing at health boards. He is a good advocate for patients and has hopes of a Senate seat, having polled well in the 2002 Seanad Election in the TCD constituency. Blowing the whistle from outside the hospital system is less fraught, but can operate as a good facilitator as he has shown.

Mr David Hickey

Mr David Hickey is director of the Kidney and Pancreas Transplant Unit at Beaumont Hospital, which is the largest such unit in these islands. In a throwaway remark during a talk at the UCD Smurfit Business School recently, he declared that Beaumont Hospital was in "lousy shape" as an edifice and showed pictures of parts of his unit being housed in portacabins, which he then contrasted with a picture of the palatial headquarters of the Northern Area Health Board in Swords. He was making the point that health spending was being wasted on fancy administration accommodation rather than on facilities for patients. It was a powerful charge but one that contained a large measure of truth.

In an interview with Conor Lally in *The Irish Times* on 19 November 2002, Mr Hickey claimed that in Beaumont the roof and windows were leaking, the air-conditioning was either non-existent or malfunctioning, and that the hospital was so chronically short of beds that vital cancer operations were regularly cancelled. He also said that the hospital was roasting in summer (it certainly was during any hot spell) and was freezing in winter. There is only one working shower for live-in male non-consultant doctors. He insinuated also that there might be morale problems in medicine by pointing out that 17 junior doctors have left Beaumont and medicine in the last five years. Twenty years ago, such an event was extremely rare.

The UK Transplant Service, which includes Ireland, issued a report in 1997 which stipulated that there should be six transplant beds per million of the population, one-third of which should be single beds. Beaumont Hospital has only four beds designated for transplant patients instead of a regulation 24, with predictable consequences. When organs become available, they are procured by Beaumont's aggressive surgeons. Consequently, patients due for urology admission, usually for prostate cancer, have their treatment postponed. Mr Hickey admitted

A Cure for the Crisis

that "we are cancelling cancer operations. I am amazed the patient takes it. I'd go ballistic if it happened to me". He also pointed out that there is only one diabetologist in Beaumont, despite the fact that around 6,000 diabetics attend the hospital: "There are no easy patients. They have blood sugar problems, eye problems, high stroke rates, higher heart-attack rates, amputation rates and huge social problems."

Mr Hickey made a naïve plea that politics needed to be taken out of the health service. He noted that decisions on where to invest in new facilities in recent years depended on the constituency of the ministers in office at the time. For example, he cited Jackie Healy-Rae's political success and joked that if Jackie was minister there would be a new facility built on Inishvickillane.

The consequences of the likely future leakage of staff from the public health service due to work pressures from underfunding, the changes in nurse education and the impact on the Indian subcontinent and poorer countries of the importation of their medical staff to fill Irish vacancies was also decried. According to Hickey, "the third world every year donates around $1 billion worth of free medical education to scavengers like ourselves. People are dying because of that".

In an interview on NewsTalk 106's *The Right Hook with George Hook,* I supported Hickey by pointing out that he is an excellent advocate for his patients and an exemplary doctor. By right he is discharging his advocacy duty. Administrators look to the guillotine as a first response to whistle-blowers. However, Hickey is entitled to a little poetic licence. After all, his is the response of a man with the highest standards who is deeply frustrated. Eight years ago, transplanted kidneys functioned an average of 7 years, whereas 14 years is the current average expectation. His arrival was a key part of this improvement and the people of Ireland are well served by his skills. At Beaumont, the one-year graft survival is 88 per cent and the five-year graft survival is 75 per cent. These figures are as good as or better than the best worldwide figures. Beaumont is world-class in medical outcomes terms but not in capacity and infrastructure. There are at least 100 beds needed at Beaumont; 35 extra beds are coming on-stream at present from a change of use of an existing staff changing area on the ground floor. The hospital is part way through a €27 million refurbishment programme which began in 2000. Beaumont is also spending €365,000 on roof waterproofing, new air conditioning in the X-ray Department and in the surgical theatres. New windows are being selected

Whistle blowing in the Irish health service

as part of a €5.3 million replacement window programme. A new 40-station dialysis unit is being designed to replace the existing 16-station unit.

RETORT I

In a letter to *The Irish Times* in response to the article, Mr John P. Lamont, CEO of Beaumont Hospital, listed the refurbishment and some of the points above. He offered no solution to the transplant bed issue and its consequence emphasised by David Hickey, but did refer specifically to the shortage of beds outside the hospital for rehabilitation and long-stay patients. Anxious to distance Hickey's views from hospital policy, he stated: "It is important to note that Mr Hickey's wide ranging views on nurse training, recruitment of doctors and various other matters are very much personal ones. They do not reflect the views of the hospital's board and management."

Word around the hospital was that a very small number of administrators were exercised by Mr Hickey's criticism, but realised that any reaction would have to be carefully measured because of the very high regard for Hickey among most staff. Two consultants remarked that they would prefer such criticisms were not made because 'it might divert patients away from Beaumont. I disagree because most people can see, experience and judge for themselves. The national units in Beaumont have an effective monopoly and local doctors are unlikely to alter their referral patterns as a result of some amusing tush in a newspaper. On the same week, the Mater Hospital was so overcrowded that it stopped taking patients. In the end, public pressure is the most effective way to correct shortfalls.

RETORT II

Almost immediately and surprisingly, David Hickey replied to Mr Lamont's letter in *The Irish Times*. He weighed in and took Lamont to task by firstly pointing out that "the administration at Beaumont is answerable to the public as to the efficacy with which it uses their money". The details in Mr Lamont's letter opened the subject to public comment and debate. Hickey wrote:

> Under the Constitution and EU law I am entitled to, and under the Hippocratic oath I am obliged to speak out publicly on the shortcomings at Beaumont, in particular, and nationally. Several reports prepared for the "normal channels" over the past 8 years have been ignored and thus compelled me to take this route.[1]

He then demanded a commission of inquiry into the current crisis in the health service, out of which a new concept of healthcare delivery could emerge. The next sentence is hilarious given the secretive, proscriptive and essentially unaccountable *modus operandi* of hospital boards:

> A commission would allow Mr Lamont and the board of Beaumont fully to express their views and philosophy more eloquently, succinctly and perhaps even more rewardingly (for the patients). Holding the commission in public would underpin the present Government's commitment to transparency, honesty and accountability.

Ironically and coincidentally, the headline in the London *Independent* on 26 November 2002, cried "Scandal of NHS and Third World nurses... Britain breaks pledge to halt recruitment from developing countries". The report claimed that Britain is systematically stripping the developing world of its nurses to shore up the NHS, despite a government ban on recruiting from the Third World. Mr Hickey is vindicated.

Mr Denis Lawlor

Shortly after David Hickey's call for a commission of inquiry by Dáil Éireann into the current crisis in the health service, Mr Denis Lawlor wrote a letter to *The Irish Times* in straight support. Speaking on behalf of the Irish Association of Plastic Surgeons, he claimed that burns facilities were adequate but the same could not be said for the rest of plastic surgery in the State. He did not expect an "operate at will' opportunity for his speciality, but highlighted the appalling service currently provided:

> ...emergencies that can take days to get into surgery, urgent procedures that take weeks or even longer to deliver and routine consultation that take up to two years or more, after which patients are placed on a never-ending waiting list, reflect an appalling service. Waiting-list initiatives are all very well but they do not in any way solve the underlying problems.
>
> We urgently require a State-wide review of our speciality and feel that the health of our people is more important than all the present inquiries into planning and such matters. Regardless of the impending draconian cuts, some things should not be sacrificed.[2]

Dr Peter Conlon

In February 2003 as described in Chapter 2, Dr Peter Conlon appeared in the press, on television and on radio following the revelation in the Dáil

Whistle blowing in the Irish health service

by the leader of the Labour Party, Pat Rabbitte TD, that the dialysis unit where he is a consultant nephrologist might be shut at night as part of a cost-saving exercise in Beaumont Hospital, with catastrophic and deadly effects for up to 80 patients. There was shock and horror at this potential development and the Irish Kidney Association was justifiably outraged.

Dr Conlon's advocacy had the positive effect of extracting a guarantee that dialysis patients would not be sacrificed. However, the publicity annoyed the administrators and not least the Taoiseach in the Dáil. Shortly afterwards, Dr Conlon had a letter published in *The Irish Times* asking why, if the ERHA had received a 7 per cent increase in funding from the Government, had the Dublin hospitals received less than a 1 per cent increase? He pointed out that 90 beds in Beaumont were due to close in the summer, while a further 90 patients were fit for discharge but needed convalescent beds which were no longer being funded. In addition, he noted "the sad fact is that hospital administrators are happy to see hospital beds occupied by patients waiting to go to nursing homes because they are relatively cheap to keep, certainly much less costly than patients having surgery, dialysis or cancer treatments".[3] The constant presence of patients waiting on trolleys was in danger of becoming the norm. On this point, Dr Conlon wrote that "we have become used to 20 to 25 patients waiting in casualty overnight. I fear we will have to get used to 50 or 60 patients waiting on trolleys each evening".

THE RETORTS

In *The Irish Times* of the following morning, Dr Conlon was admonished by John Lamont, CEO of Beaumont Hospital, for claiming that hospital administrators are happy to see patients on trolleys as above. He wrote: "No one involved in the management or provision of health services in Ireland takes any satisfaction in delivering less than the best possible service in the most appropriate setting to all patients in our care. I feel it is disingenuous and offensive for anyone to suggest otherwise."[4]

On the same day Mr Lamont wrote to Dr Conlon from Beaumont Hospital.

> Dear Peter,
>
> I refer to your letter published in this morning's Irish Times.
>
> I am not certain what the motivation in taking such a step is but from my perspective your action is extremely unhelpful to the Hospital in the current environment. I have asked on previous occasions that you do me the courtesy, as Chief Executive, of letting me know of your intentions when you choose to make public comment about

253

A Cure for the Crisis

Beaumont Hospital and the services we provide. You have ignored this request in attempting to negotiate additional funding for the Hospital. Furthermore, you have also chosen in that letter to make an outrageous claim that "hospital administrators are happy to see hospital beds occupied by patients waiting to go to nursing homes because they are relatively cheap to keep." I take personal and professional exception to that claim; it is without foundation in my experience and does not represent the position of the management of this or, indeed, any other Hospital.

Finally, your opening statement indicates that your letter is in response to a statement issued by the Eastern Regional Health Authority. While it is not my wish to suppress any member of staff from expressing personal views, I must insist that there is a clear distinction between this and engaging in media activities as a named representative of the Hospital.

In view of the comments made in your letter regarding "hospital administrators" you have left me with no alternative but to submit an appropriate response to the Editor of the Irish Times.

Kind regards, etc.

Mr Lamont's letter is open to interpretation. Undeniably, Dr Conlon gave his occupation and position and did not write as "a named representative of the Hospital". In fact, Dr Conlon was widely praised for his patient advocacy within the hospital and I am proud to say that I am a colleague. Clearly, he was doing his job ethically. Arguably, so was Mr Lamont, which is proof of my assertion that the administrators and politicians are on one side facing the doctors and their patients across the interest divide.

Assistant general secretary of the IHCA, Mr Donal Duffy, succinctly dealt with the issues in the same *Irish Times* forum:

John P. Lamont takes issue with the opinion of Dr Peter Conlon regarding hospital beds being occupied by patients awaiting placement in appropriate convalescent facilities. The record clearly shows that this problem has been in existence for many years and continues to worsen.

The Department of Health and Children, in its own study of acute hospital bed capacity, estimated that 675 hospital beds could be made available if such practices were ended. In any given year a further 35,000 patients could be treated in those hospital beds.

While hospital and health service administrators may not be jumping up and down with glee that so many beds are unavailable, the

Whistle blowing in the Irish health service

sad fact is that no administrator has taken responsibility to ensure that appropriate facilities are in place, thereby ending this practice.[5]

In November 2003, three years after a new dialysis unit was promised, 177 patients were receiving haemodialysis in a unit designed for 95. Each machine was being used by 11 patients where four would be average. Fifteen per cent were on twice weekly rather than the recommended three times per week regime with detrimental consequences. There are no slots for newly arriving patients – and should we stay SILENT?

Mr Tim Delaney

Chief pharmacist at Tallaght Hospital, Tim Delaney claimed that drug administration errors were being covered up because some staff were afraid to report mistakes due to fear of reprisal from superiors. In response, the Irish Patients Association said that there was need for change in the safety culture within the health service. Staff should learn from mistakes, rather than fear being blamed.

Clearly, the underlying problem is the pervasive medical fear of litigation where Ireland is second only to the US. However, at this stage, the patient advocacy business seems to be getting out of hand. The administrators will be seen in second-hand rag shops rummaging around for suitable gags for big mouths!

40

Change: liberalisation of the medical system

In recent years there has been an increasing call for liberalisation of the medical system. BUPA Ireland's managing director Martin O'Rourke, speaking at a Competition Authority symposium in Dublin on 25 November 2002, stated that there needs to be a liberalisation of the whole medical system, where control over the number of doctors practising is relinquished and where consumers have direct access to consultants. Mr O'Rourke cited the Spanish example where a recent liberalisation of the market has shortened waiting lists and cut treatment costs. The key to this was less control of the market: "We should… let innovation squeeze out inefficiencies."[1] In addition, BUPA marketing director Sean Murray indicated that we should double consultant numbers and allow patients direct access to consultants as, for example, in Germany.

The Irish College of General Practitioners (ICGP) would not disagree with Mr O'Rourke's assertion that GPs should be paid for cured patients, but felt it would be difficult to achieve. However, both are wrong. The only inevitability is death. Therefore, all lives will end in failure because the person dies. So what is cure? Approximately 70 per cent of acute low back pains disappears within three months. Does that mean that GPs should only be paid for the pain-free group, i.e. those cured? Clearly, this can be reduced to absurdity.

Patient registration

ICGP communications chairman Dr Brendan O'Shea called for greater patient registration: "We do believe that payments and recognition should be based on audited and documented achievements of key targets. We do support the concept of whole population register and proactive management care. Only one third of our population are registered under the General Medical Scheme."

Change: liberalisation of the medical system

However, Dr O'Shea's next comment makes me wonder: "GPs and the public now have grave reservations about the accountability, flexibility and efficiency of this system." In practice, patient registration restricts choice and is not the best way. Many patients use a plethora of doctors. For example, GPs are used for coughs, temperatures and general flop; the well woman clinic for cervical smears and the pill, usually paying higher charges than at the local GP; factory doctors for most things where there is one supplied; well man clinics; commercial executive health screens; self-referral to consultants; and widespread use of osteopaths, homeopaths, herbalists, Chinese medicine practitioners and other alternatives. I respect the right of people to make their own choices. It keeps systems honest and modest and should be preserved. It is better for patients to have knowledge of their conditions and therapy. Moreover, it is inevitable that in the future, data cards will allow people to carry their own accurate medical records, if they so wish. Many like to avoid medics as much as possible and not tie themselves down. I respect that wish also.

The NHS business of rigid registration is all right but unnecessary. The advantages of registration are clarity in the responsibility of the doctor for one's care, disease screening, convenience in trying to ensure that children and adults receive vaccinations, and follow-up of disease when there is an advantage to the patient in so doing.

Direct access

The ICGP strongly opposes direct access to consultants. On this issue, Dr O'Shea notes: "Evidence suggests that this results in a higher number of inappropriate references and inappropriate use of specialists' time overall." This is undoubtedly true but if specialist fees are advertised and specialist numbers are limited only by registration and not mainly by Comhairle na nOspidéal regulation, then the advantages of direct access will outweigh the limitations. Importantly, superspecialists can instruct their secretaries not to take appointments except where there is referral from a GP or another consultant. As it is, many patients referred from GPs for a specific condition to a consultant in a private clinic are sent around other consultants in that private clinic when the GP or referring physician routinely deals with the same condition. This is both patronising and insulting to the GP.

Dr O'Shea also opined: "I have no doubt that this would lead to increased transactions for insurance companies so I can see why they

A Cure for the Crisis

would support this." At the risk of sounding like a boring pedant, surely insurance companies increase their profits when costs are kept down not when transaction numbers by patients are increased?

41

Competition in the medical market

In May 2001, the Competition Authority decided to study competition among medical practitioners, dentists, optometrists, vets, architects, construction engineers, solicitors and barristers. This followed an OECD report which was critical of the level of competition in some professions. A list of 74 questions was sent to professional bodies with the responses due in February 2002. Economic consultants Indecon International were paid €120,000 to collate the replies. They were also commissioned to consult with professional and regulatory bodies and compare with similar professions in other countries and competition case law.

The Authority intends to report the professions separately in 2003 and make recommendations on the rules governing the professions where these are considered anti-competitive. In respect of the medical profession, the most obvious restraint is the limitation on the numbers of medical school entrants.

Meanwhile John Fingleton, chairman of the Competition Authority, wrote an article in *The Irish Times* on 7 November 2002 on whether competition could help cure the ills of the Irish healthcare system. At present, the restrictions can arise (a) if the Government supplies the service; (b) if it is the main buyer of the service; and (c) if it regulates the service or allows self-regulation. According to Mr Fingleton, the State purchases 78 per cent of all healthcare services and dominates the supply of hospital and consultant services. On the regulatory side, there are only two suppliers – BUPA and VHI; pharmacy is also restricted and the Competition Authority has argued for increased supply.

Market failure is blatant in the health sector. There are queues for OPD services, and queues for virtually every service which means that the service supply is restricted. This shoves up the price dramatically. Medical inflation continually outstrips general inflation. This will ultimately bankrupt the private insurance companies and is a reason why the VHI operates like a Health Maintenance Organisation, restricting the supply

A Cure for the Crisis

of services for which they will pay. If they were to insure patients for scans, etc. at a particular price and if they were to cover hotel charges at particular levels, then more suppliers might appear on the market, and the total amount of services would rise to the benefit of the public. Queues would diminish and ultimately vanish if the State did the same thing. The VHI has evolved in this restrictive direction but this does not necessarily have to continue. The effect is to stifle the development of private hospitals everywhere because hospital projects cannot proceed at present, if the VHI refuses to cover its subscribers in the new institution. As has been noted elsewhere, BUPA has effectively shadowed the VHI thus far in the marketplace.

The cost of scans in other countries varies considerably and an MRI scan in the private sector in France is much cheaper than in Ireland.

John Fingleton posed the question as to why the State is so involved in healthcare. He suggested that the main reason is to provide a minimum level of healthcare, especially to those that cannot afford it and wrote: "Clearly this is a worthy goal." Nevertheless, he opines that the details of the State intervention have imposed unnecessarily high costs and restrictions on all users of the system, while it fails to deliver on the objective of providing the universal service. However, Mr Fingleton does admit that competition is not the panacea for all healthcare ills but that a tincture might be no harm at all.

Irish Medical Council and the marketplace

The Irish Medical Council regulates the qualifications and medical entry requirements, patient–doctor relationships and how doctors behave towards each other in the marketplace. The State acting as buyer and seller can eliminate markets altogether, which it has in effect

I believe that the medical market should be freed up. The Medical Council should be the licensing body to guarantee the quality of specialist medical registration by determining minimum standards of training and proficiency to attain and remain on the specialty register, working in association with specialist professional bodies. It should set the standards for general medical registration and should also agree on the boundaries for determining continuing medical education. Doctors should be allowed limited advertising of their skills without saying they are number one in something. This should encompass every branch of medicine.

Competition in the medical market

Restrictive errors

The Medical Council's *Guide to Ethical Conduct and Behaviour* has some blatant restrictive errors, which must be corrected. It states in section 13.2 regarding referral: "A consultant should not normally accept a patient without referral from a general practitioner even if he/she has seen that patient in the past." This is widely honoured in the breech. It confuses etiquette with ethics. It also aims to restrict patient choice. Any doctor may determine his/her rules for acceptance of referrals. For example, the doctor may decide to deal only with kidney stones and not see anything else. Clearly, if you have an ingrowing toenail, a brain surgeon is not the most appropriate specialist. As a general rule, it is better that patients have a GP as their primary physician, seeing that it is the best way to direct access to appropriate care when needed, but such a system should not be enshrined in an ethical guide. Certainly, the Competition Authority has been concerned about this restriction and should not balk at highlighting it.

In section 13.5, the *Guide* writes about cross-referral between consultants: "In exceptional cases, cross referral between consultants may be necessary but the general practitioner must be kept informed about the patient." This stricture is also frequently breeched. The case could easily be made that many consultants run primary care in their private practices. For example, people attending cardiologists for years after bypass surgery; people with asthma attending a consultant a year after their last attack; people with arterial hypertension having their pressures controlled by a consultant only; people with routine hypothyroidism, irritable bowel syndrome, fibromyalgia, etc. Where does this leave the above 13.2 ruling in the *Guide*? If these patients were not paying, how many of them would be referred back to their GPs? The irony of the new over-70s medical card scheme is that many of these patients have now to return to their GPs to have their private prescriptions rewritten on GMS forms.

Reducing the *de facto* supply of junior doctors and forced closure of smaller hospitals

The deadline to reduce junior doctors working hours in hospitals from a maximum 65 hours to 58 hours per week is August 2004, and the maximum working hours will be 48 by 2009 under the European Working Time Directive. It will mean specific rest and break-time entitlements and a reduction in the on-call hours. The ratio of consultants to junior doctors has decreased from 1:2.39 in 1984 to 1:1.57 at present. However, two out of three patients who attend public outpatients do not see a consultant. There are just short of 4 million people in the State, yet 2.5 million people attended public outpatients in 2001. The IHCA has called for the appointment of another 1,000 consultants in order to provide a consultant-led service.

Smaller hospitals have a relatively greater reliance on junior doctors to provide a service and the European Working Time Directive is like a guillotine hanging over them, unless there is a large increase in consultant numbers. Higher medical training requires consultant supervision and specific formal training programmes which have to be authenticated so that a certificate of specialist training can be issued. The Joint Committees on Higher Medical Training will not recognise junior posts in many small hospitals and these hospitals will be unable to attract junior staff. They may have to innovate and hire "hospital practitioners" or generalists on the specialist register to allow the hospitals to remain open. Obviously, there are risk management problems in staffing hospitals with undertrained doctors in unsupervised posts.

It is claimed that resources are dissipated in smaller hospitals, but I think that is not wholly true. I admit that I am biased because I respect the will of the people as expressed at the ballot box. If the people in the Cavan Monaghan constituency vote to maintain their hospitals, I think every effort should be made to respect their wishes. It is possible to hire mobile MRI, CT and PET scan units and to service the burden of colonic, respiratory, neurological and cardiac disease in the community. Images may be downloaded to India for cheap competent reporting as already happens at some US hospitals. Outpatient specialists can be contracted on a fee-per-item basis. Also, the advantages of cross-border co-operation are obvious as many small hospitals in the Northern border counties are earmarked for closure.

Other competitive innovations and consumer choice

In the US state of Florida, radio advertisements invite people to have CT virtual colonoscopy if they had diarrhoea, constipation, abdominal pain or change in bowel habits. No reference is made to referral by any doctor, although follow-up by colonoscopy, etc., would be advisable. As technology improves in all areas and becomes cheaper and more sensitive, restrictive practices have to break down. The problem is one of assess-

Competition in the medical market

ment of the true clinical role of the investigations in an era where making profit is the first duty of equipment manufacturers to their shareholders. Lots of patients could be triaged on the phone or asked to follow a computer algorithm on a website as an indicator for the need for referral for medical attention.

In November 2003, Mr Tom Gorey, hospital manager at James Connolly Memorial Hospital, Blanchardstown, provided a current price list of scans and politely asked the consultant staff to use the most cost-effective option when referring patients. This shows commendable innovation on his part. Table 41.1 reproduces the costs, where all prices excluded VAT.

Table 41.1 Cost-effective options: price list of scans

Scan	Cappagh (€)	Bon Secours (€)	Beaumont (€)	Mater Public (€)	Mater Public (€)	Blackrock (€)	Raglan Clinic (€)
MRI	250.00	290.00	361.88	200.00	583.09	444.41	
Bone			361.88	190.00	480.07	605.00	
EMG			361.88		320.00	312.00	168.85
VQ				260.00	435.51	582.00	
EEG					216.00	202.00	
MRCP		290.00	361.88			444.00	
Mammogram				100.00	168.69	125.00	

Transnational cost-effective options exist also. According to BUPA Ireland, an MRI scan at Waterford Regional Hospital costs €612 compared to €100 in Madrid.

Non-medical clinicians

Psychologists are involved in turf wars with doctors in many places in the US. At the beginning of the 20th century, patients came to see doctors and there were no medical rivals in the conventional sense. Doctors accounted for about 1 in 3 healthcare workers. By the early 1980s, this ratio had fallen to about 1 in 16 and it is certainly much lower now. By 1997 in the US, about 36 per cent of patients visited a non-physician "clinician". Thus competition from nurse practitioners, chiropractics, homeopaths, physiotherapists and psychologists has broadened the base of medicine, but consequences for patient care and the doctor–patient interface need consideration. Who looks after the whole person? Clearly, there is a very important role for each specialist but each within context.

A Cure for the Crisis

Denturists and dentists

Martin Kenny of Denture Express in Dorset Street, Dublin, recently sued the Dental Council, the Minister for Health, the State and the Attorney General for damages of over €1 million and lost profits. He is seeking a declaration that he is entitled to provide dentures directly to the public and that the current restrictions are in breach of the European Treaty and the Competition Act.

The Dentists Act 1928 made it an offence for dental mechanics to practise dentistry. In 1978, the Irish Association for Dental Prosthesis called on the Minister to allow denturists to build, repair, and alter full and removable partial dentures. A working party of the Department of Health, the health boards and the Irish Dental Association rejected the proposals. In 1980, the Examiner of Restrictive Practices found that parts of the 1928 Act restricted competition in the provision of dental services and, following a sworn inquiry in 1982, the Restrictive Practices Commission recommended that the Act should be amended to allow denturists to supply dentures to over-18s provided they did not work on living tissue.

The 1985 Dentists Act gave the Dental Council, with the Minister's consent, the right to "make a scheme for establishing classes of auxiliary dental workers who may undertake such class or classes of dental work as shall be specified by the Council". The Minister may also set up an auxiliary dental workers scheme, however, nothing has happened to date.

Mr Kenny was refused advertising in the *Evening Herald* and the Dental Council prevented him from setting up a nationwide franchising operation. A set of chrome-cobalt palate-free dentures for €445 to €550 can be produced by Mr Kenny, whereas the dentists charge €1,200 to €1,300. At present, he is barred from publicly funded work and reckons that he is losing €500,000 per year as a consequence of this restriction.

Solutions

- Consultation fees must be displayed in waiting rooms of GPs and consultants. Add-ons should be itemised.
- Cost of scans and procedures should be advertised and a charges list should be available to potential patients.
- Hospitals should allow mobile scan companies to compete.
- VHI/BUPA should cover the procedures not the institutions.

Competition in the medical market

- Accredited laboratories should be allowed compete on price and service in/with the public sector.
- The Minister of Health should make an order freeing up competition based on training requirements for denturists and registration and quality assurance of their activities following discussion with the Dental Council.

42

Healthcare rationing

In 1984, Aaron and Schwartz defined rationing succinctly as "not all care expected to be beneficial is provided to all patients".[1] Rationing usually means sharing of a scarce resource either equally or in accordance with need. Equal distribution is possible in wartime with quantities of sugar, fruit, meat or petrol. Rationing in this context is not a response to a money supply problem. These are shortages of real resources, whereas rationing in wartime is a deliberate public policy.

Rationing in healthcare is usually taken to indicate the administrative distribution of goods that have become or are scarce. This is often done through market mechanisms. In Ireland, there is no public platform where decisions can be made on what diseases or conditions the State will cover. Hospitals throughout the country are funded to provide a limited number of services in many specialties and no service in others. For example, in November 2002, there was no rheumatologist in the Midlands, while the waiting lists in Dublin to see rheumatologists are about one year. There are no neurologists across many health board areas, despite the high incidence and prevalence of stroke and the undoubted benefits of specialist care for stroke victims in terms of reduced rates of death, disability and the need for institutional care when patients are treated in dedicated stroke units.[2]

As billions of dollars are spent on biological and healthcare-related research, doctors can do more and more for an ever-increasing number of patients. When health services are funded from central state taxation only, what can then be done for people becomes the decision of those administering the political system. The total volume of money is determined by governments and depends on their political philosophies. Decisions on resource allocation usually devolve to various officials at central and local level. The choice for the doctor and patient will often be severely constrained and the command economy with all its inefficient manifestations becomes obvious.

266

Healthcare rationing

The British National Health Service is a familiar template. Difficulties seeing GPs and prescribing guidelines based on value-for-money guidelines become the norm. The National Institute for Clinical Excellence (NICE) in the UK is intended to determine best practice in medicine regarding drugs, treatments and services. Best practice guidelines found on their website are excellent, but they have a "sell by'" date in the major specialties because of the speed with which new innovations are tested in clinical trials. However, the literature is impressively reviewed and synthesised and the complete papers can be obtained for free online.

There is an obvious political purpose to NICE, however. It is to try to get the best bang for the public buck and contain costs. This is all very earnest and good, but I am glad that I would not be judged against its standards. Its psychology of collectivisation is clear. For example, with regard to the treatment of hyperlipidaemia in type 2 diabetes, it states on page 39:

> ...The setting of a risk threshold for treatment is ultimately a value judgment informed by the cost of treatment and its effectiveness in improving outcomes. For those at higher risk of a coronary event over 10 years, the epidemiology of diabetes and the trial data suggest a substantial saving of lives at reasonable treatment costs with a possible ultimate saving of healthcare costs from lipid altering therapy. The offer of therapy is not automatically proposed for all people with abnormal lipid profiles. Potential harms as well as benefits must be taken into account in any decision to offer treatment and some people who truly have a lower risk will not always gain a large benefit from treatment.[3]

However, where does that leave the person with a relatively low risk of a coronary, i.e. the less than 1.5 per cent per year who prefer to spend money on a statin rather than booze or bet on horses?

The US has an insurance-based health service with a Medicaid programme for the very poor, jointly financed by the Federal and State Governments. They have problems with medical inflation, with health insurance premiums up by 16 per cent in 2002 preceded by an 11 per cent increase in the previous year. The average premium is now $5,700. This is now significantly impacting on take-home pay. And still 40 million have no health insurance and millions more are underinsured.[4]

A Cure for the Crisis

Referendum on treatments

Rationing is debated often inadvertently in Ireland. In the *Irish Examiner*, Dr Stephen Cusack, A&E consultant at Cork University Hospital, asserted that it was time to debate whether funding a number of small operations was preferable to one costly procedure. "As a doctor I want to treat all my patients but, faced with spiralling costs, maybe it is time to start thinking as a nation whether we would prefer five hip operations or one heart operation."[5] According to Dr Cusack, the notion of the public deciding on which treatments should be funded had already been adopted in at least one US state (Oregon): "It is one way of looking at what could be done in trying to answer questions like: 'Should we be doing operations on a smoker's heart or should we be using that money for other treatments?' "

On the subject of drugs, Dr Cusack claimed that the drug budget at Cork University Hospital had "gone through the roof". He gave the example of a thrombolytic clotbuster used for acute heart attacks. The type used three years ago cost €102 per dose, whereas the one used now costs €1,270 per dose.

Similarly, clinical oncologist Dr Seamus O'Cathain said that he would favour the setting up of a State panel of experts to decide on how money should be spent in the health services:

> The kind of thing they should be looking at is, if a lot of money is spent on one patient, how many others are going to lose out? We have a finite public purse and what we need is good management of funds.... It is quite common in parts of Britain to have a list of approved drugs rather than a free-for-all. Here we have no national agreement on what could be a useful list. There is room for negotiation on that.

However, the problem with Dr O'Cathain's view is that it could lead to the restriction of approved treatments to public patients because doctors would have the option to innovate for private patients who could afford to pay. The doctor must first of all be an advocate for his/her patients – not just for some, but for all of them. The *Guide to Ethical Conduct and Behaviour* from the Medical Council (section 4.9) is strong on the duty of doctors in the context of limited resources.

> Doctors have a place in helping to ensure the efficient and effective use of resources and in giving advice on their allocation. Lack of facilities does not excuse failure to help patients. Doctors have an

Healthcare rationing

obligation to point out deficiencies to the appropriate authorities but do not have to yield to pressure for cost savings by acting against the interests of patients.

I concur.

43

Could healthcare collapse?

Unfortunately, healthcare could collapse. Currently, the US spends $4,600 per head to total $1.3 trillion, which is 13 per cent of the US GNP per year. If the system is unchanged, costs are predicted to rise to $2.6 trillion by the end of this decade, which is 17 per cent of GDP. Yet 41 million Americans have no health insurance. On 19 November 2002, a panel from the US National Academy of Sciences, called the Committee on Rapid Advance Demonstrations, laid out proposals for change in five areas – primary care, chronic care, information technology, malpractice reform (to take it out of the courtroom to provide compensation without costly litigation), and expanded insurance coverage. There would be 40 community health centres across the US designed to improve quality and reduce costs with new technology and communications systems, improve preventive care and reward staff for waste elimination. Care in the community for chronic disease would be piloted rather than clinic-based episodic care. The record system would be paperless. Health insurance for the poor would be funded either by tax credits or direct subsidies for private insurance or an expansion of the current government-run plans. All will be supported and their outcomes contrasted for effectiveness.

Dr Lewis Sandy in December 2002 in the *New England Journal of Medicine* wrote that the US system could virtually collapse under the weight of three pressures.[1]

(1) A steady increase in real healthcare costs

In the US, the aggregate collective demand for healthcare is greater than the collective willingness to pay for it. Two of the best-managed US plans, the Federal Employees Health Benefits Program and the California Public Employees Retirement System had premium increases of 13 per cent and 21 per cent, respectively, in 2002.

Could healthcare collapse?

(2) Unabated demand for healthcare services

Three factors are pushing this, i.e. medical progress, demographic change and wealth. Aggregate demand increases even as unit costs go down. New therapies for diabetes, heart disease, depression, high blood pressure, etc. extend longevity but at a price. Basic science discoveries are quickly moved into the clinical area and cost more. Gene probes, CT, spiral CT, MRI, PET scanners all add to costs that were not there many years ago. Indeed, life without disease is the medical Utopia craved and believed in by the public.[2]

Age-specific disability rates are falling. Instead of reducing costs, this trend is likely to cost more, according to Dr Sandy, because:

> ...healthier elderly persons seek more care to improve their quality of life through joint replacements, aggressive treatment of cardiac and peripheral vascular disease and treatment of anxiety and depression.... in addition the epidemic of obesity and physical inactivity, caused by steady affluence, by changes in the nature of work and in our built environment, and by systematic alterations in the US population's caloric balance will lead to an increasing prevalence of diabetes and heart disease.

(3) Dispirited providers

There are nursing shortages worldwide. Dissatisfaction is widespread among doctors in the US. Medical school applications have decreased by 15 per cent in the past four years. Doctors foresee more years of aggravation, cost pressure and diminishing reimbursement ahead.

Rationing of care will become more explicit and will overwhelmingly involve the American poor. At the moment, it is implicit with nearly 40 million people in the US devoid of health insurance coverage. The American Medical Association has endorsed the formation of unions for collective bargaining. The possibility of strikes and white coat flu may occur in the future. Tiers of healthcare by wealth and the ability to pay will almost certainly arrive. Brutally, "the poor may just have to live with their angina while the wealthy receive coated stents and immune therapy to keep their coronary arteries clear".

Nonetheless, advances in technology, drugs and therapeutics will have dramatic effects. An example is human activated protein C, effective in the treatment of sepsis, but costing $10,000 per dose.

A Cure for the Crisis

Sandy's solutions

- Spend substantial public resources expanding insurance coverage.
- Doctors and nurses must restructure to improve quality and access.
- A general recognition of the limits of medicine and spending on health.
- A social consensus on the degree of equality in our health system to facilitate change.

Plain speaking

Self-reliance has to become a byword for common sense. It is futile to try to medicalise the vicissitudes of life. Society cannot cope if medicine is expected to cure every ill when most are self-limiting. There is no right answer to how much should be spent on health. An instantly accessible therapist for everything paid for by someone else is a recipe for institutionalised absurdity. So common sense and self-reliance should be taught in school and adverts and soap operas on television should do the mothering job.

44

Action plan for Ireland

No health system that can be devised is likely to satisfy the virtually insatiable public demands for immortality and immediate remedy for any ailment whatsoever. International experience shows that there is no level of expenditure at which all public and professional expectations can be met. So health will always remain controversial and in the political arena. Calls to take healthcare out of politics are well meaning but absurd. Details on the number of beds required are set out by Fianna Fáil in their *Quality and Fairness* document and also in the Labour Party's *Our Good Health*. Let them get on with building.

There are no free lunches

As a community we have to take responsibility for our own health. Medical Utopia is not the elimination of disease because that is impossible. The purpose of medicine is to try to ensure that people live a contented, happy and useful life, that disease or illness is postponed for as long as possible and, when it arrives, that the care given is timely and appropriate. Who pays is a matter of opinion. National longevity at present seems to revolve around Mediterranean diets, wealth and the absence of epidemics of infectious diseases.

What I suggest has to be practical and possible to implement without causing chaos and collapsing morale. There is no panacea. There are obvious faults in all the published plans but they have been honestly conceived. The exception is the over-70s medical card extension from Fianna Fáil – obvious vote buying which worked. David Wanlass's report into the NHS published in April 2002 concluded that social insurance leads to higher administrative overheads, insufficient incentives for cost control and, in places like France, large premiums for both employers and employees. I think it would not work here and would not get a single extra person treated, because there is a severe supply-side problem of

273

A Cure for the Crisis

shortages of beds, nurses, radiographers, anaesthetists and doctors. Nonetheless, it does address equity.

Oireachtas Committee on Health

The key to better services and value for money is public accountability through an effective Oireachtas Committee.

- Properly resourced TDs and Senators asking probing questions and demanding answers from service providers is the key.
- Representative members of the medical, nursing and paramedical professions from each hospital should be the primary focus for each institution. The Committee may also invite any other professional member of staff to attend to answer questions or clarify local issues.
- Costs of types of admissions categorised by speciality, disease and complexity for each institution should be available and formally scrutinised.
- **These hearings must be televised live on a national channel.** Questions as to why there are few patients in outpatient departments at 4 pm could be probed. Bottlenecks in service systems could be identified by the public through their TDs and remedied.
- When the coalface workers have finished, the hospital administration could then be questioned and asked for explanations, where such are required. The law should be changed to ensure compellability of witnesses and also extend Dáil or court-room privilege to participants.

It is worth considering why there are hospitals. The *New Oxford Dictionary of English 1998* defines a hospital as: "An institution providing medical and surgical treatment and nursing care for sick and injured people." I offer my own version: "A hospital is a building that houses overlapping and interdependent medical practices with nursing care and paramedical support." It is not an institution which doubles as a local employment agency and a place for administrators to play surreptitious power games. This is why the patients and doctors should be the prime focus of attention and inquisition. The doctors will then be seen to be true patient advocates and would also be forced to face any necessary reform of their own activities.

Action plan for Ireland

Rationing of care

> *We will reduce and then permanently end waiting lists through a combination of increased bed capacity, improved primary and secondary care and targeted reform initiatives.*
>
> An Taoiseach Bertie Ahern and Minister for Health Micheál Martin
> Fianna Fáil Health Policy Statement, 6 May 2002

> *There is a problem as long as anybody is on a waiting list, although I do not think I will ever reach the day when nobody is on a waiting list.*
>
> An Taoiseach Bertie Ahern, 7 May 2003

Medical care is always rationed. It is dishonest and untrue to pretend otherwise. For example, we have decided to prioritise accidents and emergencies and these are dealt with expeditiously 24/7, but we have also decided that some conditions are less important. For example, we do not sent 75-year-olds for a liver transplant. We ration care through waiting lists and through the market by letting money talk. Taking public consultation to the next level, it is important to let the public decide either directly through properly conducted large randomised opinion polls or through their public representatives in the Oireachtas which diseases, conditions and issues should take priority in the public provision of health services. Those in the top thousand, for example, should be fully funded and readily available in the public sector. If you want to ape American celebrities and have multiple "face jobs", then these should be at your own expense and in your own time, if you can get someone to do it. In the US, the state of Ohio took such a step many years ago.

Price transparency

It is important that elements of price transparency and competition are introduced across the health service. I believe that consultation and procedures prices should be posted in the waiting rooms of GPs, consultants, private imaging and pathology services and should be available to patients in small leaflets. Public money should follow the patients in every service.

- To ensure fairness in healthcare, patient access must be prioritised according to need. This means that there must be sufficient beds available and staffed to ensure an average bed occupancy in the mid-70

A Cure for the Crisis

percentage as in the OECD favourite, France. At present, there is greater than 100 per cent occupancy in many Irish hospitals due to patients being accommodated on trolleys. If there were sufficient beds available and staffed, then obviously queues would vanish.

- To avoid the inadvertent introduction of massive hospital inefficiency, there should be a systematic evaluation of the cost base of clinical services by specialty and disease in every hospital, both public and private.

- A National Hospital Accreditation Body should be given statutory authority to license hospitals. This agency should determine national hospital standards.

- Clinical standards should be agreed and continuously reviewed with the Royal Colleges to Western international standards.

- Outcomes of clinical audits cycles should be published. Clinical outcomes would then be published.

- As part of the accreditation process, every hospital would be obliged to have a morbidity and mortality conference, which should be confidential.

- This will require alterations to the Freedom of Information Act and Tort Laws because of the litigation risks.

- There is a need for serious investment in IT and also in financial personnel to quantify the costs in each hospital. The Department of Health and Children should be the employer and provider of these financial experts, who should ask each hospital's administration and clinical staff to provide the necessary information for appraisal, according to an agreed standard national template.

The Labour Party health policy *Our Good Health,* published in autumn 2001, claims that there is a need for an extra 4,800 beds State-wide, a need for an extra 5,000 nurses, 800 hospital consultants, 660 physiotherapists, 660 speech and language therapists and 510 occupational therapists.

Consultation charges

In Dublin, GPs usually charge in the range €32 to €40 for a basic consultation but some are higher. Procedures attract an extra charge. House calls are about €50. Perusal of the *irishhealth.com* website would indi-

276

Action plan for Ireland

cate that most people think that GP fees are excessive and have risen too quickly with the euro changeover. I agree and true competition would quickly lower the fees. Average wages for the general public range from about €25,000 per year for industrial workers, €28,000 per year for services staff employed in the private sector and €35,000 a year for public sector employees. Consultants' private fees range from €90 to €150. Others may be more. The charges for inpatients and procedures are set out in the VHI preferred provider list.

Basic acute hospital care

What should reasonably be expected from an acute hospital? Every acute hospital in the State should be able to provide A&E services for most forms of accidents and the usual emergencies at an appropriate quality of care to allow their consultant staff to remain accredited as relevant specialists with the Medical Council. All the major common diseases in medicine should be dealt with at a general physician level and specialist staff must be available to deal with life-threatening acute conditions in cardiology, respiratory medicine, gut bleeding, endocrinology, neurology (strokes), rheumatology, poisoning and paediatric emergencies, where there is no local children's hospital.

Published protocols for conventional therapy for defined acute conditions should be posted in A&E. Such protocols should be individually reviewed by a specialist protocol review team in each hospital once yearly in the autumn. Each hospital must have two geriatricians and accompanying physical and occupational therapists. All five-day ward type surgery should be available and there should be waiting-list initiative cases transferred from overextended tertiary care hospitals. In reality Irish "tertiary referral hospitals" operate simultaneously in the three tiers; walk-in self-referral patients, secondary referrals from GPs in the local area, and tertiary referrals from other hospitals.

Before hospital care can be effectively provided, there must be sufficient beds to ensure about 75 per cent occupancy at valley times of the year. There must also be sufficient outpatient facilities and suites available to service patient needs. Full costings for all clinical services must be available to allow elements of competition to effectively operate. Therefore, a major investment in IT is a baseline. The introduction of a total insurance-based system when there is a shortage of beds and queues would have little benefit as it would not increase the total numbers

A Cure for the Crisis

treated. Those with private insurance would still attend private hospitals, if the queues remained intolerable in the public hospitals. However, an insurance-based system would force money to follow the patient, which is what should happen right now but does not.

The downside is the generation of reams of paper in duplicate, requiring a plethora of personnel to process until the whole system becomes electronic. Administration costs are about 31 per cent in the US, 16.7 per cent in Canada and about 10 per cent in France. The Labour Party's *Our Good Health* policy claims that Irish administration costs will be kept at 5 per cent. There is no chance of this occurring.

- Equity would be best served in hospitals by the introduction of a universal insurance system but the public element would have to be targeted towards serious illness and not vanity surgery.
- The hospital working day should run from 8 am to 6 pm. The deleterious effects of shift work and overwork must be recognised and clinics, theatres and procedures organised accordingly. This would allow current outpatient clinics to be run in three sessions – 8 am to 11.30 am, 12 midday to 3 pm and 3.15 pm to 6 pm. Consultants would be stupid to wilfully agree to shorten their own lives through shift work, given that doctors have poor longevity statistics as it is. Service departments such as pathology, radiology and ECG will have to be organised to follow suit. That should not be too difficult.

National Hospital Accreditation Body

Hospitals should be licensed to operate by the National Accreditation Body. This should be separate from the National Hospitals Agency referred to in the Fianna Fáil Health Strategy. The same licensing rules must apply to all institutions, both public and private. Services that are best provided on a national or regional basis should have their infrastructure funded by the State. These would include neurosurgery and transplantation. Where volume allows, there should be more than one regional centre as competition is healthy.

- Audit and outcome statistics must be published from each centre.
- The validity of outcomes data must be subject to random detailed evaluation to verify their accuracy.

Release of healthcare outcomes data influences referral patterns and has led to improvements in some centres and the elimination of others. There

Action plan for Ireland

is a tacit assumption that the data are accurate. However, a survey published in 2003 has revealed that the published National Cardiac Surgery Database in England from 10 tertiary care centres is both incomplete and unreliable in its ability to yield accurate, risk-adjusted outcomes data. An independent, short process of monitoring, validation and feedback improved the quality of the database. Such databases require continuous monitoring to ensure that the quality is sufficient to be useful in improving healthcare outcomes.[1]

The Society of Cardiothoracic Surgeons of Great Britain and Ireland (SCTS) has published annual reports on mortality from cardiac surgery which have protected the anonymity of the surgical centre. In 2002, they published unadjusted mortality figures for coronary artery bypass surgery and aortic valve replacement for all UK units on their website and in its annual report for 2000–1. Full risk adjustment was not carried out because of doubts about the completeness of the data.

There is an agreement with the Society of Cardiothoracic Surgeons to proceed towards the public release on individual surgeons' outcomes in England. This follows the recommendations of the Bristol Royal Infirmary Inquiry.[2]

- Standards of practice must be set by the relevant national specialist body, i.e. the Royal Colleges and Faculties and national specialist bodies. These should be interlinked with the Medical Council's registration requirements. Standards should be set at European and US norms and must be transparent. Hospital accreditation should be affirmed by specialty in an intertwining of hospital and specialty accreditation.

Organisation

- There should be either a Hospitals Division in the Department of Health and Children or a National Hospitals Agency or Authority to share out national specialty services and to commission the building of new general hospitals and to ensure that there are enough beds to satisfy clinical demand with a 75 per cent midsummer bed occupancy rate taken as the objective. (The Hanly Report average is less than 85 per cent.)
- Each hospital should have step-down beds attached, but not necessarily onsite, run by general physicians, geriatricians and rehabilitation specialists.

A Cure for the Crisis

- Stroke units in each major hospital with consultant direction should be the norm.
- Each hospital should have an independent board consisting of ministerial appointees, local elected representatives, elected members of the medical, nursing, paramedical and other staff. Health board or Department of Health officials should not ordinarily be appointed chairman of a public hospital board. People with a track record of innovation and vision should be sought to chair the board of management and drive forward our major hospitals into the frontiers of medicine.
- With regard to controversial local hospitals such as in the North East, the democratic wishes of local people as expressed in the ballot box should be respected. However, standards must not be sacrificed and the verdict of the National Hospital Accreditation Body must be implemented in the interests of quality of care. This will mean a curtailment of some specialties such as obstetrics and paediatrics. The Medical Manpower Task Force suggests a minimum population base of 100,000, with 11,000 inpatients per year for small isolated hospitals. Each of these small hospitals should have a properly constituted A&E, with three consultants who would also have an inhouse role. Surgical and anaesthetic cover is also necessary. Hanly lists 21 doctors – 7 each in medicine, surgery and anaesthesia – as a minimum to provide basic onsite emergency care within a 48-hour working week. The hospitals should also be a hive of five-day surgical activity, taking on waiting-list patients from major centres nationally.
- Non-acute hospitals modelled on the NHS Diagnostic and Treatment Centres (DTCs) should be set up to eliminate surgical waiting lists. Hospitals like Monaghan are suitable to prototype.
- Psychiatric hospitals should be accredited separately and the Inspector of Mental Hospitals should be preserved as part of the accreditation process. General hospital laboratory services nearby should be available to the psychiatric services. Near-patient testing should be the responsibility of an outreach programme from the hospital laboratory.

Planning and lead-in times for staffing appointments

The attitude of the RCSI to the recognition of training posts in the North Eastern Health Board (NEHB) area is a bit precious. Service to the public is the first duty of medicine and training bodies should allow long lead-in times to allow for consultant staff recruitment. There are A&E staff prob-

Action plan for Ireland

lems at the hospitals in Louth and Navan. Better planning is necessary from the NEHB but the RCSI should use a little common sense too. Their recent row should have been played out in public in an Oireachtas Committee to allow the public to know where the finger should be pointed. Any similar situations should be heard in the same forum. Solutions are needed not whinges. To hold the Minister personally responsible for every personnel row in the health service is ridiculous.

Finance and activity

- **Money must follow the patient.** Each procedure and patient service should have a price tag and the Department of Health should fund hospitals on the basis of activity. There should be a national price tag on procedures and for basic routine waiting-list surgery, and private hospitals must be allowed tender for public work at the same level of payment as offered to public hospitals. The Department of Health would therefore part fund such hospitals. Teaching hospitals are more expensive than service-only hospitals and the Department should fund these through a block grant. This system is far better than the National Treatment Purchase Fund.

- The Hospital Inpatient Enquiry (HIPE) data should be made the basis for funding of public hospitals and it should be made accurate. Clinicians must be held responsible for the accuracy of their patients' HIPE data, which at present often underestimates the complexity of cases.

- Complexity of case payments. Many of the more complex procedures and ill patients are transferred to teaching hospitals, where there should be a top-up figure for such cases paid by the Department or by insurers.

- Private hospitals, all of which are smaller than voluntary teaching hospitals, should have an academic attachment to a district general hospital or a teaching hospital, so that private-only consultants do not suffer from clinical isolation. Such staff should be asked to attend and participate in specialty conferences in the bigger hospitals as part of continuing medical education. Cross-cover for leave periods should also be facilitated in small specialties.

Extra hospital beds

There needs to be about 5,000 extra hospital beds. The National Health Strategy promises to increase the number of acute beds by 3,000 over the next 10 years. Occupancy rates and usage levels for all our hospitals should be monitored to fine-tune the country's hospital bed needs.

A doubling of the size of Loughlinstown and Naas hospitals should be done and Beaumont Hospital should have 100 beds built immediately onsite. Capital investment in step-down beds must be made to increase the number by 600 in the first instance. James Connolly Memorial Hospital, Blanchardstown is an obvious place to develop, yet the rebuilding programme lacks vision and is wholly inadequate. The Eastern Health Board should never have been allowed to sell the land before the opportunity to develop a total health and exercise campus for locals had been considered.

Doctor's should act within the boundaries set out by Dr Arnold Relman, the former editor of the *New England Journal of Medicine,* in his commentaries on ethical medical practice, and ensure that they do not have a financial interest in referring patients to an institution or facility where they are co-owners.

Consultants

There are four consultants per 10,000 population in Ireland compared to the EU average of 14.' There were more than 1,731 Comhairle na nOspidéal-approved consultant posts in the Republic by mid-2003 but about 15 per cent are unfilled. All the major specialties should have new consultant appointments immediately. Some NCHD posts outside of Dublin should be suppressed as new consultants are appointed. The Cardiovascular Strategy should be implemented and manpower appointed.

The National Task Force on Medical Staffing claims that we need 3,500 extra consultants to facilitate the introduction of a 48-hour week for NCHDs. The Medical Manpower Report in *The Sunday Tribune* of 16 February 2003 proposed an increase of 1,177 consultants from a current total of 1,731 to 2,908 by 2009. The Hanly Report proposes 3,100 consultants by 2009 and 3,600 by 2013. The Royal College of Physicians in London claims that there is a need for 13,000 new consultants in the NHS by 2008 to realise the government's targets. So there is a medical manpower crisis of considerable proportions. Like any shortage, the price will inevitably rise or the employers will insist that anyone finishing a training course, who is eligible for inclusion on the specialist register, must be

Action plan for Ireland

appointed to a consultant post. At any rate, the role and cachet of the consultant will be immutably changed.

- The only medical grade whose members have clinical autonomy is the consultant. The roles of the clinical nurse specialist, the advanced nurse practitioner (ANP), top grade biochemists, chief medical scientists, physiotherapists and other professions allied to medicine will have to be further clarified. Where does their responsibility lie in relation to the consultant? The level of autonomy of advanced nurse practitioners as set out and defined in the Report of the Forum on Medical Manpower is dangerously diffuse in my view. This is less so with clinical nurse specialists. The definitions that particularly concern me are:

- "The ANP receives clients with undifferentiated and undiagnosed problems and initiates treatments according to agreed protocols and within agreed expanded parameters."

- "The ANP practises an advanced nursing or midwifery role – makes professionally autonomous decisions taking responsibility within agreed protocols."

- "The ANP works independently, but closely, with other professionals and respects professional boundaries."

How can you respect professional boundaries when you have trampled all over them? Autonomous decisions on whose patients? I think this is a minefield and most likely a legal one too.

- Compulsory retirement at 65 should be abolished and be replaced by an option to retire as at present or to continue part-time or full-time without pension loss or penalty. Such a reform is necessary because of the oncoming consultant manpower crisis.

- A candid consultant will know that every patient should be private. If every patient were private, there would be equity in care and freedom of conscience for the doctor. It would also mean that the doctor would be paid for seeing each patient. The objective should be to make the public health system effective enough to make private health provision pointless. Until that happens, then money will buy something extra and there is no point in pretending otherwise.

A Cure for the Crisis

Organisation of general hospital care

1. Appoint or allow into practice sufficient consultants to have patient choice and some competition.

2. Elegibility for specialist registration at the Medical Council should be the minimum requirement for a consultant.

3. The medical directorates in each hospital in association with a reformed Comhairle na nOspidéal/Department of Health should determine the number of specialists needed to deal with patient volume in each hospital. There are international norms recommended for specialties. These need not be blindly accepted as a degree of special pleading and padding of numbers is obvious. A senior official in the Department of Health should be responsible for groups of specialties countrywide. For example, a principle officer should look after neurology, neurosurgery, neurophysiology, psychology, neuropathology, neurological imaging, rehabilitation and long-term care like Headways.

4. The admitting physician must be the primary carer for each patient. "Consultants working in teams" (Hanly Report) or collectivisation will inevitably lead to professional conflict.

5. Hospital medical boards should also be allowed appoint general physicians where there is a demonstrable need.

6. General physicians would facilitate true superspecialists to really concentrate on their area of expertise, including time for research and the introduction of new developments.

7. Consultant appointments should share junior doctors within a specialty. The issue of NCHDs should not be used as an excuse to postpone consultant appointments.

8. The common contract for consultants should be changed to allow the appointment of consultants who would be paid a retainer and a fee-per-patient. The fee should be specialty dependent. Clearly, a neurology and psychiatry consultation, for example, will usually take much longer than a cardiology consult. Therefore, a weighting fee multiplier would have to be agreed, taking cognisance of the specialty and complexity. The fee for a new patient should be greater than for a return. The current scheduling of throughput in private clinics could be used as an initial template for negotiation. This would set the template for a universal hospital insurance system which would

Action plan for Ireland

allow competition within the public sector and between the private and public sectors.

9. Fees for procedures would have a professional and technical element.

10. Audits should temper overuse, underuse or inappropriate use of procedures.

11. These consultants would have visiting and admission rights.

12. Their remuneration would have to be pensionable in the usual way.

13. Consultants in private hospitals could then be appointed part-time to public hospitals.

14. Current common contract holders could opt into the retainer plus fees system, but the pension consequences would have to be clarified.

15. Merit awards of significance such as €50,000 to €200,000 should be payable for excellence. The criteria for such payments should be academic work, teaching commitment, medical work at the Royal Colleges or on State boards and after peer review. Such awards should only be available to new, retained contract holders, so that they would not be inhibited from making a full professional contribution.

16. Radiologists could be included in the new contract dispensation.

17. Histopathologists and neuropathologists should similarly be included, but there would have to be a time and complexity payment factored in to their remuneration, which would differ according to subspecialty.

18. Haematologists, clinical microbiologists, immunologists and chemical pathologists should be treated as clinicians in the clinical sphere and have a volume and complexity adjustment added for laboratory work. There should also be a laboratory management component. Professional fees should only be paid to those on the relevant specialist register. Hospitals without a medical consultant specialist pathologist in any subspecialty must not be allowed bill for professional fees in that area.

19. A version of the Medicare/Medicaid payment scheme for doctors using the Harvard Relative Values for procedures, etc. could be used as a payment template.

20. Part-time and job-sharing arrangements must be made flexible and family-friendly for consultants who wish to participate.

A Cure for the Crisis

21. A consultant-provided clinical service would need a change of common contract and some rostering of work time, which has serious implications for manpower. Any roster would have to be tapered towards a lessening of late hours with age and length of service.

22. Clinical directorates and teamwork would likely become part of such a system to ensure continuity of care. This has implications for clinical autonomy because not all consultants agree on the details of care for every patient.

23. The thrust of the measures to place administrator control on consultants in public hospitals as set out in the Commission on Financial Management and Control Systems in the Health Service (January 2003) is a recipe for morale collapse and interminable industrial trouble for at least 20 years until the present medical cohort has retired. You cannot monitor and control the core activities of consultants without undermining professionalism. The motives of the originators of such activities must be open to question. In my system, dilettante doctors would not get paid for not seeing patients.

24. Consultants must be allowed to manage their own practices. Pathologists and radiologists must be allowed to effectively direct their disciplines.

25. In the longer term, equity would be best served by the introduction of an insurance-based system for hospitals, which should include an extra payment element for teaching hospitals and high-tech institutions. Fianna Fáil would be well advised to steal Labour's clothes on this issue.

Working time

A recent survey of 504 specialist registrars found that 92 per cent felt that teamwork and continuity of care were reduced by shift work when compared to an on-call system. Seventy-five per cent also thought that on-call was better for training, 53 per cent felt it was better for the quality of care and 55 per cent said it was better for their quality of life. In the *Irish Medical Journal,* Dr MF Geoghegan wrote that shift work promoted a "caretaker" and clocking-off culture.[3] The overnight doctor has no responsibility for the patient the next day. An attitude of "do the minimum and let someone else get on with the rest" prevails. There is reduced feedback on cases, reduced learning as a consequence, less socialising with peers and more isolation and poorer morale.

Action plan for Ireland

A shift-work system must be avoided as there is ample objective evidence of its ill effects on health. And it might not be the best for medicine either. There is no way that current consultants will do or should work a 24-hour shift, no matter what the Department of Health demands. The advantages of the European Working Time Directive 1998 of a maximum 56-hour week are less stress, more leisure time, less tired doctors and better clinical care. Disadvantages may include reduced teamwork and continuity of care, reduced time for training, less patient exposure and less experience, reduced quality of care and perhaps reduced quality of life for doctors. The 24/7 tenor of the Hanly Report[4] is absurd. Hospitals are not branches of Tesco's. Only A&E and invasive cardiology should have 24-hour onsite cover (assuming primary angioplasty as the optimal standard of care for heart attacks). The Hanly Report is best read sceptically; but the data presented are an addition to this book. However, the costings are most likely aspirational.

Public health doctors and public health

Public health consultants should have their salaries tied to the average consultant salary under the common contract without salary abatement by location. Roster payments should be in line with the common contract.

Resources should be targeted at socioeconomic disadvantage in particular in children. Protecting children from poverty in childhood could reduce the burden of disease experienced by adults. This arbitrary fact is not left-wing fiction. All physical health measures at age 26 years, except systolic blood pressure, show a graded relation with childhood socioeconomic status. As socioeconomic status increased, body mass index and waist–hip ratio decreased and cardiorespiratory fitness increased. All dental health measures also show a graded relation to childhood socioeconomic status. Depression and smoking were not linked but alcohol abuse was weakly linked and related more to adult social conditions. The downwardly socially mobile also have poor cardiovascular fitness and tooth cleanliness.

- Public policy should divert resources from the wealthy to improve the schooling, nutrition and parenting of children in lower socioeconomic areas. Children's allowances should be tapered away from well-to-do professionals and diverted to where the societal impact will be most beneficial.

A Cure for the Crisis

- The 130,000 voluntary carers who save the State about €2 billion annually in services to the handicapped and the elderly get a paltry €129.60 per week, but only 19,000 get the full-time allowance. Comprehensive assessment guidelines must be introduced to take the discretionary element away from the payment and ensure fairness and clarity.

Accident and Emergency

The improvements in emergency care over the past two decades are enormous. Clearly, there is a need for more consultants and for more part-time consultants and medical assistants. The Manpower Forum is calling for 88 A&E consultants by 2009. The appointment of general physicians to the front of the house and the use of medical assessment units may reshape the current concepts of casualty services and the role and number of A&E consultants. It is likely that nurses will be involved in managing minor injuries and other specific conditions.

Television advertising campaigns should be used to educate the public into what is a real accident or an emergency. Convenience self-referral of primary care problems can only be discouraged by public education programmes and by using the price mechanism.

- Patients should be charged for the use of A&E along the present lines. Otherwise A&E would be used as a convenience store and life for staff would become unbearable.

- A list of diagnoses should be exempt from charges, such as road traffic accident victims, acute asthma, acute chest pains, etc. to facilitate appropriate medical interventions. At present, some of the triage effect ensures that unnecessary attenders are kept waiting for a sufficiently long period to make primary care obviously more attractive.

- Group general practices will facilitate the proper use of hospital facilities because there is a need for the public to be able to access GPs out-of-hours *appropriately*.

- There should be three A&E consultants in each large general hospital appointed to cover an extended day. Proper supervision of junior doctors and nurses is necessary for good practice. Patients should be educated to use the service appropriately. For major accidents, the plan to call in extra consultants should be operated. This may also be necessary during the throes of an epidemic. The widespread closure of A&E departments in small hospitals is simply wrong.

288

Action plan for Ireland

- Diversion of appropriately triaged patients to a medical assessment unit to be seen by medical registrars and consultants should be arranged. This seems to be a better arrangement for patients and for the hospital medical staff. Some but not all of these patients may require admission. The physical spaces for such a unit would have to be appropriately designed. It will be interesting to see and read reports on how the unit at St James's Hospital works in 2003.
- General internal medicine consultants should play a role in A&E as consultants and trainers. If this was organised properly, then there may not be the need for three A&E consultants. Two would suffice with another two general internal medicine consultants giving better value for money. Consultants' work schedules would be dictated by local demands.
- GPs should not be working in A&E. If general practice is about holistic patient care, then once-off spot cases are not the best model, and patients should not be trained to regard hospitals as convenient primary care drop-in centres.
- Chest Pain Evaluation and Therapy Units (CPETU) should be developed to process all patients with chest pains definitively within one day. This is well worked out in the United States where there are ready-made protocols. Primary angioplasty must be available in all general hospitals. Heart attack patients within a two-hour transfer time should be sent for invasive treatment.

General practitioners

GPs are a success story in Irish life and have a tradition of dutiful service over generations. Life has become fast moving and market driven and old values of community and caring are to an extent being replaced by "How much is in it for me?" Good GPs are the caring general physicians of the future. We should be careful not to demoralise that group as there is no ready alternative.

The World Organization of National Colleges, Academies and Academic Associations of General Practitioners/Family Physicians (WONCA) Europe set out the key characteristics of general practice in 2002. These are:

- The point of first medical contact within the healthcare system.
- The GP makes efficient use of healthcare resources.

A Cure for the Crisis

- A person-orientated approach.
- A unique consultation process and a long-term relationship with the patient.
- Uses a decision-making process determined by the prevalence and incidence of illness in the community.
- Manages simultaneously acute and chronic illness in the patient.
- Promotes preventive health.

GPs care for individuals in the context of their family, community and their culture, always respecting the autonomy of the patient. Six core competencies are regarded as essential:

- Primary care management.
- Person-centred care.
- Specific problem-solving skills.
- Comprehensive approach.
- Community orientation.
- Holistic modelling.

There are at present a number of different types of general practice and each has a niche. Both the Health Strategy and the Primary Care Strategy, published by the Department of Health and Children, offer models. In relation to the Health Strategy, it is important for GPs to identify the exclusive preserve of the GP, what can and should be the responsibility of the primary care team and where the GP responsibility stops.[5] In primary care – a new direction from the Government – there is a clear emphasis in declaring a team approach. To this end, the IMO and the ICGP published *A Vision of General Practice*, which is their agreed basis for development.

Currently over 50 per cent of the ICGP membership is in single-handed practices. There are about 2,200 GPs in the country, some of whom work part-time. The ICGP suggests that there is a shortage of 1,500. There are five GPs per 10,000 population compared to the EU average of nine. There are three times more GPs in wealthy areas than in poorer areas in the State. General practice is almost certain to develop differently in deprived communities than in wealthy areas. Doctors in the latter areas will continue to provide a humane, patient-orientated individual service based on an evolving best practice. In deprived areas,

Action plan for Ireland

doctors are likely to have a different workload and a different set of priorities driven by a different set of patient demands and expectations.

A poll of the requirements of people in poorer areas listed the following priorities. This is a move away from the personal and continuing care towards multidisciplinary services.[6]

- Out-of-hours GP service.
- Accident and emergency services.
- Maternity services.
- Contraceptive and psychological services for adults.
- Services for the elderly, women, men and adolescents.
- Counselling.
- Drug and alcohol services.
- Social work services.

Early teamwork is evident in the newer health services between GPs and public health nurses. A key question for GPs is whether they are providing care for the individual or service to a community.

Pilot primary care teams

The primary care teams consist of GPs, nurses, midwives, healthcare assistants, home helps, occupational therapists, physiotherapists, social workers and administrative people. As outlined in the Primary Care Strategy, 10 centres have been established involving about 80,000 patients. As the new model is developed, a wider primary care network of other primary care professionals will also provide services. Public subvention of €8.4 million has been allocated for 2002 and 2003. The areas involved are Lifford, Co Donegal; the South Inner City, Dublin; Virginia, Co Cavan; Ballymun, Dublin; the Dingle Peninsula, Kerry; Portarlington, Co Laois; West Limerick; Erris, Co Mayo; Cashel, Co Tipperary; and Arklow, Co Wicklow.

Out-of-hours GP service

Lifestyle changes have downgraded the tradition of house calls in general practice. Convenience house calls are a thing of the past. Now most GPs only do house calls where the patient cannot physically attend the surgery. Demand for house calls is still high and there is a need to educate the public as to the function of the service. Clearly, where do house calls

A Cure for the Crisis

fit in? – if a GP who starts at 8.30 am and works all morning seeing patients one after another relentlessly, then has a break from somewhere between 12.30 and 1.30 pm, before starting again from 2.30 to 5 pm or from 3 to 6 pm or from x to 7 or 7.30 pm. Each house call would take at least 30 minutes when transportation is factored in. The true cost of a house call is much more expensive than a surgery visit. Now there are also the demands of CME with hospital teaching meetings often at lunchtime. Time has become a precious commodity. General practice is quickly feminising and this too has consequences. Unreasonable patients will be avoided and part-time and session work will become more common.

GP co-ops are in place, for example, North East DOC, KDOC and others. These are subvented by the health board and the GPs do about 11 sessions every three months. One doctor sees people who go to a central clinic and there is also a mobile doctor with a driver doing house calls. Nearly all GPs in Drogheda do not take appointments after 5.30 pm, whereby the calls are forwarded to the locum service at 6 pm. If perchance a GP sees a patient after hours, the GP cannot claim a fee from the GMS if relevant, because the payment system is routed through the on-call service payments agreement. Private patients' income is managed by a financial manager and is used to top up a fixed payment which is agreed with the health board. It is also used to cover the cost of the management of the system. The number of GMS calls is not directly relevant to payment, as there is a health board deal for a fixed payment per session. The GPs have found it satisfactory so far, making their lives easier. It does take away from the personal service of one doctor/one patient. WESTDOC will cover Galway city and environs. The co-op is being allocated €2 million in 2003 and will be run on a fee-per-item basis.

The price mechanism does play some role in tempering the demand for house calls. The charge in Dublin is about €50 per call, unless there is extra mileage involved. Hotel calls are in the range €70 to €90 depending on the hotel. This is not excessive when you consider that the usual surgery visit basic charge ranges from about €32 to €40 in Dublin, with most GPs on about €35. Immediate follow-up visits usually cost less. Note the €20 charge in France and the GP basic consultation fee in Melbourne, Australia of AUS$35 (€18), of which AUS$25 is reimbursed by the state Medicaid and there is a AUS$10 co-payment! Pathology and procedures attract an extra charge.

Action plan for Ireland

Solutions

1. GPs must be the personal physician of the patient.

2. GPs should be gatekeepers for consultants. There are primary care consultants in private clinic practice who accept self-referrals; CME and audit for them will be interesting. The coming consultant short-fall will lead to many of these entering the public system. Then these consultants will be properly utilised.

3. There are other consultants who run primary care private rooms and refer to other consultants. Unless the GMS rules are changed, patients over 70 years must have private consultant prescriptions rewritten by their GPs or the patients will have to pay for their medication. After a while the patients may opt to attend the GP only.

4. Where there is a particularly heavy burden of social and socioeconomic problems, the GP's role will require team leadership, liaison with other professionals and advocacy.

5. GP practical procedure work will be influenced by the age profile of the practice, distance from hospitals and the services that hospitals provide.

6. Good liaison with community pharmacists is important. It reduces prescription errors and facilitates better patient care.

7. Minor surgical procedures, cryotherapy, insertions of intrauterine contraceptive devices (IUCDs), diaphragms and mirena coils are often part of group practices. This is less likely where there are convenient well-publicised specialist clinics operating such as the Well Woman Centre.

8. Lone GPs in rural areas should inter-refer to allow the retention of expertise in a chosen subject.

9. Compulsory retirement from the GMS must be abolished. GPs should be allowed opt for retirement at 65 or be allowed continue to practise as long as they remain licensed under the specialist register rules of the Medical Council. There should be a loyalty bonus paid in rural areas and pensions must be unaffected or enhanced for those who continue to work after the age of 65 years.

10. Restrictions on entry to the GMS should be limited to being a fully specialist trained and registered GP. How long you have been at a practice site should be irrelevant. Many businesses fail. Do the pub-

A Cure for the Crisis

lic benefit by restraints of trade? I doubt it. Why not allow all patients full freedom of choice?

11. GPs should take the lead in cardiovascular medicine, preventive medicine and in screening for disease as part of their normal remit.

12. The ICGP should invite all its members to make sure that every patient is screened for disease at the appropriate age. Such screening programmes should be modified in the light of new trial evidence. This is an issue suitable for CPD accreditation.

13. GPs should have ICGP check lists for common disease therapies, such as statins in secondary prevention, B_{12}, folate and pyridoxine for homocystinaemia and vascular disease, niacin for low HDL cases, ACE inhibitors, betablockers and spironolactone in heart failure, and ACE inhibitors in renal failure. Furthermore, they should get the blood pressure down where possible when above 140/90 or 130/80 mmHg in diabetics, give statins anyway, normalise the TSH, etc. and keep reading the *New England Journal of Medicine*, even if they only have time for the abstracts. The *British Medical Journal* is the best journal for general medical practice.

14. The ICGP should have printed lists of therapies and explanations for patients covering common diseases which could be handed out in GP surgeries. These must be reviewed yearly. The master copy should include references for the doctor.

15. In Dublin, where there is an excellent service from hospitals, GPs have open access to endoscopy, radiology, blood tests, microbiology, smear testing and exercise ECGs. **There should be direct access to 24-hour blood pressure monitoring, dieticians, physiotherapists and all the services enjoyed by hospital consultants on the same basis as consultants.** In other words, there should be closer links between primary care and hospitals for routine services which can more efficiently be provided in the hospital.

In England, there are primary care endoscopy services and a survey revealed 13 providing upper and lower gastrointestinal endoscopy services.[7] The definition of primary care was a little fanciful and the endoscopists had between 6 and 25 years (average 16) endoscopy experience. I am not in favour of this because of the consequences of ruptured varices, perforations or other problems. These operators would be better having sessions in a local hospital unit staffed by consultants with full paraphernalia.

294

Action plan for Ireland

16. Shared care protocols should be agreed and regularly reviewed at a formal hospital/GP interface. Shared IT systems are crucial to their success.

17. The times and programme of specialty meetings in hospitals should be notified by email to local and interested GPs. Attendance at such a meeting should qualify automatically for CME points.

18. Courier services should be made available to collect specimens from GP surgeries in cities and near county hospitals.

19. Where GPs are using near-patient testing services, the liaison hospital should supply quality control and technical assistance.

20. The current discriminatory practice of funding certain types of practices only for disease campaigns should be stopped.

21. Sophisticated IT links to all GPs should be developed, so that the GPs can access any hospital information system pertaining to their patients and practice results, whereby reports can be sent directly by email on a daily basis when validated in the hospital.

22. IT for video conferencing to local hospitals and for CME should be used. Such activity should be recognised for CME points.

23. Practice nurses and other ancillary staff should have their roles more clearly defined. Clinical responsibility lies with the GP, and medical indemnity and insurance cover issues will need to be reviewed. Nurses are insured through the Irish Nurses Organisation.

24. Nurses may replace much of the GP work in protocol-driven hypertension, antenatal, diabetes, obesity and other clinics. However, it is important that doctors continue to see the bulk of these patients because if they do not, skill levels will fall over time.

25. It is unlikely that there will be inroads by nurse protocol clinics into private practice because money will dictate otherwise.

26. Public health nurses play a crucial role in local communities. GPs should have formal liaison with the district nurses and should be in regular contact, especially with difficult patient management problems.

27. Home helps should be available for patients when the GP and district nurse considers this appropriate.

28. GPs would be wise to retain their autonomy. It would be short-sighted to allow the health boards to employ them. The question of practice ownership will also arise.

295

29. Group practices are likely to become more common. In concert with feminisation, out-of-hours co-ops and the demands of CME and registration, it is likely that GP surgeries outside of the conventional 9 am to 5 pm opening hours will become unusual. Political attempts to buck this will prove futile.

30. Should primary care come to be regarded by the public as just another resource devoid of personal relationships, it is likely that big health clinics will be opened in shopping centres that will do acute-item GP work on demand. This might include "well woman" and "well man" clinics. Boots or a similar organisation are likely candidates.

31. Audits should be undertaken in association with the ICGP as part of quality assurance, education and outcomes improvement for patients.

32. For quality assurance, the ICGP suggests that the *Australian Model Standards for General Practices* (2nd edition), RACGP and the requirements of Australian GP accreditation might be suitable for adaptation for Irish use. Issues like a vaccine cold chain for the storage of vaccines and fridge thermometers are part of GP accreditation.[8]

33. GP out-of-hours co-ops may be useful.

34. Refugees and foreigners: the local faculty of the ICGP should organise discussions about haemoglobinopathies, Mediterranean fever, tropical diseases such as malaria and leishmaniasis, Lime disease, unusual tuberculosis, infectious diseases and others where there are new influxes of ethnic migrants. Recognition of these conditions, where present, is important.

GP fees and the GMS

Because there is a considerable degree of overvisiting of GPs by patients when there is no payment or co-payment, innovative methods of extension of the publicly funded element of GP services should be carefully considered. It is wasteful, stupid and sometimes cynical not to target scarce resources on those who need them most. It is easy to say extend the GMS to cover an increasing number of people with lower incomes, for example the 200,000 promised by Fianna Fáil. This would require detailed negotiations with GPs, who are unlikely to accept a cheap deal especially after the over-70s' result.

Action plan for Ireland

- Alternatives include means testing the wasteful over-70s free scheme to see how much could be saved and diverting the money to the real needy, just above the current income cut-off levels. To reduce the political storm, the threshold levels could be kept above the level of €300 per week per person.
- Or, the whole over-70s new scheme could be changed to a voucher system with the Drug Payments Scheme also used.
- The voucher scheme would entail the issuance of GP vouchers of €30 each in value, which could be taken and used to pay for services at any practice. The GP can then encash these by submission to the GMS Payments Board. These vouchers could be distributed at post offices or by mail. They would be means tested. In private practice, expenses consume about 50 per cent of practice income.
- GPs could require a co-payment or accept one voucher as a full settlement.
- At least five vouchers would be issued per eligible person per year.
- The number of vouchers could be increased by need after application and assessment.
- The voucher scheme could be extended to those on low incomes.
- The budget implications are easy to calculate because the tax system will accurately reveal the numbers at any given income cut-off.
- Everyone with chronic diseases, such as severe asthma as defined by the experts, cystic fibrosis, diabetes, etc., should be eligible for totally free medical care at the point of contact.

Palliative care

- Hospice care should be available to all who wish it.
- Hospices should be fully publicly funded.
- Hospice homecare teams should be linked to groups of GPs. They should act in concert and not independently of the GP.
- A pain relief guarantee should be issued to each patient.
- Palliative care should be extended to patients with muscular dystrophy, motor neurone disease and similar conditions.

Medical schools

There should be no limitation on the number of Irish entrants to medical schools, even if some are privately funded. If the Government wants to limit the numbers publicly funded, then the colleges should be free to take fee-paying students. This would increase competition in practice by increasing the supply of doctors and would ultimately reduce the fees charged to patients.

Pharmacy

There should be open competition in the supply of pharmacy services, but a qualified pharmacist must be onsite during trading hours. Parallel drug importing from other EU countries must be allowed. Spain and Portugal have much cheaper proprietary drug prices than Northern Europe, including Ireland. The wholesale price fixing arrangement by the Department of Health is not beneficial to consumers and must be abolished. Large chains should be prevented from gaining a monopoly.

Health boards

After removing hospital management from the health boards, they should be slimmed down to subserve public health, primary care, geriatrics and social medicine functions. The Prospectus Plan to have four Regional Health Service Executive Bodies, with a heavy professional presence and a consumer's interest, is unwise. It reinforces the anonymity of remote decision-makers and takes away local accountability. The most responsive people to consumer opinion are local politicians elected by the public. Once again, I have to reaffirm my faith in democracy.

Talented officials could be moved into hospital management but responsible to the new hospital boards. Most definitely, the ERHA supertanker deserves abolision. A health board or executive should be sited in Cork, Galway, the Midlands, Sligo and Waterford. Another (East Coast) should be sited in Bray to cover services south of the River Liffey down to include Wicklow and Kildare, and a seventh should cover the territory north of the Liffey all the way to the border.

Complementary and alternative medicine

Complementary and alternative medicine – such as homeopathy, chiropractic, osteopathy, naturopathic doctors, acupuncturists, herbal medi-

Action plan for Ireland

cine and other complementary medical services – must come under statutory regulation, in particular the pills and potions element to ensure public safety. *A Report on the Regulation of Practitioners of Complementary and Alternative Medicine in Ireland* published by the Institute of Public Administration is available on the website of the Department of Health and Children. It should be read by all doctors who should also remember that many patients attend alternative medicine with all sorts of ailments. The power of the placebo and the benefit of concern and niceness must never be forgotten.

The American requirements for training vary from four to five years or 4,200 hours for chiropractors to 500 hours for massage therapists in most states. State legislatures can grant licences to practise alternative medicine, even if science has not vindicated the theory. There are large variations in the rigour of the training programmes. Chiropractors' training includes basic medical sciences as well as clinical experience. For homeopaths, Nevada and Arizona specify six months and 300 hours of postgraduate training, respectively, but Connecticut does not specify any educational requirements. In complete contrast, naturopathic physicians are examined in basic sciences, and undergo clinical examinations in clinical, physical and laboratory diagnosis, pharmacology, diagnostic imaging, botanical medicine, nutrition, physical medicine, minor surgery, psychology, lifestyle counselling and emergency medicine.[9]

Herbal remedies are exempt from rigorous regulation in the US. These herbs can cause serious health risks. Adulterants such as bacteria, toxins, metals and drugs may contaminate the potions and have been well described. Cardiac, liver, nerve and kidney toxicity have been listed and interactions with prescribed drugs may be lethal.[10]

The cure – immediate steps

Healthcare is in crisis in every country in the world. Rationing of care is an irreducible fact. How this is done is a matter of opinion and philosophy. The results of medical research change clinical practice by the month at greater and greater expense. (The US NIH spends $28 billion annually on research.) Therefore, no model will satisfy the public's demand for universal mistake-free medical care. The public must take more responsibility for their own lives and welfare. The immediate crisis in Ireland can be alleviated by putting in 600 nursing home step-down beds and by organising acute medical investigation and treatment units alongside A&E departments. Buy MRI scanners. Implement the continuous audit of all institutional medical prac-

A Cure for the Crisis

tices with all audit cycles subjected to scrutiny by the Oireachtas. This will re-establish the primacy of the doctor–patient relationship and ensure that minimal standards are maintained in all specialties. The centralised control and command of medical practices by administrators would therefore be rendered impossible. Irrespective of whether the system of hospital care is wholly insurance-based or remains the present public–private mix, money must follow the patient. My preference is that everyone be made a private patient with different levels of cover. Finally, medical incomes will fall as numbers and competition increase.

Glossary

ACB	Association of Clinical Biochemists
ACBI	Association of Clinical Biochemists in Ireland
ACE inhibitor	angiotensin-converting enzyme inhibitor
ADRs	adverse drug reactions
AED	automated external defibrillator
AIDS	acquired immune deficiency syndrome
ANP	advanced nurse practitioner
A&E	Accident & Emergency
BHF-HPS	British Heart Foundation Heart Protection Study
BMA	British Medical Association
BMJ	British Medical Journal
BTSB	Blood Transfusion Service Board
BUPA	British United Provident Association
CAO	Central Admissions Office
CEO	chief executive officer
CMA	Canadian Medical Association
CME	continuous medical education
COPD	chronic obstructive pulmonary disease
CPD	continuous professional development
CPETUs	Chest Pain Evaluation and Therapy Units
CSM	Committee on the Safety of Medicines
CSO	Central Statistics Office
CSSD	central sterile supply department
CT	computed tomography
DALYs	disability adjusted life years
DATH	Dublin Academic Teaching Hospitals
DOHC	Department of Health and Children
DPS	Drug Payment Scheme
DTCs	Diagnostic and Treatment Centres
EAHB	Eastern Area Health Board
ECG	electrocardiogram
ECHO	echocardiogram
ECT	electroconvulsive therapy
EHB	Eastern Health Board

EMG	electromyogram
ENT	Ear, Nose and Throat
ERHA	Eastern Regional Health Authority
ESRI	Economic and Social Research Institute
EU	European Union
FCTC	Framework Convention on Tobacco Control
FDA	Food and Drugs Administration
FDG	18 fluorodeoxyglucose
FCTC	Framework Convention on Tobacco Control
GDP	gross domestic product
GMC	General Medical Council
GMS	General Medical Services
GNP	gross national product
GP	general practitioner
HbA1c	haemoglobin A1c
HDL	high-density lipoprotein
HEA	Higher Education Authority
HIA	Health Insurance Authority
HIPE	Hospital Inpatient Inquiry Data
HIV	human immunodeficiency virus
HK	Hong Kong
HMO	Health Maintenance Organisation
HNCC	Haemophilia National Co-ordinating Committee
HPV	human papilloma virus
HR	human resources
HSE	Health Services Executive
IBTS	Irish Blood Transfusion Service
ICGP	Irish College of General Practitioners
ICU	intensive care unit
IHCA	Irish Hospital Consultants' Association
IHS	Irish Haemophilia Society
IMB	Irish Medicines Board
IMC	Irish Medical Council
IMO	Irish Medical Organisation
INO	Irish Nurses Organisation
INR	international normalised ratio
ISPCC	Irish Society for Prevention of Cruelty to Children
IT	information technology
ITUs	intensive therapy units

Glossary

IUCD	intrauterine contraceptive device
JAMA	Journal of the American Medical Association
JCMH	James Connolly Memorial Hospital, Blanchardstown
LAC	Local Appointments Commission
LDL	low-density lipoprotein
MACs	medical assistants in caring
MCA	Medicines Control Agency
MCQs	multiple choice questions
MDU	Medical Defence Union
MIMS	Monthly Index of Medical Specialities
MPS	Medical Protection Society
MRC	Medical Research Council
MRCP	magnetic resonance cholangiopancreatography
MRI	magnetic resonance imaging
NAHB	Northern Area Health Board
NACD	Natinal Advisory Committee on Drugs
NCHD	non-consultant hospital doctor
NEHB	North Eastern Health Board
NHS	National Health Service
NICE	National Institute for Clinical Excellence
NIH	National Institutes of Health
NMH	National Maternity Hospital
NTPF	National Treatment Purchase Fund
ODDs	one disease doctors
OECD	Organisation for Economic Co-operation and Development
OPD	outpatient department
PDs	Progressive Democrats
PET	positron emission tomography
PSA	prostate specific antigen
PTCA	percutaneous transluminal coronary angioplasty
QC	quality control
RACGP	Royal Australian College of General Practitioners
RCP	Royal College of Physicians
RCPath	Royal College of Pathologists
RCPI	Royal College of Physicans of Ireland
RCSI	Royal College of Surgeons in Ireland
RTÉ	Radio Telefís Éireann
SCA	State Claims Agency

A Cure for the Crisis

SCTS	Society of Cardiothoracic Surgeons
SENs	state enrolled nurses
SHARP	Southern Heart Attack Response Project
SRNs	state registered nurses
SSRIs	selective serotonin reuptake inhibitors
SRSV	small round structured virus
TCD	Trinity College Dublin
TSH	thyroid-stimulating hormone
UCD	University College Dublin
UCHG	University College Hospital Galway
UK	United Kingdom
UKHAS	United Kingdom Heart Attack Study
UN	United Nations
US	United States
USI	Union of Students in Ireland
VHI	Voluntary Health Insurance
VLDP	very low density lipoprotein
VQ	ventilation perfusion lung scan
WHO	World Health Organization
WONCA	World Organization of National Colleges and Academies, Academic Associations of General Practitioners/Family Physicians [World Organization of Family Doctors]

References

2 National Health Strategy

[1] Wall M. Medical cardholders may have to pay for treatment. *The Sunday Tribune* 2003 Jan 5; p. 12.

[2] Shanahan C. Check up time for health strategy. *Irish Examiner* 2002 Dec 2; p. 6.

[3] McCarthaigh S. €500,000 for sick children's hospital. *Irish Examiner* 2002 Dec 2; p. 5.

[4] Making patients the first priority [editorial]. *The Irish Times* 2002 Dec 23.

5 The Health Boards

[1] Health crisis bureaucratic excess must be eliminated [editorial]. *Irish Examiner* 2002 Nov 19.

6 The General Medical Services (GMS)

[1] Howe A, Parry G, Pickvance D, Hockley B. Defining frequent attendance: evidence for routine age and sex correction in studies from primary care settings. *Br J Gen Pract* 2002;**52**:561–565.

[2] Barry M. Drug expenditure in Ireland 1991–2001. *Ir Med J* 2002;**95**:294–5.

[3] Cooke N. GPs slam Health Department claims they were paid for 20,000 ghost payments. *Irish Examiner* 2002 Nov 21.

[4] Halloran C. Students' healthcare cash crisis. *The Irish Star* 2002 Nov 20.

[5] Stewart P, O'Dowd T. Clinically inexplicable frequent attenders in general practice. *Br J Gen Pract* 2002;**52**:1000–01.

[6] O'Dowd TC. Five years of heartsink patients in general practice. *Br Med J* 1988;**297**:528–30.

[7] Cooke N. Low income families face rise in illness. *Irish Examiner* 2002 Nov 19; p. 8.

A Cure for the Crisis

7 Nursing

[1] Abel-Smith B. *A History of the Nursing Profession*. New York: Springer, 1960.

[2] O'Dowd T. Is the primary care strategy the way to go? *Forum* 2002;**19**(19):21–2.

[3] Needleman J, Buerhaus P, Mattke S, et al. Nurse staffing levels and the quality of care in hospitals. *N Engl J Med* 2002;**346**:1715–22.

[4] Steinbrook R. Nursing in the crossfire. *N Engl J Med* 2002;**346**:1757–65.

[5] Kinley H, Czoski-Murray C, George S, et al. Effectiveness of appropriately trained nurses in preoperative assessment: randomised controlled equivalence/non-inferiority trial. *Br Med J* 2002;**325**:1323–6.

[6] Melleney EM-A, Willoughby CP. Audit of a nurse endoscopist based one stop dyspepsia clinic. *Postgrad Med J* 2002;**78**:161–4.

[7] Eisemon N, Stucky-Marshall L, Talamonti MS. Screening for colorectal cancer: developing a preventive heathcare program utilizing nurse endoscopists. *Gastroenterol Nurs* 2001;**24**:12–19.

[8] Horrocks S, Anderson E, Salisbury C. Systematic review of whether nurse practitioners working in primary care can provide equivalent care to doctors. *Br Med J* 2002;**324**:819–2.

[9] Costello R. Another systematic review. *Br Med J* 2002; 9 April [eletters].

[10] Laurance J. Hospitals cut back on doctors' night cover. *The Independent* 2003 Jan 4; p. 1.

[11] Aiken LH. Achieving an interdisciplinary workforce in healthcare. *N Engl J Med* 2003;**348**:164–6.

8 Self-preservation for administrators

[1] Donnellan E. Heads of health boards see need for structural reforms. *The Irish Times* 2002 Dec 6; p. 11.

[2] Lyons M. Reducing the number of health boards is not the real issue in reform of services. *The Irish Times* 2002 Nov 25.

[3] Donnellan E, Holland K. Plan calls for radical shake-up of health boards. *The Irish Times* 2002 Dec 23; p. 1.

[4] Lyons M. Black hole? No, the money's right here. *The Irish Times* 2003 May 19; p. 11.

References

5 Audit of Structures and Functions in the Health System (Prospectus Report on behalf of the Department of Health and Children). Dublin: Stationery Office, 2003.

6 Commission on Financial Management and Control Systems in the Health Service (Brennan Report on behalf of the Department of Finance). Dublin: Stationery Office, 31 January 2003 [released publicly in June 2003].

9 Waiting lists and treatment plans

1 Donohoe M. Hospital waiting list pledge to be broken. *The Irish Times* 2002 Dec 4; p. 7.

2 O'Regan E. Waiting list shoots up by 10,000. *Irish Independent* 2002 Dec 5.

3 Shanahan C. Martin accused over hospital lists. *Irish Examiner* 2002 Dec 5; p. 2.

4 Health services [editorial]. *Irish Examiner* 2003 May 23; p. 16.

5 Donnellan E. 29,000 patients on waiting lists last December. *The Irish Times* 2003 May 23; p. 3.

6 Donnellan E. Consultants deny boycott of treatment programme. *The Irish Times* 2002 Dec 6; p. 4.

7 O'Regan E. Doctors slow to use new €10 million surgery scheme. *Irish Independent* 2002 Dec 5; p. 4.

8 McDowell M. Charlie's not solely to blame for runaway spending craze. *Irish Independent* 2002 Nov 19.

9 Moore A. The cost of exporting health care in Europe. *Medicine Weekly* 2002 May 8; p. 12.

10 Castle S, Linton L. EU opens borders for health treatment. *The Independent* (London) 2002 Dec 4; p. 1.

11 Private health insurance

1 Wall M. State hits out at "self-serving" BUPA. *Sunday Tribune* [Business section] 2002 Dec 1; p. 2.

2 MacCarthaigh S. VHI bonanza is no certainty. *Sunday Business Post* 2002 Dec 1; p. 6.

3 O'Regan E. BUPA may pay €20 million a year under equalisation plan. *Irish Independent* 2003 May 16; p. 7.

A Cure for the Crisis

12 Medical indemnity

[1] O'Sullivan J, Donnellan E. Consultants oppose changes to medical negligence claims. *The Irish Times* 2003 Jan 3; p. 1.

[2] Rennie D. US doctors strike over lawsuits. *The Daily Telegraph* 2003 Jan 3; p. 16.

13 Prescription medicines

[1] Byrne D. Prescription medicine costs. *The Irish Times* 2002 Nov 29; p. 21.

[2] O'Brien C. Pharmacists object to drug scheme. *Irish Examiner* 2002 Dec 6; p. 2.

[3] Orellana C. Germany's generic-drug law prompts concern among doctors. *Lancet* 2002;**359**:1498.

[4] Shepherd J. Resource management in prevention of coronary heart disease: optimizing prescription of lipid-lowering drugs. *Lancet* 2002;**359**:2271–3.

[5] West of Scotland Coronary Prevention Study Group. Influence of pravastatin and plasma lipids on coronary events in the West of Scotland Coronary Prevention Study. *Circulation* 1998;**97**:1440–45.

[6] Collier J, Iheanacho I. The pharmaceutical industry as an informant. *Lancet* 2002;**360**:1405–09.

[7] Abraham J. The pharmaceutical industry as a political player. *Lancet* 2002;**360**:1498–1502.

[8] Moynihan R. The making of a disease: female sexual dysfunction. *Br Med J* 2003;**326**:45–47.

[9] Laumann E, Paik A, Rosen R. Sexual dysfunction in the United States: prevalence and predictors. *JAMA* 1999;**281**:537–544.

[10] Berman J, Berman L, Goldstein I. Female sexual dysfunction: incidence, pathophysiology, evaluation and treatment options. *Urology* 1999;**54**:385–391.

[11] Revill J. Health claims for new pill are 'bogus'. *The Observer* 2002 Dec 8; p. 5.

14 Impact of advances in technology

[1] International Subarachnoid Aneurysm Trial (ISAT) Collaborative Group. International subarachnoid aneurysm trial (ISAT) of neurological clipping versus endovascular coiling in 2,143 patients with rup-

308

tured intracranial aneurysms: a randomized trial. *Lancet* 2002;**360**:1267–74.

2 Nichols DA, Brown RD Jr, Meyer FB. Coils or clips in subarachnoid haemorrhage? *Lancet* 2002;**360**:1262–3.

3 Van Tinteren H, Hoekstra OS, Smit EF, et al. Effectiveness of positron emission tomography in the preoperative assessment of patients with suspected non-small-cell lung cancer: the PLUS multicentre randomized trial. *Lancet* 2002;**359**:1388–92.

16 National Health Service (NHS)

1 Marshall M, Roland M. The new contract: renaissance or requiem for general practice. *Br J Gen Pract* 2002;**52**:531–2.

2 Carvel J, Baker M. Doctors to get US-style assistants. *The Guardian* 2003 Jan 15; p. 10.

3 Doctors in distress. No more national deals for consultants [editorial]. *The Guardian* 2002 Nov 1.

4 Kivimaki M, Leino-Arjas P, Luukkonen R, et al. Work stress and risk of cardiovascular mortality: prospective cohort study of industrial employees. *Br Med J* 2002;**325**:857.

5 Jones G, Martin N. Consultants reject new contract. *Daily Telegraph* 2002 Nov 1; p. 1.

6 Thomson A. Private hospitals can be bad for your health. *Daily Telegraph* 2002 Dec 20; p. 25.

7 Dalrymple T. Consultants would rather have freedom to operate than gold. *Daily Telegraph* 2002 Nov 1; p. 26.

8 Abel-Smith B. *The Hospitals 1800–1948*. London: Heinemann, 1964.

9 Wales J. Strategy to combat obesity epidemic. *The Times* 2002 Dec 26; p. 19.

10 Norfolk A. One in three hospitals fiddles waiting lists. *The Times* 2002 Dec 23; p. 1.

11 Dixon J. Foundation hospitals. *Lancet* 2002;**360**:1900–1.

17 Best healthcare system: France

1 Cahill A. France has best health care in EU but workers pay 20% of wages for it. *Irish Examiner* 2002 Dec 11; p. 19.

2 Duranf de Bousingen D. New French government solves doctors' long-standing grievances. *Lancet* 2002;**359**:2258.

A Cure for the Crisis

3 Report of the National Task Force on Medical Staffing (Hanly Report). Appendix 8. Working Time Legislation for Doctors in Training: International Review. Dublin: Department of Health, 2003; pp. 179–186.

18 Healthcare systems of selected countries

1 Watts J. Japan tries again to contain health costs. *Lancet* 2002;**359**:2260.

2 Van Kolfschooten F. Dutch government announces large cuts in health spending. *Lancet* 2003; **263**:1048.

20 Health inequalities

1 Class I: professional, etc. occupations; Class II: managerial and technical occupations; Class III: skilled occupations (N) non-manual (M) manual; Class IV: partly-skilled occupations; Class V: unskilled occupations.

2 Power C, Matthews S. Origins of health inequalities in a national population sample. *Lancet* 1997;**350**:1584–89.

3 Lynch JW, Kaplan GA, Shema SJ. Cumulative impact of sustained economic hardship on physical, cognitive, psychological, and social functioning. *N Engl J Med* 1997;**337**:1889–95.

4 Ezzati M, Lopez AD, Rodgers A, et al. Selected major risk factors and global and regional burden of disease. *Lancet* 2002;**360**:1347–60.

5 *World Health Report 2002. Reducing risks, promoting healthy life.* Geneva: WHO, 2002.

6 *Against All Odds – Family Life On a Low Income in Ireland.* Dublin: Combat Poverty Agency/IPA, 2002.

21 Immigrants and the Irish nation

1 Goldenberg S. Greatest wave of migrants drives US engine. *The Guardian* 2002 Dec 3.

2 O'Toole F. Law with a dangerous edge of racism. *The Irish Times* [Weekend Review] 2003 Jan 25; p. 1.

3 O'Doherty G. The right to citizenship. Shutting the gates. *Irish Independent* 2003, Jan 25.

4 Park A, Curtice J, Thomson K, Jarvis L, Bromley C (eds). *British Social Attitudes: 19th Report.* London: Sage, 2002.

5 Meikle J. Health recruits to face compulsory HIV tests. *The Guardian* 2003 Jan 3; p. 6.

310

References

22 Disturbed children

[1] Special care unit fails to meet needs, court hears. *Irish Examiner* 2002 Nov 28; p.11.

[2] Lamb H. Public Voices. High anxiety and stacks of back-covering forms. *The Guardian* 2002 Nov 27; p. 21.

23 People with disabilities

[1] Ring E. Poor economy no excuse, says DFI. *Irish Examiner* 2002 Nov 13; p. 7.

[2] Shanahan C. Disabled people treated unequally in and outside work. *Irish Examiner* 2002 Dec 3; p. 7.

24 Depression and suicide

[1] Phillips MR, Li X, Zhang Y. Suicide rates in China. *Lancet* 2002;**359**:835.

[2] O'Regan E. Sharp rise in number of under-25s' suicides. *Irish Independent* 2003 Feb 12; p. 6.

[3] Report of the National Task Force on Suicide. Dublin: Stationary Office, 1998.

[4] Department of Health. National Suicide Prevention Strategy for England. London: Department of Health, 2002.

[5] Centres for Disease Control and Prevention, National Institute of Mental Health, Office of the Surgeon General. Reporting on suicide: recommendations for the media. *Suicide Life Threat Behav* 2002;**32**:vii–xiii

[6] Hawton K, Williams K. Influences of the media on suicide. *Br Med J* 2002;**325**:1374–5.

25 Drugs of abuse and recreational drug use

[1] Van Kolfschooten F. Dutch investigators recommend prescription of heroin to addicts. *Lancet* 2002;**359**:590.

[2] *Working Group on a Courts Commission, Fifth Report.* Dublin: Government Publications, 1998.

[3] Mukamal KJ, Conigrave KM, Mittleman MA, et al. Roles of drinking pattern and type of alcohol consumed in coronary heart disease in men. *N Engl J Med* 2003;**348**:109–18.

A Cure for the Crisis

26 Alcohol and tobacco

[1] Hong M-K, Bero LA. How the tobacco industry responded to an influential study of the health effects of secondhand smoke. *Br Med J* 2002;**325**:1413–6.

[2] Who has the power over tobacco control? [editorial]. *Lancet* 2002;**360**:267.

[3] Williamson DF, Madans J, Anda RF, et al. Smoking cessation and severity of weight gain in a national cohort. *N Engl J Med* 1991;**324**:739–45.

[4] Cabanac M, Frankham P. Evidence that transient nicotine lowers the body weight set point. *Physiol Behav* 2002;**76**:539–42.

[5] Jung RT. Obesity as a disease. *Br Med Bull* 1987;**53**:307–321

[6] Hodmun KS, Gritz ER, Clayton S, Nisenbaum R. Eating orientation, postcessation weight gain, and continued abstinence among female smokers receiving an unsolicited smoking cessation intervention. *Health Psychol* 1999;**1**:29–36.

[7] Borrelli B, Spring B, Niaura R, et al. Weight suppression and weight rebound in ex-smokers treated with fluoxetine. *J Consult Clin Psychol* 1999;**1**:124–31.

[8] Anderson JE, Jorenby DE, Scott WT, Fiore MC. Treating tobacco use and dependence: an evidence-based clinical practice guideline for tobacco cessation. *Chest* 2002;**121**:932–41.

27 Mental Health Act Ireland

[1] O'Shea B. The Mental Health Act, 2001: a brief summary. *Ir Med J* 2002;**95**:153.

[2] Kelly BD. The Mental Health Act 2001. *Ir Med J* 2002;**95**:151–2.

[3] Daly A, Walsh D. *Irish Psychiatric Services: Activities 1999*. Dublin: The Health Research Board, 2000.

[4] Kelly, The Mental Health Act, 2001.

28 Exercise and obesity

[1] McCarthy SN, Gibney MJ, Flynn A, Livingstone MBE. Overweight, obesity and physical activity levels in Irish adults: evidence from the North/South Ireland Food Consumption Survey. *Proc Nutr Soc* 2002;**61**:3–7.

References

[2] Krause WE, Houmard JA, Duschos BD, et al. Effects of the amount and intensity of exercise on plasma lipoproteins. *N Engl J Med* 2002;**347**:1483–92.

[3] Manson JE, Willett WC, Stampfer MJ, et al. Body weight and mortality among women. *N Engl J Med* 1995;**333**:677–85.

[4] Jung RT. Obesity as a disease. *Br Med Bull* 1997;**53**:307–321.

[5] Ebbeling CB, Pawlak DB, Ludwig DS. Childhood obesity: public-health crisis, common sense cure. *Lancet* 2002;**360**:473–82.

[6] Tuomilehto J, Lindstrom J, Eriksson JG, et al. Prevention of type 2 diabetes mellitus by changes in lifestyle among subjects with impaired glucose tolerance. *N Engl J Med* 22001;**344**:1343–50.

[7] Armstrong J, Reilly JJ and the Child Health Information Team. Breastfeeding and lowering the risk of childhood obesity. *Lancet* 2002;**359**:2003–04.

29 Cardiovascular Strategy: Building Healthier Hearts

[1] Clancy L, Goodman P, Sinclair H, Dockery DW. Effect of air-pollution control on death rates in Dublin, Ireland: an intervention study. *Lancet* 2002;**360**:1210–14.

[2] Kraus WE, Houmard JA, Duscha BD, et al. Effects of the amount and intensity of exercise on plasma lipoproteins. *N Engl J Med* 2002;**347**:1483–92.

[3] American Diabetes Association. Standards of Medical Care for patients with Diabetes Mellitus. *Diabetes Care* 2002;**25**:213–229.

[4] Heart Protection Study Collaborative Group. MRC/BHF Heart Protection Study of cholesterol lowering with simvastatin in 20,536 high-risk individuals: a randomised placebo-controlled trial. *Lancet* 2002;**360**:7–22.

[5] Schnyder G, Roffi M, Pin R, Flammer Y, et al. Decreased rate of coronary restenosis after lowering of plasma homocysteine levels. *N Engl J Med* 2001:**345**:1593–600.

[6] Brown BG, Zhao X-Q, Chait A, et al. Simvastatin and niacin, antioxidant vitamins, or the combination for the prevention of coronary disease. *N Engl J Med* 2001;**345**:1583–92.

[7] Van Es RF, Jonker JJC, Verheugt FWA, et al. Aspirin and coumarin after acute coronary syndromes (the ASPECT-2 study): a randomised controlled trial. *Lancet* 2002;**360**:109–13.

A Cure for the Crisis

8 Gaspoz J-M, Coxson PG, Goldman PA, et al. Cost effectiveness of aspirin, clopidogrel, or both for secondary prevention of coronary heart disease. *N Engl J Med* 2002;**346**:1800–6.

9 Yusuf S. Two decades of progress in preventing vascular disease. *Lancet* 2002;**360**:2–3.

10 Hall M, McGettigan M, O'Callaghan P, Graham I, Shelley E, Feely J. Comparison of secondary prevention of heart disease in Europe: Lifestyle getting worse, therapy getting better in Ireland. *Ir Med J* 2002;**95**:272–4.

11 EUROASPIRE II Study Group. Life style and risk factor management and use of drug therapies in coronary patients from 15 countries; principal results from EUROASPIRE II Heart Survey Programme. *Eur Heart J* 2001;**22**:554–572.

12 The United Kingdom Heart Attack Study Collaborative Group. Effect of time from onset to coming under care on fatality of patients with acute myocardial infarction: effect of resuscitation and thrombolytic treatment. *Heart* 1998;**80**:114–20

13 Norris RM, for the Southern Heart Attack Response Project (SHARP) investigators. A new performance indicator for acute myocardial infarction. *Heart* 2001;**85**:395–401.

14 Boersma E, Maas ACP, Simoons ML, et al. Early thrombolytic treatment in acute myocardial infarction: reappraisal of the Golden Hour. *Lancet* 1996;**348**:771–75.

15 GREAT Group. Feasibility, safety, and efficacy of domiciliary thrombolysis by general practitioners. *Br Med J* 1992;**305**:548–53.

16 Bonnefoy E, Lapostolle F, Leizorovicz A, et al. Primary angioplasty versus prehospital fibrinolysis in acute myocardial infarction: a randomised study. *Lancet* 2002;**360**:825–29.

17 Keeley EC, Boura JA, Grines CL. Primary angioplasty versus intravenous thrombolytic therapy for acute myocardial infarction: a quantitative review of 23 randomised trials. *Lancet* 2003;**361**:13–20.

18 Stone GW. Primary angioplasty versus "earlier" thrombolysis – time for a wake-up call. *Lancet* 2002;**360**:814–16.

19 Anderson HR, Nielsen TT, Rasmussen K, et al. A comparison of coronary angioplasty with fibrinolytic therapy in acute myocardial infarction. *N Engl J Med*;**349**:733–42.

20 Morice M-C, Serruys PW, Sousa JE, et al. A randomised comparison of a sirolimus-eluting stent with a standard stent for coronary revascularization. *N Engl J Med* 2002;**346**:1773–80.

References

[21] Caffrey SL, Willoughby PJ. Pepe PE, Becker LB. Public use of automated external defibrillators. *N Engl J Med* 2002;**347**:1242.

[22] Weaver WD, Peberdy MA. Defibrillators in public places – one step closer to home. *N Engl J Med* 2002;**347**:1223–4.

[23] O'Neill JO, Nash PJ, Bourke W, McGarry K, Bedford D. The management of acute myocardial infarction – practical problems in implementing the evidence. *Ir Med J* 2002;**95**:270-2.

[24] Pate GE, Curtin R, Talbot A, et al. Audit of acute myocardial infarctions at St James's Hospital, Dublin, from 1996 to 1999. *Ir Med J* 2002;**95**:274–6.

30 Screening for disease

[1] Grimes DSA, Schulz KF. Uses and abuses of screening tests. *Lancet* 2002;**359**:881–4.

[2] Laderson PW, Singer PA, Ain KB, et al. American Thyroid Association guidelines for detection of thyroid dysfunction. *Arch Intern Med* 2000;**160**:1573–5.

[3] Helfand M, Redfern CC. Clinical guidelines part 2. Screening for thyroid disease: an update. American College of Physicians. *Ann Intern Med* 1998;**129**:144–58.

[4] Mazhar D, Waxman J. Prostate cancer. *Postgrad Med J*. 2002;**78**:590–5.

[5] Tannock IF. Eradication of a disease. *Lancet* 22002;**359**:1341–2.

[6] Barry MJ. Prostate Specific Antigen testing for early diagnosis of prostate cancer. *N Engl J Med* 2001;**344**:1373–7.

[7] Chodak GW, Thisted RA, Gerber GS, et al. Results of conservative management of clinically localized prostate cancer. *N Engl J Med* 1994;**330**:242–8.

[8] Frankel S, Davey Smith G, Donovan J, Neal D. Screening for prostate cancer. *Lancet* 2003;**361**:1122–28.

[9] Gøtzsche P, Olsen O. Is screening for breast cancer with mammography justifiable? *Lancet* 2000;**355**:129–134.

[10] Miller AB. The Canadian National Breast Study 2. *J Natl Cancer Inst* 2000;**92**:1490–99.

[11] Nyström L, Anderson J, Bjurstam N, et al. Long-term effects of mammography screening: updated overview of the Swedish randomised trials. *Lancet* 2002;**359**:909–19.

[12] Gøtzsche PC. Update on effects of screening mammography. *Lancet* 2002;**360**:338–39.

A Cure for the Crisis

[13] Fletcher SW, Elmore JG. Mammographic screening for breast cancer. *N Engl J Med* 2003;**348**:1672–80.

[14] Tabar L, Yen M-F, Vitak B, et al. Mammography service screening and mortality in breast cancer patients: 20-year follow-up before and after introduction of screening. *Lancet* 2003;**361**:1405–10.

[15] Fenlon HM, Nunes DP, Schroy PC, et al. A comparison of virtual and conventional colonoscopy for detection of colorectal polyps. *N Engl J Med* 1999;**341**:1496–503.

[16] Gollub MJ. Virtual colonoscopy. *Lancet* 2002;**360**:964.

[17] Chapman AH, Blakeborough A. United States has recommended screening for colon cancer. *Br Med J* 1997;**314**:1624.

[18] Mulcahy HE, Farthing MJG, O'Donoghue DP. Screening for colorectal cancer. *Br Med J* 1997;**314**:285–91.

[19] Johnson J. Media focus on failures of screening programme. *Br Med J* 1997;**314**:1630.

[20] Wright TC, Schiffman M. Adding a test for human papillomavirus DNA to cervical-cancer screening. *N Eng J Med 2003*;**348**:489–90.

[21] Quinn M, Babb P, Jones J, Allen E. Effect of screening on incidence of and mortality from cancer of cervix in England: evaluation based on routinely collected statistics. *Br Med J* 1999:**318**:904.

[22] Crum CP. The beginning of the end for cervical cancer? *N Engl J Med* 2002;**347**:1703–5.

34 Continuing medical education/continuing professional development

[1] Haman H. Regulation – a matter of trust. *GMC News* 2002 Dec 15; p. 2.

[2] General Medical Council. Appraisal and revalidation. http://www.revalidationuk.info

35 Salaries and economic incentives

[1] Relman AS. Salaried physicians and economic incentives. *N Engl J Med* 1988;**319**:784.

[2] Relman AS. Practising medicine in the new business climate. *N Engl J Med* 1987;**316**:1150–1.

[3] Irvine D. The performance of doctors: the new professionalism. *Lancet* 1999;**353**:1174–7.

[4] Kondro W. Threats to medical professionalism tackled in Canada. *Lancet* 2002;**360**:316.

References

36 Medical errors

[1] Lee T. A broader concept of medical errors. *N Engl J Med* 2002;**347**: 1965–7.

[2] Blendon RJ, DesRoches CM, Brodie M, Benson JM, et al. Views of practicing physicians and the public on medical errors. *N Engl J Med* 2002;**347**:1933–40.

[3] Studdert TEJ, Burstin HR, Orav EJ, et al. Incidence and types of adverse events and negligent care in Utah and Colorado. *Med Care* 2000;**38**:247–9.

[4] Thomas EJ, Brennan TA. Incidence and types of preventable adverse events in elderly patients: population based review of medical records. *Br Med J* 2000;**320**:741–4.

[5] John S. Litigation improves safety. *Daily Telegraph* 2002 Dec 20; p. 25.

[6] *Expert Group on Learning from Adverse Events in the NHS. An Organization with a Memory.* London: Department of Health, 2000.

[7] Dean B, Schachter M, Vincent C, Barber N. Causes of prescribing errors in hospital inpatients: a prospective study. *Lancet* 2002;**359**: 1373–78.

[8] O'Regan E. Medical chiefs probe only 6% of complaints about doctors. *Irish Independent* 2003 June 2; p. 4.

[9] Studdert DM, Brennan TA. No-fault compensation for medical injuries: the prospect for error prevention. *JAMA* 2001;**286**:226–8.

[10] Vincent C. Patient safety: Understanding and responding to adverse events. *N Engl J Med* 2003;**348**:1051–56.

[11] Orellana C. New law in Germany compensates patients for drug side-effects. *Lancet* 2002;**360**:471.

[12] Petersen LA, Orav EJ, Teach JM, et al. Using a computerized sign-out program to improve continuity of inpatient care and prevent adverse events. *Jt Comm J Qual Improv* 1998;**24**:77–87.

[13] Coulehan J, Williams PC. Vanquishing virtue: the impact of medical education. *Acad Med* 2001;**76**:598–605.

[14] Leape LL. Reporting of adverse events. *N Engl J Med* 2002;**347**:1633–38.

A Cure for the Crisis

37 Organ retention inquiry

[1] Ring E. Parents for Justice take organ cases to Gardai. *Irish Examiner* 2002 Nov 25; p. 1.

[2] O'Doherty C. Organ scandal parents dig in heels. *Irish Examiner* 2002 Nov 26; p. 17.

[3] Hall C. Fears after organs scandal delay child cancer studies. *Daily Telegraph* 2002, Dec 17; p. 9.

38 Aberrant clinical behaviour

[1] Donnellan E. 'He told me to go home and get on with my life.' *The Irish Times* [Weekend Review] 2002 Nov 16.

[2] Donnellan E. 37 complaints to Medical Council about obstetrician. *The Irish Times* 2002 Dec 21; p. 10.

[3] Houston M. How did it happen – and could it happen now? *The Irish Times* [Weekend Review] 2002 Nov 16.

[4] Murphy JFA. The Lindsay Tribunal into HIV and hepatitis infection in haemophiliacs. *Ir Med J* 2002;**95**:260–1.

[5] *Report of the Tribunal of Inquiry into the Infection with HIV and Hepatitis C of Persons with Haemophilia and Related Matters*. Dublin: Government Publications, 2002.

[6] Opinion: The Lindsay Tribunal. *The Bar Review* 2002;**7**(7).

[7] Newman C. Article backing Lindsay assailed by group. *The Irish Times* 2003 Jan 3; p. 6.

39 Whistle blowing in the Irish health service

[1] Hickey DP. Beaumont Hospital. [Letters] *The Irish Times* 2002 Nov 27.

[2] Lawlor DL. Crisis in the health service. [Letters] *The Irish Times* 2002 Dec 6.

[3] Conlon P. Shortage of hospital beds. [Letters] *The Irish Times* 2003 May 9.

[4] Lamont JP. Shortage of hospital beds. [Letters] *The Irish Times* 2003 May 10.

[5] Duffy D. Shortage of hospital beds. [Letters] *The Irish Times* 2003 May 20.

References

40 Change: liberalisation of the medical market

[1] Cooke N. Change health system urges BUPA chief. *Irish Examiner* 2002 Nov 22; p. 13.

42 Healthcare rationing

[1] Aaron HD, Schwartz WB. *The Painful Prescription: Rationing Hospital Care*. Washington, DC: Brookings Institution, 1984.

[2] Stroke Unit Trialists' Collaboration. Collaborative systematic review of the randomised trials of organized inpatient (stroke unit) care after stroke. *Br Med J* 1997;**314**:1151.

[3] National Institute for Clinical Excellence (NICE). http://www.nice.org.uk

[4] Greenberg DS. Surge continues in US health-care spending. *Lancet* 2002;**360**:700.

[5] Shanahan C. Call for health referendum. *Irish Examiner* 2002 Nov 19; p. 8.

43 Could healthcare collapse?

[1] Sandy LG. Homeostasis without reserve – The risk of health system collapse. *N Engl J Med* 2002;**347**:1971–5.

[2] Schwartz WB. *Life Without Disease: The Pursuit of Medical Utopia*. Berkeley: University of California Press, 1998.

44 Action plan for Ireland

[1] Fine LG, Keogh BE, Cretin S, Orlando M, Gould MM. How to evaluate and improve the quality and credibility of an outcomes database: validation and feedback study on the UK Cardiac Surgery Experience. *Br Med J* 2003;**326**:25–28.

[2] Bristol Royal Infirmary Inquiry. The inquiry into the management of care of children receiving complex heart surgery at the Bristol Royal Infirmary. http://www.bristol-inquiry.og.uk

[3] Geoghegan MF. Is the EU working time directive making teamwork obsolete? *Ir Med J* 2002;**95**:151.

[4] *Report of the National Task Force on Medical Staffing* (Hanly Report, dated June 2003). Dublin: Department of Health and Children, released publicly 15 October 2003.

A Cure for the Crisis

[5] Brennan R. Setting strategies and priorities for 2003–2008. *Forum* 2002;**19**(11):17–20.

[6] O'Dowd T. Is the Primary Care Strategy the way to go? *Forum* 2002;**19**(11):21–22.

[7] Galloway JM, Gibson J, Dalrymple J. Endoscopy in primary care – a survey of current practice. *Br J Gen Pract* 2002;**52**:536–38.

[8] Wilson H. Cold chain requirements. *Irish Medical News* 2002 Nov 18; p. 38.

[9] Eisenberg DM, Cohen MH, Hrbek A, et al. Credentialing complementary and alternative medical providers. *Ann Intern Med* 2002;**137**:965–973.

[10] De Smet P. Herbal remedies. *N Engl J Med* 2002;**347**:2046–56.

Selected bibliography

Books

Abel-Smith B. *A History of the Nursing Profession*. New York: Springer, 1960.

Abel-Smith B. *The Hospitals 1800-1948*. London: Heinemann, 1964.

Barrington R. *Health, Medicine and Politics in Ireland 1900–1970*. Dublin: Institute of Public Administration, 1987.

A Guide to Ethical Conduct and Behaviour. 5th edn. Dublin: Irish Medical Council, 1998.

Hensey B. *The Health Services of Ireland*. 4th edn. Dublin: Institute of Public Administration, 1988.

Schwartz WB. *Life Without Disease: The Pursuit of Medical Utopia.* Berkeley: University of California Press, 1998.

Tormey WP. "Two-speed Public and Private Medical Practice in the Republic of Ireland" in *Ireland Develops – Administration and Social Policy 1953–2003*. Fanning B, McNamara T (eds), Vol. 51 Nos. 1–2. Dublin: Institute of Public Administration, 2003; pp. 191–200.

Journals/Periodicals

Annals of Clinical Biochemistry
Annals of Emergency Medicine
Annals of Internal Medicine
Archives of Internal Medicine
British Journal of General Practice
British Medical Bulletin
British Medical Journal
Chest
Circulation
Clinical Chemistry
Diabetes Care
Forum
Gastroenterology Nursing
Health Psychology

A Cure for the Crisis

Heart
Irish Medical Journal
Joint Commission Journal on Quality Improvement
Journal of Consulting and Clinical Psychology
Journal of the National Cancer Institute
Medical Care
New England Journal of Medicine
Postgraduate Medical Journal
Proceedings of the Nutrition Society
Suicide and Life-Threatening Behavior
The Bar Review
The Lancet
Urology

Reports/Strategies

Against All Odds: Family Life on a Low Income in Ireland. Dublin: Combat Poverty Agency/IPA, 2002.

Audit of Structures and Functions in the Health System (Prospectus Report on behalf of the Department of Health and Children. Dublin: Stationery Office, 2003.

A Vision of General Practice 2001–2006. Dublin: IMO/ICGP, 2001.

Building Healthier Hearts, the Report of the Cardiovascular Health Strategy Group 1999, Dublin: Stationary Office, 1999.

Commission on Financial Management and Control Systems in the Health Service (Brennan Report). Dublin: Stationery Office, 2003.

Daly A, Walsh D. *Irish Psychiatric Services: Activities 1999*. Dublin: The Health Research Board, 2000.

Expert Group on Learning from Adverse Events in the NHS. An National Organisation with a Memory. London: Department of Health, 2000.

National Health Strategy: Quality and Fairness – A Health System for You. Dublin: Department of Health and Children, 2001.

Park A, Curtice J, Thomson K, Jarvis L, Bromley C. (eds) *British Social Attitudes: 19th Report*. London: Sage, 2003.

Prevention of Coronary Disease in Clinical Practice 1998, Second Joint Task Force of European and Other Societies on Coronary Prevention.

Selected bibliography

Report of the Commission on Health Funding. Dublin: Stationery Office, 1989.

Report of the Tribunal of Inquiry into the Infection with HIV and Hepatitis C of Persons with Haemophilia and Related Matters. Dublin: Stationery Office, 2002.

Report of the National Task Force on Medical Staffing (Hanly Report). Dublin: Department of Health and Children, 2003.

Report of the National Task Force on Suicide. Dublin: Stationary Office, 1998.

World Health Report 2002. Reducing Risks, Promoting Healthy Life. Geneva: WHO, 2002.

Newspapers

Evening Herald
The Irish Examiner
The Irish Independent
The Irish Star
The Irish Times
The Sunday Business Post
The Sunday Independent
The Sunday Times
The Sunday Tribune

The Daily Telegraph
The Guardian
The Independent (London)
The Observer

Medical newspapers

Irish Medical News
Irish Medical Times
Medicine Weekly
GMC News

Index

A

A Vision of General Practice 290
Academy of Biomedical
  Sciences 212
accident & emergency medicine
  25, 288
Addenbrooke's Hospital,
  Cambridge 99, 115
Administration 20
administrationism 15
Administrators 3, 55
advanced nurse practitioner
  (ANP) 283
Advertising Standards
  Authority of Ireland 163
Ahern, Bertie 63, 70
AIB Better Ireland Programme
  163
AIDS/HIV 141
alcohol 161
Alder Hay Hospital 232
Alder Hay organ scandal 235
Aliens Act 138
American Cancer Society 196,
  203, 204
American College of
  Obstetricians and
  Gynaecologists 84
American College of Physicians
  193
American Diabetes Association
  182
American Gastroenterology
  Society 203
American Society for Clinical
  Oncology 202
American Thyroid Association
  193
An Bord Altranais 53
Annals of Clinical Biochemistry
  216
Annals of Emergency Medicine
  30
Anti-competitive practices 76
Armour Pharmaceuticals 245
Association of Clinical
  Biochemists in Ireland
  (ACBI) 212
ASTMS 212
audits 59
*Australian Model Standards for
  General Practices* 296

B

Ballydowd Special Care Unit
  145
Bancroft, Dr John 92
Bantry General Hospital 25
Bar Review 244, 245
Barrett, Dr Sean 20
Beaumont Hospital 2, 3, 5, 12,
  14, 15, 30, 45, 48, 50, 60, 63,
  65, 70, 72, 96, 98, 148, 173,
  189, 205, 206, 241, 249, 251,
  253, 282
Bed pressures 65
Benchmarking 44, 69
Berman, Dr Jennifer 93
Bevan, Aneurin 106
Beveridge Report 106
biochemists 211
Blackrock Clinic 98
Blair, Tony MP 156
Blood Bank scandal 225
Blood Transfusion Service
  Board (BTSB) 242
Bogle, Dr Ian 111
Boland, Dr Ronan 42
Bolkovac, Kathryn 247
Bonnar, Prof John 239, 240
Bons Secours Hospital, Cork 83
Bons Secours Hospital,
  Glasnevin 14
Bowers, Fergal 235
BreastCheck 9, 201
Brennan Report 6, 61
Bristol Inquiry 236
British Committee on the Safety
  of Medicines (CSM) 91
British Dental Association 143
*British Journal of General
  Practice* 108
British Medical Association 51,
  106, 111, 143
British Medical Journal 50, 57,
  92, 108, 152, 205, 294
British Social Attitudes 143
Browse, Prof Norman 113
BUPA 66, 73, 127, 256, 259
Byrne, Des 87
Byrne, Gary 239
Byrne, Gay 30, 209

C

California Public Employees
  Retirement Scheme 270
Canadian Medical Association
  222

Canadian National Breast Study
  2 200
Cancer Research UK 236
capitation 36
Cardiovascular Strategy 9, 14,
  179, 282
Cavan General Hospital 225
Caulfield, Helen 51
Center for Labor Market
  Studies, Northeastern
  University 139
Central Admissions Office 47
Central Statistics Office 103
CEO Group of the Health
  Boards Audit 60
Chest Pain Evaluation and
  Treatment Units 30, 289
Chisholm, Dr John 108
Circuit Court 174
Circulation 56
Clancy, Dr Luke 179
Clinical Chemistry 216
clinical nurse specialist 45
Clinton, Bill 209
Clonmel General Hospital 25
Coghlan, Eamonn 13
Collier, Dr Joe 90, 93
Combat Poverty Agency 135
Comhairle na nOspidéal 14, 257,
  282, 284
Commission on Financial
  Management and Control
  Systems in the Health Service
  61, 286
Commission on Health Funding
  Report 1989 66
Committee on Rapid Advance
  Demonstrations 270
common contract 59, 61, 78, 81,
  216, 284, 285, 286, 287
Company magazine 162
Competition Authority 95, 256,
  259
Complementary & alternative
  medicine 298
Comptroller and Auditor
  General 16, 72
Conlon, Dr Peter 71, 252
consultant salaries 129
consultants 62, 78, 109, 128,
  208–210, 213, 282
Control of Clinical Trials Act,
  1987 174
Coombe Women's Hospital 240
Cooper, Cynthia 247

324

Index

Corbally, Martin 31
Cork Blood Bank 248
Cork University Hospital 72, 268
Costello, Dr Richard 16, 50
Cowley, Dr Gerry 197
Cronin, Norma 167
Crown Indemnity 83
Cunningham, Cecily 245
Cusack, Dr Stephen 268
cutbacks 69

D

Dalrymple, Dr Theodore 114
Delaney, Tim 255
Denham, Mrs Justice Susan 158
Dentists Act 1928 264
Denture Express 264
Department of Finance 7, 10, 34
Department of Health and
 Children 7, 17, 20, 24, 27, 31,
 42, 55, 59, 67, 70, 78, 83, 98,
 163, 179, 186, 201, 204, 233,
 235, 284, 290
depression 150
Diagnostic and Treatment
 Centres (DTCs) 116, 280
disabilities 147
disturbed children 145
disability adjusted life years 134
Disability Federation of Ireland
 147
Dobson, Frank MP 116
doctor substitutes 49
Donnellan, Eithne 64
Drogheda obstetric cases 225
Drug and Therapeutics Bulletin
 90
Drug Payment Scheme (DPS) 87
Drug Refund Scheme 8
Drug Treatment Centre 153, 154,
 155
Drug use
 – Britain 157
 – Italy 157
 – Netherlands 156, 157
 – Portugal 157
 – Spain 157
 – Switzerland 157
drugs 153
Drug Court 158, 159
Dublin Academic Teaching
 Hospitals (DATH) 64
Dublin City University 48
Dublin Voluntary Teaching
 Hospitals 28
Duffy, Donal 254
Dundalk RTC 47
Dunne Inquiry 232
Dunne, Judge Anne 233, 234
Dunphy, Eamon 18

E

Eastern Health Board (EHB) 3,
 28, 157
Eastern Health Shared Services
 31
Eastern Regional Health
 Authority (ERHA) 14, 27, 28,
 32, 61, 253
Employment Equality Act 1998
 147, 148
Ennis General Hospital 25
enterprise indemnity 79
enterprise liability 78, 85
Equality Authority 147, 148
Equal Status Act 2000 148
ERHA Public Health
 Department 194
ESRI 57, 147
EU Commission 76
EU healthcare systems 125
EU transnational border 67
EUROASPIRE II Study 2000
 186
European Union 124
European Working Time
 Directive 22, 50, 107, 229,
 261, 262, 287
Evening Herald 18, 264
exercise 175
Expert Group Report on
 Medical Laboratory
 Scientists 2001 211

F

Federal Employees Health
 Benefits Programme 270
Feely, Seamus 87
Fell, Frank 169
female sexual dysfunction 92
Fianna Fáil 7, 30, 63, 64, 130, 273
Fielding, Prof John 242
Fine Gael 9, 130, 131
Fingleton, John 259, 260
Finlay Tribunal 242, 246
Finlay, Mr Justice Thomas 242
Finlayson, Belinda 109
Finnish Diabetes Prevention
 Group 177
Fitzpatrick, Finbarr 65
FitzPatrick, Tony 46
Flynn, Dr Kate 242
Forum on Medical Manpower 22
Foster, Andrew 113
foundation hospitals 115
Fox, Dr Liam MP 51, 116
Freedom of Information Act 231
Freeman Hospital, Newcastle 66
Freeman, John MP 106

G

Galwey, Mick 209
General Medical Council (GMC)
 83, 109, 214, 226

General Medical Services (GMS)
 8, 9, 11, 32, 35–42, 256
general practice 35, 107
general practitioner 9, 23, 35,
 289
generic drugs 88
Geoghegan, Dr MF 286
Geoghegan, Tony 157
Georgopoulis, Mr Cristos 242
German Medical Association
 122
Gesetzliche
 Krankenversicherungen
 (GKV) 121
Gilligan, Paul 162
GMC News 228
Gorbachev, Mikhail 209
Gorey, Tom 263
Gøtzsche, Dr Peter 197, 200
Gough, Alison 238, 239
GP fees 36, 296
Grampian Study (GREAT) 188
Gray, Dr Diane 109
Grogan, Dr Liam 15
*Guide to Ethical Conduct and
 Behaviour* 220, 261, 268

H

Hanly Report 6, 10, 280, 279, 287
Harney, Mary 179
Haughton, Mr Justice Gerard
 158
Health Act 1970 27
Health and Safety Authority 168
health boards 27–34, 280, 298
 – Canada 58
 – Greater Manchester,
 England 58
 – New Zealand 58
 – Scotland 58
Health Boards Chief Executive
 Officers' Group 55, 57
Health Care Guarantee 133
health inequalities 134
Health Information Evaluation
 Agency 33
Health Insurance (Amendment)
 Bill 2000 76
health insurance 73, 126
Health Insurance Authority
 (HIA) 76
Health Maintenance
 Organisation 74
health rationer 74
Health Service Employers
 Agency 48
health service employment 20
Health Service Executive 34, 61
healthcare systems
 – Canada 123
 – EU 124
 – France 118
 – Germany 121

325

A Cure for the Crisis

– Hong Kong 122
– Japan 121
– The Netherlands 122
– United Kingdom 106
Heartwatch Programme 179
Hennessy, Mark 7
Hickey, Mr David 249, 250, 251, 252
Higher Education Authority (HEA) 26, 207
Horgan, Prof John H. 30
Hospital Inpatient Enquiry (HIPE) 16, 281
Houston, Dr Muiris 9, 88, 241
human resources 5

I
Iheanacho, Dr Ike 90
immigrants 138
IMPACT 71, 212
Indecon International 259
indicative drug budgeting 38, 220
Inspector of Mental Hospitals 280
Institute of Obstetricians and Gynaecologists 84, 239
Intoxicating Liquor Act 2003 162
Irish Association of Plastic Surgeons 252
Irish Blood Transfusion Service (IBTS) 238, 244
Irish Cancer Society 13, 167
Irish Cardiac Society 192
Irish College of General Practitioners (ICGP) 24, 34, 179, 218, 224, 256
Irish Committee for Higher Medical Training 241
Irish Dental Association 264
Irish Dental Council 264
Irish Examiner 13, 25, 33, 64, 65, 71, 234, 268
Irish Haemophilia Society 243, 244
Irish Heart Foundation 179, 187, 192
Irish Hospital Consultants' Association (IHCA) 22, 65, 66, 67, 254, 262
Irish Independent 10, 22, 27, 64
Irish Kidney Association 253
Irish Labour Party 130, 132, 253, 273, 278
Irish Medical Council 17, 30, 59, 82, 214, 228, 240, 260, 268
Irish Medical Directory 249
Irish Medical Journal 171, 217, 242, 286
Irish Medical Organisation (IMO) 23, 34, 180, 206
Irish Medical Times 17

Irish Medicines Board 57, 88
Irish National Cancer Registry 98
Irish Nurses Organisation (INO) 4, 46
Irish Patients Association 255
Irish Pharmaceutical Union 87
Irish Society for the Prevention of Cruelty to Children (ISPCC) 162
Irish Universities Nutrition Alliance 175
irishhealth.com 235
Irvine, Dr Donald 222

J
James Connolly Memorial Hospital, Blanchardstown 2, 3, 13, 30, 71, 173. 206, 263, 282
Jervis Street Hospital 5
Johns Hopkins Hospital, Baltimore 32
Johnson, Dr Michael 228
Johnson, Mr Justice Richard 238, 239
Jordan, Colm 40
Joseph Rowntree Foundation 150
Journal of the American Medical Association (JAMA) 57, 92
Journal of the National Cancer Institute 200

K
Karzai, Hamid 156
Kearns, Adrian 80
Kelly, Dr BD 172
Kelly, Michael 201
Kelly, Mr Justice Peter 145
Kenny, Martin 264
Kiberd, Damian 69
Kinsey Institute, Indiana University 92
Kirby, Michael 124

L
Laffoy Commission 146
Lamb, Hazel 145
Lammy, David 114
Lamont, John P 251–254
Lansdowne Market Research 161
Late Late Show 30
Lawlor, Denis 252
league tables 113
Leen, Dr Eamonn 14
legislation 147
Lenihan, Brian TD 79
Licensed Vintners Association 169
life expectancy 100
Lindsay Tribunal 245
Lindsay, Judge Alison 243, 245

litigation 81, 84
Livingstone, Denise 17
Local Appointments Commission (LAC) 210
Louth County Hospital, Dundalk 25, 56, 281
Lyons, Michael 55, 57, 58, 61

M
Madden, Dr Michael 234
Maher, Dr Vincent 187
Mallow General Hospital 25
Malone, Beverley 44
Mandela, Nelson 209
Maresh, Dr Michael 239
Martin, Micheál TD, Minister for Health and Children 7, 17, 10,19, 33, 64 66, 72, 74, 75, 87, 130, 169, 235
Mater Hospital 2, 8, 14, 30, 48, 63, 65, 72, 85, 251
McCarthy, Dr 239
McCracken, Mr Justice Brian 239
McCreevy, Charlie TD, Minister for Finance 7, 10, 19, 21, 59, 70, 74
McDowell, Michael, Minister for Justice and Law Reform 245
McDowell, Moore 10, 11, 66
McGeehan, Terry 8
McKenna, Dr Peter 140
McManus, Liz TD 88, 132
McNeice, George 206
Medicaid 267
medical assistants in caring (MACs) 53
Medical Defence Union 78–86
medical errors 225
medical incomes 126
medical indemnity 78
medical manpower 14, 107
Medical Manpower National Task Force 11, 280
Medical Protection Society 78–86
medical schools 26
medical scientists 211
Medicare/Medicaid 285
Medicine Weekly 248, 249
Medicines Control Agency 93
Mental Health Act 171
Mental Health Commission 172
Mental Health Tribunal 172, 173
Merchant's Quay Project 157
Mid Western Health Board 204
Midgeley, Dr Adrian 50
migration 138
Milburn, Alan MP 116, 168
Mitchell, Olivia TD 9, 131
Monaghan General Hospital 17, 280
Moon, Chae 221

326

Index

Morgan, Prof D. Brian 93
Moriarty Tribunal 70
Morning Ireland 11
Moroney, Dr Joan 16
Morris Tribunal 70
Moussaoui, Zacarias 247
MRI Ireland Limited 74
Mulcahy, Prof Risteard 209
Murphy, Dr John 242

N

Naas General Hospital 30, 282
National Advisory Committee
  on Drugs (NACD) 153
National Alcohol Awareness
  Campaign 163
National Association of
  Insurance Physicians 121
National Cancer Institute 202
National Cancer Registry 166
National Centre for
  Pharmacoeconomics 95
National Cholesterol Education
  Programme 184
National Disability Authority
  148, 149
National Disease Surveillance
  Centre 141
National Health Service (NHS)
  18, 19, 90, 106–117, 129, 267,
  273
National Health Strategy 7, 11,
  12, 63, 65, 281, 290
National Hospitals Authority 11
National Hospitals Plan 56, 60
National Institute for Clinical
  Excellence (NICE) 33, 267
National Institutes of Health 1
National Maternity Hospital,
  Holles Street 12, 140, 240
National Programme in General
  Practice for the Secondary
  Prevention of Cardiovascular
  Disease 179
National Suicide Prevention
  Strategy for England 152
National Task Force on Medical
  Staffing 282
National Treasury Management
  Agency 80
National Treatment Purchase
  Fund 8, 65, 86, 281
Nationwide Drug and Alcohol
  Prevention Programme 163
Navan General Hospital 281
NCHDs 5, 23, 67, 282, 284
Neary, Dr Michael 238, 239, 240
Neligan, Prof Maurice 209
Nenagh General Hospital 25,
  173
*New England Journal of
  Medicine* 52, 56, 200, 216,
  219, 228, 270, 282, 294

NewsTalk 106 250
Noonan Walsh, Dr Patricia 148
North Eastern Health Board
  (NEHB) 152, 239, 240, 280
North/South Ireland Food
  Consumption Survey 175
Northern Area Health Board
  (NAHB) 3, 14, 249
nurse retention 48
nurse shortages 43
nursing 3, 43–54
Nursing Recruitment and
  Retention Report 48, 52
Nyström, Dr Lennarth 200

O

O'Cathain, Dr Seamus 268
O'Connell, Dr Paul 16
O'Connor, Sheila 240
O'Dea, Willie TD 148
O'Donoghue, Dr Diarmuid 203
O'Higgins, Mr Justice Kevin 145
O'Higgins, Prof Niall 197
O'Laoire, Mr Sean 242
O'Mahony, Brian 244, 245
O'Neill, Mr Padraig 242
O'Neill, Prof Shane 15, 17, 71
O'Regan, Eilish 27, 64
O'Reilly, Fionnuala 234, 235
O'Rourke, Martin 256
O'Shea, Donal 29, 71
O'Shea, Dr Brendan 257, 258
O'Shea, Dr Brian 171
O'Sullivan, Dr Tony 241
O'Toole, Fintan 18
obesity 175
Oberstown House 145
OECD 100, 118, 151
Oireachtas Committee on Health
  168, 274
Olsen, Dr O 197, 200
one disease doctors 49, 53
organ retension 232
Our Good Health 273, 276, 278
Our Lady of Lourdes Hospital,
  Drogheda 238, 240
Our Lady's Hospital for Sick
  Children, Crumlin 2, 30, 31,
  232, 235, 237
Our Lady's Hospital, Navan 191
out-of-hours GP service 291
over-70s medical card 35, 41,
  126, 273

P

palliative care 297
Parents for Justice 233, 235
party policies 126, 130
patient categories 126
Patient Focus 240
pay and expenditure 69
pharmaceutical industry 90
pharmacy 298

Pharmacy Act, 1875 95
Pharmacy Review Group 95
physician's assistants 110
pilot primary care teams 291
Portiuncula Hospital,
  Ballinasloe 173
Portlaoise General Hospital 96,
  99, 173
Postgraduate Medical and
  Dental Board 23
Powell, Enoch MP 138
prescribing 221
prescription medicines 87
Prescriptions Medicines Code of
  Practice Authority 93
Prevention of Coronary Disease
  in Clinical Practice 1998 181
Primary Care Strategy 290
private health insurance 73
Progressive Democrats 7, 20
Prompt Payment of Accounts
  Act 1997 34
Prospectus Report 6, 10, 33
public health 287
public health doctors 287
public–private partnership 16

Q

*Quality and Fairness – a Health
  System for You* 10, 273
Queen's University Belfast 26
Quinn, Niall 13
Quinn, Ruairí TD 247

R

Rabbitte, Pat TD 70, 253
Reader's Digest 40
Realyvasquez, Fidel 221
Redmond, Mr Mark 31
Relman, Dr Arnold 112, 219,
  220, 282
Report of the Alder Hay
  Children's Hospital,
  Liverpool 232
Report of the National Task
  Force on Suicide, 1998 151
Report on the Health Effects of
  Environmental Tobacco
  Smoke 168
Report on the Regulation of
  Practitioners of
  Complementary and
  Alternative Medicine in
  Ireland 299
Restrictive Practices
  Commission 264
Review Body on Higher
  Remuneration in the Public
  Sector (Buckley Review) 69
Reynolds, Albert 247
risk equalisation 75
risk management 84
Romanow, Roy 123

327

A Cure for the Crisis

Rotunda Hospital 78, 140
Rotunda Sexual Assault Unit 225
Rowley, Coleen 247
Royal College of Nursing 44, 51
Royal College of Pathologists (RCPath) 211, 218, 232, 233, 237
Royal College of Physicians 51, 107, 214, 282
Royal College of Physicians of Ireland (RCPI) 30, 84, 216, 234
Royal College of Surgeons in Ireland (RCSI) 25, 26, 30, 48, 56, 85
Royal Commission on the Future of Health Care 123
Royal Infirmary, Edinburgh 203
Royal Victoria Hospital, Belfast 236
RTÉ 11
Ryan, Eoin TD 158

S
Sandy, Dr Lewis 270–272
Saunders, Dr Michael 83
scanning equipment 98
Scottish Blood Transfusion Service 243
screening for disease 19
Shelley, Dr Emer 186
SIPTU 71, 212
Skeen, Michael 221
Sligo General Hospital 173
Smurfit, Michael 209
Society of Cardiothoracic Surgeons of Great Britain and Ireland (SCTS) 279
South Eastern Health Board 64
South Infirmary Hospital, Cork 201
Southern Heart Attack Response Project (SHARP) 186, 187, 188
St Andrew's School, Dublin 154
St Columcille's Hospital, Loughlinstown 30, 282
St George's Hospital Medical School, UK 110
St James's Hospital, Dublin 3, 72, 95, 191, 194, 248, 289
St John's Hospital, Sligo 46
St Luke's General Hospital, Kilkenny 25
St Michael's House 54, 149
St Thomas' Hospital, London 99
St Vincent's Private Hospital 86
St Vincent's University Hospital 14, 30, 46, 48, 86, 173, 203
State Claims Agency 80
state enrolled nurses 53
state indemnity 83
state registered nurses 53

Stone, Dr Gregg 189
suicide 150
Sullivan, Dr Richard 236
Sunday Business Post 75
Sunday Tribune 12
Sutton Park School, Dublin 154
Swords, John 31

T
Tallaght Hospital 3, 72, 255
Task Force on Alcohol 164
Task Force on Medical Staffing 22
Trinity College Dublin 26
technology 96
Temperley, Prof Ian 243, 244
The Children's Hospital, Temple Street 2, 30
The Daily Telegraph 113
The Guardian 106, 111, 112, 145
The Independent, London 51, 252
The Irish Examiner 235
The Irish Star 7, 8
The Irish Times 7, 8, 17, 20, 28, 45, 59, 61, 64, 65, 88, 235, 241, 249, 251, 252, 253, 254, 256, 257, 259
The Joint Committees on Higher Medical Training 262
The Lancet 56, 90, 91, 116, 184, 189, 197, 200, 216, 217, 222
The Last Word 18
The Right Hook with George Hook 250
The Sunday Times 10, 69
The Sunday Tribune 21, 33, 72, 282
Thompson, Dr Chris 45
tobacco 161
Travellers 103
treatment plans 63
Turning Vision into Reality in 2000 206

U
University College Cork 26
University College Dublin 26, 148
University College Galway 26
UK Department of Health 143, 236
UK National Cancer Registry 205
UK Transplant Service 249
Underwood, Prof JCE 232
Union of Students in Ireland (USI) 40, 153
United Kingdom Heart Attack Study (UKHAS) 187
United Nations (UN) 137
University College Hospital Galway (UCHG) 201

University of Sheffield 67
University of York 155
US Department of Justice 221
US Food and Drugs Administration 91
US Institute of Medicine 225
US National Academy of Sciences 270

V
Viani, Dr Laura 32
Voluntary Health Insurance (VHI) 12, 73, 127, 261

W
waiting lists 63
Wales, Dr John 114
Walsh, Dr Terry 245
Wanlass, David 273
Wanless Report 19, 106
warfarin and INR service 38
Waterford Regional Hospital 46, 194
Watkins, Sherron 247
West of Ireland Cardiology Foundation 190
Western Health Board 201
Which? magazine 117
Whistle blowing 247
White, Dan 18
White, Dr Martin 42
WHO 135, 136
Whyte, Christina 148
Wilson, Harold 106
Wingfield, Dr Mary 239
WONCA 289
Woodlock, Michael 145
World Health Organization 118, 136, 169
Wren, Maev-Ann 6

Y
Young Adults in Action 154

328

For anyone thinking, talking, writing about or experiencing the Irish healthcare system, this book is a must have. It presents an insider's view of medicine today and the wider healthcare scenario in Ireland. The picture is one of seemingly unsolvable crises, despite massive Government funding and recommendations from a plethora of task forces and commissions.

It exposes the culture of "administrationism" that threatens to destroy the professional autonomy of doctors, forcing them to publicly advocate for their patients.

Avoiding the empty rhetoric of other responses, this book clearly presents practical solutions and remedies for the current ills in the Irish health system, such as hospital waiting lists, cutbacks, health insurance, and the staffing and equipping of hospitals. Moreover, it promotes a vision of Irish healthcare for the 21st century, where dignity of the patient and professional autonomy are assured, yet underpinned by accountability and fairness.

For the subject that won't go away, *A Cure for the Crisis – Irish Healthcare in Context* will change the way you think about health.

Dr Bill Tormey is a consultant at Beaumont Hospital and James Connolly Memorial Hospital, Blanchardstown, and is registered as a specialist in Chemical Pathology and General Internal Medicine. A graduate of UCD Medical School, he holds a PhD from TCD. He is a Fellow of the Royal College of Physicians of Ireland and the Royal College of Pathologists. Committed to improving the Irish political system through accountability, he is experienced in losing elections.

All royalties from the sale of the book will be donated to the Dublin Simon Community and the Irish Heart Foundation.

ISBN 1-84131-629-6

9 781841 316291

Blackwater Press
c/o Folens Publishers
Hibernian Industrial Estate
Greenhills Road
Tallaght, Dublin 24

www.folens.ie

Cover photo:
imagefile